OBSTETRICIANS SPEAK

On Training, Practice, Fear, and Transformation

The Anthropology of Obstetrics and Obstetricians:
The Practice, Maintenance, and Reproduction of a Biomedical Profession

Editors:
Robbie Davis-Floyd, Rice University
Ashish Premkumar, Northwestern University

Obstetricians are the primary drivers of the research on and the implementation of interventions in the birth process that have long been the subjects of anthropological critiques. In many countries, they are also primary drivers of violence, disrespect, and abuse during the perinatal period. Yet there is little social science literature on obstetricians themselves, their educational processes, and their personal rationales for their practices. Thus, this dearth of social science literature on obstetricians constitutes a huge gap waiting to be filled. These groundbreaking edited collections seek to fill that gap by officially creating an "anthropology of obstetrics and obstetricians" across countries and cultures—including biopolitical and professional cultures—so that a broad and deep understanding of these maternity care providers and their practices, ideologies, motivations, and diversities can be achieved.

Volume I
Obstetricians Speak:
On Training, Practice, Fear, and Transformation
Edited by Robbie Davis-Floyd and Ashish Premkumar

Volume II
Cognition, Risk, and Responsibility in Obstetrics:
Anthropological Analyses and Critiques of Obstetricians' Practices
Edited by Robbie Davis-Floyd and Ashish Premkumar

Volume III
Obstetric Violence and Systemic Disparities:
Can Obstetrics Be Humanized and Decolonized?
Edited by Robbie Davis-Floyd and Ashish Premkumar

Obstetricians Speak
On Training, Practice, Fear, and Transformation

Edited by
Robbie Davis-Floyd and Ashish Premkumar

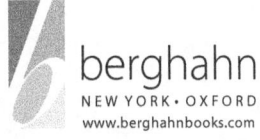

First published in 2023 by
Berghahn Books
www.berghahnbooks.com

© 2023 Robbie Davis-Floyd and Ashish Premkumar

All rights reserved. Except for the quotation of short passages for the purposes of criticism and review, no part of this book may be reproduced in any form or by any means, electronic or mechanical, including photocopying, recording, or any information storage and retrieval system now known or to be invented, without written permission of the publisher.

Library of Congress Cataloging-in-Publication Data

Names: Davis-Floyd, Robbie, editor. | Premkumar, Ashish, editor.
Title: Obstetricians speak : on training, practice, fear, and transformation / edited by Robbie Davis-Floyd, and Ashish Premkumar.
Description: New York : Berghahn Books, 2023. | Series: The anthropology of obstetrics and obstetricians: the practice, maintenance, and reproduction of a biomedical profession; vol 1 | Includes bibliographical references and index.
Identifiers: LCCN 2023001066 (print) | LCCN 2023001067 (ebook) | ISBN 9781800738287 (hardback) | ISBN 9781800738300 (paperback) | ISBN 9781800738294 (ebook)
Subjects: LCSH: Obstetrics. | Obstetricians—Biography.
Classification: LCC RG101 .O19526 2023 (print) | LCC RG101 (ebook) | DDC 618.2—dc23/eng/20230307
LC record available at https://lccn.loc.gov/2023001066
LC ebook record available at https://lccn.loc.gov/2023001067

British Library Cataloguing in Publication Data

A catalogue record for this book is available from the British Library

ISBN 978-1-80073-828-7 hardback
ISBN 978-1-80073-830-0 paperback
ISBN 978-1-80073-829-4 ebook

https://doi.org/10.3167/9781800738287

Robbie Davis-Floyd dedicates this book to its chapter authors, all of whom have demonstrated great courage in the face of the multiple adversities that have challenged them along their transformative journeys.

Ashish Premkumar dedicates this book to his wife, Natalie, and his two children, James and Jude, and to his entire family for their guidance and support throughout his training.

Contents

List of Illustrations	ix
Acknowledgments	xi

Series Overview. The Anthropology of Obstetrics and Obstetricians: The Practice, Maintenance, and Reproduction of a Biomedical Profession   xii
Robbie Davis-Floyd and Ashish Premkumar

Introduction to Volume I. Obstetricians Speak   1
Robbie Davis-Floyd and Ashish Premkumar

Chapter 1. On Becoming an Abortion Provider in the United States: An Autoethnographic Account   10
Scott Moses

Chapter 2. Abortion, Professional Identity, and Generational Meaning Making among US Ob/Gyns   32
Rebecca Henderson, Chu J. Hsiao, and Jody Steinauer

Chapter 3. My Transformation from an Obstetrician to a Maternal-Fetal Medicine Subspecialist: Autoethnographic Thoughts on Situated Knowledges and Habitus   54
Ashish Premkumar

Chapter 4. Cold Steel and Sunshine: Ethnographic and Autoethnographic Perspectives on Two Obstetric Careers in the United States from across the Chasm   72
Kathleen Hanlon-Lundberg

Chapter 5. An Awakening   93
Jesanna Cooper

Chapter 6. Repercussions of a Paradigm Shift in the Professional and Personal Life of a Brazilian Obstetrician   101
Rosana Fontes

Chapter 7. The Bullying and Persecution of a Humanistic/Holistic Obstetrician in Brazil: The Benefits and Costs of My Paradigm Shift   123
Ricardo Herbert Jones

Chapter 8. Hungarian Birth Models Seen through the Prism of Prison: The Journey of Ágnes Geréb   144
Ágnes Geréb and Katalin Fábián

Chapter 9. Adopting the Midwifery Model of Care in India   171
Evita Fernandez

Chapter 10. "Birth with No Regret" in Turkey: The Natural Childbirth of the 21st Century   192
Hakan Çoker

Chapter 11. Attempting to Maintain a Positive Awareness about Vaginal Breech Birth in Australia   210
Andrew Bisits

Chapter 12. Mixing Modalities in My Technocratic/Humanistic Obstetric Practice: Ideology and Rationales   228
Marco Gianotti

Chapter 13. How an Obstetrician Promoted Respectful Care in Canada and in the World   245
André Lalonde

Conclusions. What Have We Learned from Obstetricians?   262
Robbie Davis-Floyd and Ashish Premkumar

Index   294

Illustrations

Figures

8.1. Ágnes's chair inside, surrounded by supporters inside her home during her house arrest, April 2013. © Éva Ágnes Molnár   151

8.2. Ágnes' symbolic empty chair outside, surrounded by her supporters during her house arrest, April 2013. © Éva Ágnes Molnár   151

8.3. Protest in front of Ágnes's prison cell with hundreds of participants, December 20, 2010. © István Csintalan   153

8.4. "Flowers of Gratitude," January 2018, Freedom Bridge, Budapest. © Jakab Erdély   164

9.1. Birth days are the greatest risk to mothers and newborns. © Evita Fernandez   172

9.2. Andy with a midwife in India. © Fernandez Foundation   175

9.3. PROMISE campaign. © Evita Fernandez   176

9.4. Episiotomy rates in spontaneous vaginal births from 2011 to 2021 at Fernandez Hospital. © Evita Fernandez   179

9.5. Midwife-attended births displayed a lower incidence of episiotomies compared with obstetrician-attended births. © Evita Fernandez   179

9.6. Reduction in use of epidural analgesia for vaginal births at Fernandez Hospital, due to midwifery support throughout labor and birth. © Evita Fernandez   180

9.7. The drop in CB rates in Karimnagar between December 2017 and May 2018. © Evita Fernandez   184

9.8. A midwife from Telangana ensures that the mother is comfortable during the antenatal check-up. © Fernandez Foundation — 185

9.9. Midwife-led births and choice of birthing positions during preceptorship. © Evita Fernandez — 186

13.1. *The International Childbirth Initiative* (ICI): *12 Steps* (summary version) *to Safe and Respectful MotherBaby-Family Maternity Care.* — 255

Tables

0.1. The 12 Tenets of the Technocratic, Humanistic, and Holistic Paradigms of Birth and Health Care Compared. © Robbie Davis-Floyd — xviii

0.2. The Stages of Cognition and Their Anthropological Equivalents. © Robbie Davis-Floyd and Charles D. Laughlin — xxi

2.1. Demographic characteristics of participating abortion care providers, N=34. © Rebecca Henderson — 36

9.1. Eight key questions addressed to mothers birthing at Fernandez Hospital with a midwife as their primary caregiver. The questions were carefully curated to gauge how the mothers felt and whether or not they had a positive birth experience. © Evita Fernandez — 177

9.2. Maternal satisfaction grades. © Evita Fernandez — 178

10.1. Our "Birth with No Regret" Statistics on 450 Births (2010–2021). © Hakan Çoker — 206

13.1. Facility partners in the ICI network (as of October 2022). © André Lalonde and Michelle Therrien — 257

Acknowledgments

We thank our chapter authors for their willingness to reflect on their practices and their career journeys, for their courage in telling their stories in print, for the hard work they put into the writings of their chapters, and for the sometimes brutal honesty they offer in those chapters. We also thank our Berghahn Books editors Tom Bonnington and Keara Hagerty for answering our endless questions and for shepherding this book through to production.

Series Overview
The Anthropology of Obstetrics and Obstetricians
The Practice, Maintenance, and Reproduction of a Biomedical Profession

Series Editors: Robbie Davis-Floyd PhD, medical and reproductive anthropologist, and Ashish Premkumar MD, maternal-fetal medicine specialist and medical anthropologist.

We begin this Overview with a list of the three volumes in this series.:

Volumes I, II, and III

Volume I. *Obstetricians Speak: On Training, Practice, Fear, and Transformation* (Davis-Floyd and Premkumar 2023a).

Volume II. *Cognition, Risk, and Responsibility in Obstetrics: Anthropological Analyses and Critiques of Obstetricians' Practices* (Davis-Floyd and Premkumar 2023b).

Volume IIII. *Obstetric Violence and Systemic Disparities: Can Obstetrics Be Humanized and Decolonized?* (Davis-Floyd and Premkumar 2023c).

Creating the Anthropology of Obstetrics and Obstetricians

Can a book create a field? We respond with a resounding "Yes!" The broader field of the anthropology of reproduction, within which we situate the field we intend to create with this series—the anthropology of obstetrics and obstetricians—was, by scholarly consensus, founded by Faye Ginsburg and Rayna Rapp with their 1995 publication of *Conceiving the New World Order: The Global Politics of Reproduction*. Yet much scholarly work was done within that field and its subfields long before it existed by name. How pregnant and birthing people are treated has been subject to a variety of critiques and analyses over the past five decades. Since the seminal work of various anthropologists and others in the 1970s and 1980s, there have long existed the anthropologies of birth and of midwifery. Nurses and doulas as well have been the subject of a great deal of social science consideration. Analyses of abortion, amniocentesis, fetal surveillance methods (e.g., ultrasound, electronic fetal monitoring), and assisted reproductive technologies—inclusive of surrogacy and in vitro fertilization—have also found their home within the anthropology of reproduction. And the field of obstetrics in its broadest sense—defined as the branch of biomedicine concerned with perinatal care given by obstetricians—has been the subject of multiple analyses and radical critiques by social scientists, maternity care practitioners, mothers, and birth activists. Obstetricians are the primary drivers of the research on and the implementation of interventions in the birth process that have been the subjects of those critiques since the 1950s. In many countries, they are also primary drivers of forms of violence, disrespect, and abuse during the intrapartum period. Yet there is little social science literature on obstetricians themselves, their educational processes, and their personal rationales for their practices. Thus, this dearth of social science literature on obstetricians constitutes a huge gap waiting to be filled.

This groundbreaking edited collection seeks to fill that gap by officially creating an "anthropology of obstetrics and obstetricians" across countries and cultures—including biopolitical and professional cultures—so that a broad and deep understanding of these maternity care providers, their practices, ideologies, motivations, and diversities can be achieved. This is our central organizing theme for all three volumes. Thus the subfield of the anthropology of reproduction that we seek to create with this book series includes both the profession of obstetrics as it is practiced, maintained, and reproduced, and the individuals who practice within that profession (and within its sub-specialty—maternal-fetal medicine, or perinatology); these are the practitioners who have been understudied by social scientists, while, again, the wider field of obstetrics in general has been heavily studied. That is why we do not name this field simply "the anthropology of obstetrics" but rather "the anthropology of obstetrics and obstetricians."

Some few books we can point to that, retrospectively, fit into this field include, in chronological order:

- Diana Scully's *Men Who Control Women's Health: The Miseducation of Obstetrician Gynecologists* (1980);
- William Ray Arney's *Power and the Profession of Obstetrics* (1982);

- Jo Murphy-Lawless's *Reading Birth and Death: A History of Obstetric Thinking* (1998);
- Parts of Deborah K. McGregor's *From Midwives to Medicine: The Birth of American Gynecology* (1998);
- Parts of Monica J. Casper's *The Making of the Unborn Patient: A Social Anatomy of Fetal Surgery* (1998);
- Parts of G. J. Barker-Benfield's *The Horrors of the Half-Known Life: Male Attitudes toward Women and Sexuality in Nineteenth-Century America* (2000);
- Jacqueline Wolf's *Cesarean Section: An American History of Risk, Technology, and Consequence* (2020);
- Vania Smith-Oka's *Becoming Gods: Medical Training in Mexican Hospitals* (2021).

We follow these excellent works with humility.

Some Notes on Language

First, we note that throughout this series, we use the term "cesarean births" instead of "cesarean sections" to honor the fact that these are births. We have left the use of terms for people who gestate and give birth to babies up to each chapter author; they tend to alternate between terms such as "birthing people," "childbearers," and "women," yet mostly use "woman" and "women" because that is what most individual interlocutors wished to be called (see Gribble et al. 2022 for a discussion on this issue).

Also throughout this series, we and our chapter authors use "biopolitical" in the Foucauldian sense, in which "biopolitics" refers to a way of regulating populations through "biopower"—the applications and impacts of political power on human biology in all aspects of human life. Obstetrics as a profession tends to be biopolitically engaged, silo-oriented, and narrowly defined—only medical doctors with a specialization in obstetrics during residency may call themselves obstetricians; beyond that there are maternal-fetal medicine (MFM) specialists, also called perinatologists, who, already obstetricians, require three years of additional training to perform fetal procedures, for example, and to care for extremely ill childbearers.

We concentrate in all three volumes on obstetricians (obs) and perinatologists (who must become obs before they undertake their training in Maternal-Fetal Medicine) in their multiple aspects, including their relationships—or lack thereof—with the childbearers they attend, and with midwives, nurses, doulas, and other types of maternity care providers. We also address their almost universally negative opinions of home birth and community midwives (midwives who attend births only in homes and freestanding birth centers), and why some of our ob chapter authors and interlocutors disagree and choose to work with community midwives, and also with hospital-based midwives. Our chapters deal with the gynecological aspects of obs' practices only minimally, focusing primarily on their roles in pregnancy and birth. We leave the creation of the anthropologies of gynecology, pediatrics, and other specialties to future researchers.

Scholars argue that there is a large potential for collaboration between social science researchers and biomedical professionals, and for the integration of ethnography into biomedicine (see Long et al. 2008). Those are also goals that this series achieves, especially as many of its authors are both obstetricians and social scientists; most of the latter are medical anthropologists, and their chapters are deeply informed by anthropological perspectives. Some of our chapter authors are sociologists—when sociological works are qualitative, not quantitative, they tend to closely resemble anthropological works. Thus, in this series, we elide sociology into anthropology or speak of "social science" research.

The Hidden Curriculum, and Questions Asked

Many of our chapters ask: How are today's obstetricians trained, and what is the "hidden curriculum" behind that training? As Lydia Dixon, Vania Smith-Oka, and Mounia El Kotni describe it (2019:40):

> A large portion of knowledge can be transmitted in unintended ways, in what has been termed the "hidden curriculum" . . . defined as the gap between what people are *taught* (through direct means) and what they *learn* (through indirect means). In some cases what is transmitted is the opposite of what is intended. So, while clinicians might *speak about* patient-centeredness as an important goal, their *actions* might emphasize . . . [their] authority, or even attitudes of contempt for patients.

We also ask: Have obstetric training and its hidden curriculum changed in recent years to teach more humanistic ways of treating people in labor? If so, how and why? If not, why not? How do obstetricians—

who certainly do not constitute a homogeneous group whose members share the same perspectives—conceptualize the processes of pregnancy and childbirth, and what are the differences in those conceptualizations? What are the politics of research and intervention in labor and birth, and why don't many obstetricians emphasize low-intervention birth practices that prioritize normal, physiologic birth? (See ACOG 2019a.) What are the cross-cultural differences in all of the above, and how do obstetrician's practices reflect cultural values and beliefs? Many of these issues have been explored in the literature, yet rarely from obstetricians' points of view. All of them will be addressed in our chapters.

For its theoretical underpinnings, our series heavily relies on Robbie Davis-Floyd's (2018a, 2022) description and comparison of "the technocratic, humanistic, and holistic paradigms of birth and health care," because many of our chapter authors use this terminology, because the technocratic model forms a large part of the hidden curriculum of obstetricians' training, and because the "paradigm shifts" made by some of our chapter authors need to be understood in these terms. Thus, here we present a brief overview of these three paradigms as Davis-Floyd has delineated them (for full descriptions, see Davis-Floyd 2018a, 2022).

The Technocratic, Humanistic, and Holistic Paradigms of Birth and Health Care

A Brief Overview

Robbie (Davis-Floyd 2003, 2018a, 2022) defines a "technocracy" as a post-industrial, capitalistic, hierarchical, bureaucratic, institution-laden, socially stratified and racialized, and (still) patriarchal society that "supervalues" (Robbie's invented term; 2003, 2018, 2022) an ideology of progress through the development of ever-higher technologies and the global flow of information via such technologies. The technocratic paradigm of birth and health care, which reflects the core values and social structures of technocracies, is based on the *principle of separation*—of mind and body, practitioner and patient, body parts from the whole body. It metaphorizes the body as a machine that can be reduced to its component parts, and views the birthgiving body as a dysfunctional machine and the patient as an object. And it charters an alienated, depersonalized physician-patient relationship (e.g., referring to a patient as "the gall bladder in Room 212" or "the cesarean in 313").

In contrast, the humanistic paradigm is based on the *principle of connection*—of mind and body, practitioner(s) and patient, body parts to the bodily whole, encompassing the influence of emotional and psychological states on the body, and vice versa. This humanistic model defines the body as an organism (which, of course, it is), views the patient as a relational subject—for example, Louellen Jackson, the woman with two children who just lost her husband—and sees the uterus not as a dysfunctional machine but as a responsive part of the whole person. Other essential aspects of a humanistic approach to birth include relationship, communication, and caring between patient and practitioner, and shared decision-making. The humanistic paradigm could also be called a "bio-psycho-social" approach, as it encompasses the biology/physiology, the psychology, and the sociality of pregnancy, birth, and the postpartum period.

Robbie (Davis-Floyd 2018a, 2022) has been careful to distinguish between *superficial humanism*, which is a kind and compassionate overlay on technocratic practice and includes the admission of partners and doulas into the labor room right along with the performance of multiple technocratic interventions, and *deep humanism*, which consists of practices that facilitate what Robbie calls "the deep physiology of normal birth," such as movement, eating and drinking at will during labor, and the use of upright or all-fours positions for labor and birth (this latter position opens the pelvic outlet to its maximal diameter). Deeply humanistic practitioners are also aware of and committed to honoring childbearers' human rights. Because of the extreme importance of the differences between superficial and deep humanism, Robbie (Davis-Floyd 2022) has redefined the spectrum "technocratic–humanistic–holistic" as "technocratic–superficially humanistic–deeply humanistic–holistic." For it is a spectrum, as practitioners can move back and forth along this spectrum, depending on the circumstances of an individual birth and their own career trajectories.

The holistic paradigm/model of birth and health care, which fully encompasses the deeply humanistic approach, is based on the *principles of connection and integration*, defines the body as an energy field, insists that body, mind, and spirit are one, employs spirit and energy in the treatment process, and views patient and practitioner(s) as part of one unified energy field, so that each can affect the other, for better or for worse. Thus, holistic practitioners pay close attention to the *psychosphere* of birth (Jones 2009)—the environmental ambience surrounding the birth scene—and work to keep that psychosphere clear and clean, perhaps by encouraging the laboring woman and/or her partner to release their negative emotions/fears through words or tears, or by sending away people whose own worries and fears—or blocked energies—may be impeding the birth.

For a brief and very funny example, world-famous holistic midwife Ina May Gaskin once told Robbie about a birth that was proceeding well until pushing started, and then stalled. "Sussing out" the energy in the room, Ina May asked if anyone was holding something back? And the husband, upon whose lap his wife had been sitting, said that for the last 30 minutes, he had been desperately needing to pee, so of course he had been holding something back! That accomplished, they resumed their former positions, and the baby was born quickly. For another example of holism in action, if a baby is born and not breathing, holistically inclined midwives—whether community- or hospital-based—will immediately ask the parents to "call the baby," asking that baby's spirit or soul to choose to come into the body. According to many of the midwives Robbie has interviewed over the years, and to some neonatologists, often this practice works so well that resuscitation is not needed (see Table 0.1, and for a complete description of these paradigms, please see Davis-Floyd 2018a, 2022.)

Table 0.1. The 12 Tenets of the Technocratic, Humanistic, and Holistic Paradigms of Birth and Health Care Compared. © Robbie Davis-Floyd. This table is adapted and updated from Davis-Floyd 2018a with the permission of Waveland Press.

The Technocratic Model	The Humanistic (Bio-psycho-social) Model	The Holistic Model
1. Mind/body separation	1. Mind-body connection	1. Oneness of bodymindspirit
2. The body as machine	2. The body as an organism	2. The body as an energy system interlinked with other energy systems
3. The patient as object	3. The patient as relational subject	3. Healing the whole person in whole-life context
4. Alienation of practitioner from patient	4. Connection and caring between practitioner and patient	4. Essential unity of practitioner and client (a more egalitarian term than "patient")

The Technocratic Model	The Humanistic (Bio-psycho-social) Model	The Holistic Model
5. Diagnosis and treatment from the outside in (use of technologies for diagnosis; curing disease; repairing dysfunction)	5. Diagnosis and healing from the outside in and from the inside out (combining technological diagnosis with active listening)	5. Diagnosis and healing primarily from the inside out (reliance on intuition, intuitive diagnosis; may include use of high technologies but not total reliance on them)
6. Hierarchical organization and standardization of care	6. Balance between the needs of the institution and the individual	6. Lateral networking organizational structure that facilitates individualization of care
7. Authority and responsibility inherent in practitioner, not patient; patient's human rights dishonored by practitioners	7. Information, decision-making, and responsibility shared between patient and practitioner; patient's human rights often honored	7. Authority and responsibility inherent in each individual; client's human rights honored
8. Supervaluation of science and technology	8. Science and technology counterbalanced with humanism	8. Science and technology placed at the service of the individual
9. Aggressive intervention with emphasis on short-term results	9. A long-term focus on disease prevention	9. A long-term focus on creating and maintain health and wellbeing
10. Death as defeat	10. Death as an acceptable outcome when appropriate	10. Death as a step in a process
11. A profit-driven system	11. Compassion-driven care	11. Healing as the focus
12. Intolerance of other modalities	12. Open-mindedness toward other modalities	12. Embrace of multiple healing modalities
Basic underlying principle: Separation	*Basic underlying principle:* Connection	*Basic underlying principles*: Connection and integration
Type of thinking: unimodal, left-brained, linear	*Type of thinking:* bimodal	*Type of thinking:* fluid, multimodal, right-brained, gestaltic

The 4 Stages of Cognition and "Substage"

We turn now to another of the theoretical underpinnings of this series—a cognitive framework developed by Robbie, which she fully explicates in Chapter 1 of Volume II of this series (Davis-Floyd 2023b). We provide a description here, as some of our authors in this present volume make use of this conceptual framework in their chapters. In her chapter, Robbie describes the differences between "open" and "closed" ways of thinking and delineates "4 Stages of Cognition" originally developed by others, correlating each with an anthropological concept. She correlates Stage 1—rigid or concrete thinking—with *naïve realism* ("Our way is the only way, or the only way that matters"), *fundamentalism* ("Our way is the right way and should be the only way for everyone"), and *fanaticism* ("Our way is so right that everyone who disagrees with it should be assimilated or eliminated"). Robbie notes that many technocratic obstetricians can be coded as any one of these, and that fundamentalist and fanatical obs often persecute those who step out of their Stage 1 silos. She correlates Stage 2 thinking with *ethnocentrism* ("There are other ways out there, and that's ok, but our way is best"), and demonstrates that technocratic obstetrics is a relatively rigid Stage 1 or 2 system, depending on how it is practiced.

The next two Stages represent more open and fluid types of thinking—Robbie correlates Stage 3 thinking with *cultural relativism* ("All ways have value; individual behavior should be understood within its sociocultural context"), suggesting that cultural relativists are very open to providing culturally competent and culturally safe care. Yet she also suggests that cultural relativism has severe limitations, as it can and has been used to justify behaviors that are fully acceptable within their cultural contexts yet also violate human rights—of which she provides various examples in her chapter. Thus, Robbie relates Stage 4 thinking to *global humanism* ("We must search for higher, better ways that can support cultural integrity while also supporting individual human rights").

Robbie goes on to show how ongoing stress can cause even the most fluid of thinkers to shut down cognitively and operate at a Stage 1 level, or to degenerate into "Substage"—a condition of cognitive breakdown, or "losing it," which can include treating birthing people and other practitioners below them in the obstetric hierarchy with disrespect, violence, and abuse. Thus she demonstrates how rituals, which "stand as a buffer between cognition and chaos," can be used for cognitive stabilization. She also draws attention to the ongoing battles between fundamentalists and global humanists, and to the persecutions that Stage 4 globally humanistic birth practitioners, including obstetricians, often experience from fundamentalist or fanatical Stage 1 obstetricians and officials, as several of the chapters in this volume describe. Table 0.2 delineates these differences among Stages 1-4 thinkers, and describes Substage.

Table 0.2. The Stages of Cognition and Their Anthropological Equivalents © Robbie Davis-Floyd and Charles D. Laughlin. This Table was created by Robbie Davis-Floyd with the help of Charles D. Laughlin; it originally appeared in *The Power of Ritual* (2016), on which Davis-Floyd and Laughlin hold the copyright, so we present it here with Laughlin's permission. This Table also appears in the recently abridged version of that book, called *Ritual: What It Is, How It Works, and Why* (Davis-Floyd and Laughlin 2022).

Stages of Cognition	Anthropological Equivalents
Stage 4: Fluid, open thinking	**Global humanism**: "All individuals have rights that should be honored, not violated."
Stage 3: Relative, open thinking	**Cultural relativism**: "All ways have value; individual behavior should be understood within its cultural context."
Stage 2: Self- and culture-centered semi-closed thinking	**Ethnocentrism**: "Other ways may be OK for others, but our way is best."
Stage 1: Rigid/concrete closed thinking, intolerance of other ways of thinking	**Naïve realism**: "Our way is the only way that matters"; **Fundamentalism**: "Our is way is the only *right* way"; **Fanaticism**: "Our way is so right that all others should be assimilated or eliminated."
Substage: Non-thinking; inability to process information; lack or loss of compassion for others	**Cognitive regression**: Intense egocentrism, irritability, inability to cope, burnout, breakdown, hysteria, panic, "losing it," abusing or mistreating others

And now we proceed to a brief overview of the global childbirth scene as background and context for our three volumes.

The Global Childbirth Scene: A Brief Overview

For millennia, the primary birth practitioners around the world were traditional midwives trained by apprenticeship or simply by experience. Today in most low-to-middle-income countries (LMICs) where traditional midwives still exist, they are being rapidly phased out of practice by their governments or have simply died off, leaving no one to fill the valuable community roles these honored midwives played. In rural areas in many LMICs, where women face major problems in accessing maternity care, traditional midwives still attend large numbers of births. And yes, maternal and fetal mortality rates in those countries are high: traditional midwives, who usually recognize life-threatening complications yet sometimes miss them, need training in identifying these complications and in lifesaving procedures such as the use of misoprostol (Cytotec) to stop postpartum hemorrhages; and they need access to transport to prevent the well-known "three delays": delay in decision to transport, delay in finding transport, and delay in getting effective care upon arrival at the biomedical facility (Thaddeus and Maine 1994); these are all major causes of many unnecessary fetal and maternal deaths. Yet many deaths also occur in biomedical facilities in LMICs due to understaffing, under-resourcing, insufficient staff training, and the resultant poor quality of care.

Thus the most notable differences in the contemporary biomedical treatment of birth have little to do with the specific customs of particular cultures, but much to do with the vast disparities between resource-rich and resource-poor countries (see Cheyney and Davis-Floyd 2020a, 2020b, 2021). In many high-resource nations, laboring people routinely receive multiple technological interventions, such as epidurals and electronic fetal monitoring, in attractive and humane hospital settings. In many low-resource nations, childbearers routinely receive less expensive interventions, such as pubic shaving, enemas, episiotomies, the Kristeller maneuver (pushing down hard on the abdomen to expel the baby more rapidly—a dangerous practice), and (extremely painful) manual uterine cavity revisions (see the chapter by Smith-Oka and Dixon [2023] in Volume II of this series)—all now mostly considered outdated in technocratic birth—without the superficially humanistic benefits of expensive interior decorating or even of a birthing companion. LMICs in general have experienced the massive importation of Westernized industrial modes of birth, including delivering in the dorsal lithotomy (flat on the back) position—which narrows the pelvic outlet, making it harder to push—the withholding of food and drink, and the overuse of synthetic oxytocin (Pitocin) to induce or speed labor—all this without the pain relief provided by epidurals, which are too costly for most LMIC hospitals and clinics to employ. Although episiotomy rates are now relatively minimal in most high-resource nations, obstetricians Robbie has interviewed or simply spoken with in many LMICs fully believe that "the perineum will explode" if an episiotomy is not performed; the vast majority of obs in LMICs have never seen a vaginal birth without an episiotomy (see the chapter by Davis-Floyd and Georges (2023) in Volume III of this series). Another reason given by many LMIC obs in support of episiotomy is to maintain vaginal tightness for the enhanced pleasure of a male sexual partner—that extra stitch placed during the repair of a perineal laceration or a mediolateral episiotomy (an episiotomy cut at an angle instead of straight down) is often called "the husband stitch." During Robbie's travels to give talks, she has learned that in such countries, which include Romania, Croatia, Bulgaria, Turkey, and almost all Latin American nations, among many others, women will inevitably receive either "the cut above" (a cesarean) or "the cut below" (an episiotomy).

In both rich and poor countries, cesarean rates are rising without concomitant improvements in maternal and perinatal health outcomes (Belizán et al. 2018). And iatrogenic morbidity (Villar et al. 2006; Liu et al. 2007; Villar and Carroli 2007) and maternal mortality disproportionately affect poor women and Women of Color (Davis 2018, 2019a, 2019b; Krisberg 2019; Liese et al. 2021). The national cesarean rates in many LMICs are astronomical. The transnational range throughout Latin America is 30%–56%, with public hospitals showing cesarean birth (CB) rates of 20%–40% and private hospitals, 70%–95% (Dixon, Smith-Oka, and El Kotni 2019; Williamson and Matsuoka 2019). In 2018, the regional rate for Latin America and the Caribbean was 44.3% (Boerma et al. 2018).

Globally, in 1990, roughly 1 in 15 babies was born via CB, in what has long been called the "cesarean epidemic." By 2014, this global rate had risen to almost 1 in 5—18% (Betran et al. 2015), and to 21.1% in 2015 (Boerma et al. 2018) and continues to increase. The lowest rates (around 4%) cluster in West and Central African countries where access to CB is limited and women and babies die due to its lack. In Western Europe, where births are primarily attended by professional midwives, the 2015 CB rate was 26.9% (Boerma et al. 2018). The highest rates are found in Brazil, Egypt, Turkey, the Dominican Republic, and Venezuela, where the CB rates hover between 52% and 56% (Boerma et al. 2018), and most especially in Greece, where the rate is 65% (see Georges and Daellenbach 2019, and the chapter by Robbie Davis-Floyd and Eugenia Georges [2023] in Volume II of this series). For wealthier women globally, CB rates are five times higher than for economically poor women, who in LMICs often prefer to give birth at home with traditional midwives, due to the maltreatment they receive in public hospitals, where, again, CB rates are generally lower than in private hospitals. Sadly, the increases in CB rates *are not accompanied by improved mortality outcomes for either mothers or babies, or, where there are improvements, these are not necessarily attributable to the increase in cesareans* (Betran et al. 2015; Boerma et al. 2018).

As the World Health Organization (WHO) has long stressed, a CB rate under 10% results in higher rates of maternal mortality, whereas a CB rate of well above 15% means that some women are dying from massive overuse of cesareans (WHO 2015). This cesarean epidemic is largely doctor-driven, as many of our Volume II chapters show. Strong beliefs about the dangerous and dysfunctional nature of birth are widely held by obstetricians, who also generally make more money by doing cesareans over vaginal births, due either being paid more to do them, and/or to the time-saving nature of cesareans, which can take less than an hour to perform, while physiologic vaginal births can take many hours. (Latent labor—before six cm of cervical dilation—can even safely take two to three days before active labor sets in [see Lewis 2020; Mayo Clinic Staff 2020]). Yet in some countries, these high CB rates are also consumer-driven; for example, many Greek women, who are under the influence of what Georges (2008) has called "the symbolic domination of modernity," are culturally conditioned to perceive CB as beneficial to themselves and their babies, because their vaginas remain intact and their babies' heads are round and not peaked, as they often are after vaginal births (Georges and Daellenbach 2019). And Taiwanese women often prefer cesareans to avoid having to "suffer twice"—meaning suffering from the pain of labor, then also suffering from the pain of the operation, which more than a third of them receive (Kuan 2014). In the United States, elective (woman's choice) cesareans account for only 2.5% of cesarean births (ACOG 2019b). Of course, in litigious nations like the United States, CBs can result from fear of lawsuit, as performing a cesarean is considered the most a doctor can do to prevent fetal harm.

Robbie has toured many hospitals in many countries, and the most positive global development she can see is the spreading adoption of the UNICEF Baby-Friendly Hospital Initiative (BFHI), launched in 1991, which has resulted in major changes, such as mothers and newborns being separated for only a few moments after birth or not at all. Entering a baby- friendly postpartum maternity unit in an LMIC, as Robbie has often done, is an otherworldly experience: mothers sleep with their babies in the same bed or have them in bassinets close by, fathers are often present, breastfeeding is the norm, and an atmosphere of cheer and joy pervades.

Such hospitals, of which there are more than 20,000 around the world, are often just a few steps away from humanistic "mother-friendly" care, which involves the full range of choices in childbirth, and is heavily promoted by the *International Childbirth Initiative* (ICI): *12 Steps to Safe and Respectful MotherBaby-Family Maternity Care*. The ICI Principles and 12 Steps provide a template that any birthing facility or practice can implement in order to provide fully humanistic care; they can be found at www.icichildbirth.org, or in Lalonde et al. (2019). They are being put to work in increasing numbers of birth facilities and practices around the world, both small and large. (The specific facilities that are currently engaged in ICI implementation are listed in André Lalonde's chapter, this volume.) We strongly recommend their implementation in all birth practices everywhere. And we call for researchers to study the barriers to and effects of ICI implementation; if you are interested, please contact Robbie at davis-floyd@outlook.com.

As LMICs continue to overadopt Western biomedical approaches to birth and to devalue and eliminate Indigenous practitioners, "the Western biomedical model" (described in Gaines and Davis-Floyd 2003) turns out to be full of cultural variations, even in the high-resource countries that supposedly share common obstetric technologies and knowledge bases. These variations have been thoroughly documented in multiple volumes, importantly including:

- Brigitte Jordan's classic *Birth in Four Cultures: A Cross-Cultural Investigation of Childbirth in Yucatan, Holland, Sweden, and the United States* ([1978] 1993);
- *Childbirth and Authoritative Knowledge: Cross-Cultural Perspectives*, edited by Robbie Davis-Floyd and Carolyn Sargent (1997);
- *Birth by Design: Pregnancy, Maternity Care, and Midwifery in North America and Europe*, edited by Raymond DeVries, Cecilia Benoit, Edwin van Teijligen, and Sirpa Wrede (2001);
- *Maternities and Modernities: Colonial and Postcolonial Experiences in Asia and the Pacific*, edited by Kalpana Ram and Margaret Jolly (1998);
- *Birthing in the Pacific: Beyond Tradition and Modernity?* edited by Vicki Lukere and Margaret Jolly (2002);
- *Childbirth across Cultures: Ideas and Practices of Pregnancy, Childbirth and the Postpartum*, edited by Helaine Selin and Pamela K. Stone (2009);
- *Birth in Eight Cultures*, edited by Robbie Davis-Floyd and Melissa Cheyney (2019).

In most European countries, the Philippines, Malaysia, Japan, and many others, the majority of births are attended by midwives in hospitals; in most high-resource countries, home births stand at around only 1%. Despite recent changes in the Dutch obstetric system that include a major reduction in home births between 2009, when the homebirth rate stood at 30% as it had for decades, and the present, the Dutch still have the highest homebirth rate in the high-resource world: 13% (Davis-Floyd and Cheyney 2019), followed by New Zealand (3.6%), where midwives in danger of becoming extinct decades ago have revitalized their profession, and now are chosen by 94% of childbearers as their primary caregivers (Georges and Daellenbach 2019). In many high-resource countries, births at home or in freestanding birth centers are on the rise; and there was a significant rise in the United States and other countries—high, middle, and low resource alike—during the coronavirus pandemic as many childbearers fled potential hospital contagion and separation from their newborns, and in higher resource countries, forced separation from their partners and/or doulas (Davis-Floyd, Gutschow, and Schwartz 2020; Gutschow and Davis-Floyd 2021). For example, from 2019 to 2020 in the United States, out-of-hospital births increased by 19.5%, reaching a total of 2%, up from their previous 1.26% (Eugene Declerq, epidemiologist, personal communication with Robbie, January 2022). In low-resource countries, many women returned to the still-remaining traditional midwives (see for examples Ali et al. 2021).

Thus we have the inescapable irony that as low-resource countries continue to lose their homebirth practitioners and traditions, actively seeking to replace them with modern biomedical hospitals, technologies, and technocratically trained practitioners, childbearers in high-resource countries are engaged in a slow and ongoing process of rediscovering the value of community birth (births at home and in midwife-led freestanding birth centers) and recreating it as a viable option. And around the globe, the fight for autonomy is a crucial issue for midwives, both professional and traditional (see Davis-Floyd et al. 2018), as it is primarily when a midwifery (humanistic/holistic) model prevails that women can receive respectful and culturally appropriate care that supports the deep physiology of normal births.

Globally, a curious phenomenon prevails, which Melissa (Missy) Cheyney and Robbie have called the *obstetric paradox* (Cheyney and Davis-Floyd 2019:8): intervene in birth to keep it safe, thereby causing harm—identified in various chapters in this series, following Amali Lokugamage (2011), as "obstetric iatrogenesis." Birth around the world is generally characterized by interventions that are "too much too soon" (TMTS) or "too little too late" (TLTL) (Miller et al. 2016). Missy and Robbie have recommended the replacement of the iatrogenic TMTS and TLTL dichotomy with care given in "the right amount at the right time in the right way" (RARTRW) (Cheyney and Davis-Floyd 2020b, 2021)—for *how* care is provided matters as much what kind of care is provided and when.

Although humanism has made inroads into maternity care in many countries, the Stage 1 technocratic paradigm remains hegemonic in most hospitals, but usually only in high-resource countries, due to its heavy reliance on expensive technologies such as electronic fetal monitoring/cardiotocography (EFM/CTG). In low-resource countries, the older, also Stage 1 industrial model of medicine, which tends to work in assembly-line fashion, especially for birth, still prevails; low-resource hospitals generally do not have the technologies that facilitate and characterize the application of the technocratic model (see Davis-Floyd 2022 for descriptions of the differences between the industrial and technocratic models of birth). In hospitals around the world, this technocratic model (or its industrial predecessor) is daily enacted through "standard procedures" such as, for examples, the "prep," during which the laboring woman is separated from her support person(s), dressed in a hospital gown, and often hooked up to the EFM/CTG; routine, often-painful cervical examinations to make sure the laboring person's body-machine is producing on time; artificial labor induction or augmentation; and far too often, cesarean "sections," which, again, we refer to throughout this series as "cesarean births" (CBs) to emphasize that these are not just "sections," but births. Many of these also characterize low-resource industrialized births.

Robbie (Davis-Floyd 2003, 2018b, 2022) has long identified such standard procedures as rituals that enact the core value systems of technocratic societies, which tend to center around science, technology, institutions, and the preservation of paternalism and patriarchy, even by female obstetricians (see the chapter by Deborah McNabb in Volume III of this series). Rituals as Robbie has long defined them (see Davis-Floyd 2003; 2018b; Davis-Floyd and Laughlin 2022) are patterned, repetitive, and symbolic enactments of cultural—or individual—values and beliefs. Hospitals are both institutions and societal microcosms in which these core values are enacted and transmitted by practitioners via the rituals/standard procedures of hospital birth, and are often accepted as the status quo by laboring "patients" (see Soliday 2012; Davis-Floyd 2022).

And we note here that all standard obstetric procedures/rituals are examples of what anthropologist Peter Reynolds (1991) has called "the 1–2 Punch": Punch 1: mutilate/deconstruct a natural process like birth, then prosthetize/reconstruct it with technology. Reynold's brilliant insight was that usually Punch 2 is the point. Those of us who live in industrial or technocratic societies tend to believe that we have improved on natural processes by mutilating/deconstructing them—like damming a river to build a power plant, no matter the environmental cost. And so it is with technocratic birth: practitioners dam the natural river of the birth process with multiple interventions, thereby deconstructing/mutilating it, believing, in the obstetric paradox, that they have improved on it via these interventions.

Foregrounding Obstetrics as a Practice and a Profession: Theoretical and Ethnographic Gains

Once upon a time, Robbie was asked by a frustrated Latin American epidemiologist who worked for PAHO (the Pan American Health Organization/WHO [World Health Organization]):

> Why don't obstetricians get it? We epidemiologists understand that the vast majority of what they do during labor and birth is just plain wrong. Lots of pediatricians do too. Like—cutting the umbilical cord immediately, and using the EFM instead of manual auscultation, is just stupid! So why don't obs act according to the evidence, as we have long been insisting that they do? Instead they just blindly follow obstetric traditions—why can't they learn to think for themselves?

And indeed, some do, as Robbie Davis-Floyd and Eugenia Georges (2023) describe in their Volume III chapter on the self-named "good guys and girls" of Brazil, who have consciously made a paradigm shift to humanistic or holistic practice, based on the scientific evidence and their understanding that pregnant people must be the protagonists of their own births for both their physical and psychological well-being. How do humanistic and holistic obstetricians, some of whom attend home births, respond to the multiple forms of persecution directed against them by Stage 1 fundamentalist and often fanatical obstetricians? The chapters by obstetricians Rosana Fontes, Ricardo Jones, Jesanna Cooper, Kathleen Handlon-Lundberg, and Ágnes Geréb in this volume have much to say on this topic.

Foregrounding obstetrics as a practice and profession and obstetricians as a group of practitioners worthy of anthropological inquiry, as our three volumes do, has much to uncover regarding obs' perceptions of risk and of the stratified and racialized constructions of maternal treatment and responsibility (Ginsburg and Rapp 1995; Roberts 1999; Bridges 2011; Murphy 2017). Various chapters in this series directly address the systemic racial disparities in obstetric practices in various countries and obstetricians' views on these. Many have also critiqued obstetricians around the world for perpetrating obstetric iatrogenesis in the forms of obstetric disrespect, violence, and abuse (DVA) (see Pérez D'Gregorio 2010; Sadler et al. 2016; Bohren et al. 2019), yet few have directly observed obstetricians committing these acts nor interviewed obstetricians about why they do so, why they feel justified in doing so, and whether or not they perceive acts of overt DVA as such. Several of our chapter authors in Volumes II and III have done precisely that.

Given that overt DVA is rampant in many countries, especially in LMICs, but also in high-resource nations like the United States, some of our chapter authors have addressed this issue at its roots by seeking to understand the obstetric training that produces the mentality, motivations, and structural maintenance of DVA and obstetric iatrogenesis—which Liese and colleagues (2021) place along a UHDVA (unintentional harm, disrespect, violence, and abuse) spectrum. This UHDVA spectrum ranges from invisible forms of UH, such as standard procedures that are not intended to cause harm, yet do—in the obstetric paradox mentioned above—to overt and obvious DVA. Around half of the chapters in Volume III address these issues; the other half are dedicated to answering the complex questions in the book subtitle: *Can Obstetrics Be Humanized and Decolonized?* Additionally, some of our chapter authors address the "evidence–discourse–practice gap" (so-named in 2002 in a class paper by Kyra Kramer, one of Davis-Floyd's former students), asking why many obstetricians know and talk about the evidence, yet fail to implement it in practice. Others of our chapters address policy creation by or in conjunction with obstetricians, and the biopolitical aspects of the obstetric profession.

Clearly, a fully-fledged anthropology of obstetrics and obstetricians is needed, and that is what we hope to create, for the first time ever, via this international collection, which includes chapters focusing on obstetricians, their ideologies and practices, and their contestations and critiques in 19 countries: New Zealand, Australia, Nigeria, South Africa, Russia, Hungary, Switzerland, Ireland, the UK, Greece, Turkey, India, Chile, Brazil, Peru, the Dominican Republic, Mexico, the United States, and Canada.

Now we turn to brief descriptions of each of the three volumes in this series on *The Anthropology of Obstetrics and Obstetricians: The Practice, Maintenance, and Reproduction of a Biomedical Profession.*

Brief Description of Volume I

Obstetricians Speak:
On Training, Practice, Fear, and Transformation

In this present volume, we present 13 chapters written by obstetricians, some of whom are also medical anthropologists or are in the process of getting their PhDs in medical anthropology. Most provide autoethnographic accounts of their opinions about their profession and their medical training and its hidden curriculum—of which they became aware as they became anthropologists. They describe their practice styles and the ideologies that underlie them; their awakenings to awareness of those ideologies and, for some, the challenging paradigm shifts they undertook from technocratic to humanistic or holistic practice. Two chapters examine the difficulties of being abortion providers, and why some obstetricians do so despite those hardships. Another two examine the differences between obs and perinatologists. Five obstetricians describe the persecutions they experienced due to their shifts to humanistic or holistic practice, including famed Hungarian obstetrician/midwife Ágnes Geréb. One Turkish ob, Hakan Çoker, describes the deeply humanistic model he has developed and its basic principles. An Australian ob describes his efforts to reclaim breech delivery skills; an ob from India, Evita Fernandez, details how she and her colleagues are introducing professional midwives in their country; and a US ob, Marco Gianotti, describes how he mixes modalities in his technocratic/humanistic private practice. A Canadian ob, André Lalonde, describes his global efforts to create policies that effect positive change. And in our Conclusions to this volume, we discuss what we have learned from its chapters and describe the theoretical concepts and frameworks that its authors have found most useful in analyzing their own practices. This is the first volume ever to consist entirely of autoethnographically informed accounts by obstetricians themselves.

Brief Description of Volume II

Cognition, Risk, and Responsibility in Obstetrics: Anthropological Analyses and Critiques of Obstetricians' Practices

In this 11-chapter volume, we begin with Robbie's chapter on the "4 Stages of Cognition," described above as a theoretical framework that is carried out in various chapters in this series. We proceed to social science examinations and analyses of the cultures of Swiss, Chilean, Mexican, US, and Irish obstetrics and obstetricians, most especially around their over-performance of cesareans. The chapter on Ireland describes the international hegemony of the Irish text *Active Management of Labour: The Dublin Experience* (O'Driscoll, Meagher, and Robson 2003). Other chapters in the volume examine how Mexican obs develop and come to embody their skills through their senses—sight, hearing, and touch; US obstetricians' accounts of caring for substance-using patients; and contraceptive provision (or the lack thereof) by obs in the United States. The final chapter describes the benefits of home birth and why obstetricians fear it. What ties all these chapters together and makes this volume unique are the authors' analyses—and sometimes radical critiques—of obstetricians' practices based on observing and interviewing obstetricians themselves, and the fact that their authors stay focused on obstetricians, rather than critiquing the wider field of obstetrics in general, as many others have done. In the Conclusions to this volume, we address key concepts and theoretical frameworks used in its chapters, ask why obstetricians in multiple countries over-perform cesareans and other interventions, and describe the answers that our chapter authors provided.

Brief Description of Volume III

Obstetric Violence and Systemic Disparities: Can Obstetrics Be Humanized and Decolonized?

In our third and final volume, with 12 chapters, we split our chapters into three Parts, with Part 1 focusing on the powerful and heated subjects of obstetric violence and systemic (systematic and endemic) racial, ethnic, gendered, and socio-structural disparities in obstetricians' practices. Scholars and activists around the world have long pointed out and railed against such destructive disparities and their negative effects on women's childbearing experiences, but again, they have not been investigated from obstetricians' perspectives, as these chapters do. Our authors ask the brave questions of obstetricians from the United States, the Dominican Republic, Mexico, and Peru: are they aware of the violence, disrespect, and abuse they often perpetrate on their patients? Do they perceive these as such? How do they justify their disrespect and abuse to themselves and to others? Are they aware of the racial and ethnic biases that often heavily influence their practices? Do they understand the socio-structural embeddedness and root causes of these biases, both in the history of their profession and in society at large? Do they seek to eliminate these in their own practices?

And with the practical question—"What can be done about these damaging issues by obstetricians themselves?"—we move to Part 2 of Volume III, "Decolonizing and Humanizing Obstetric Training and Practice? Obstetricians, Midwives, and Their Battles against 'The System.'" Here our chapters, written by both obstetricians and social scientists, address decolonizing obstetric education in the UK; efforts to change obstetric training and practice by teaching humanistic and holistic practices in Russia and the former Soviet nations; a new model for collaboration among obstetricians and midwives in New Zealand; and how the face of US obstetrics has changed as more women enter that field. One chapter addresses how obstetricians in Russia struggle to "go against the system" by humanizing and personalizing their care, with varying degrees of success, while another chapter details the profound paradigm shifts made by some Brazilian obstetricians, their processes, and their effects.

Part 3 of this third volume, entitled "The Ethnographic Challenges of Gaining Access to Obstetricians for Surveys, Interviews, and Observations" contains only one chapter, which addresses that topic based on our chapter authors' own experiences of dealing with those challenges. Our Conclusions to this final volume, like those of the other volumes, describe some of the theoretical concepts and frameworks that the chapter authors found most useful, and also describe lessons learned from those chapters. Our Series Conclusions provide some brief reflections on our findings from all three volumes, yet focus primarily on our chapter authors' and our own suggestions for future research. Students and other researchers are always looking for new topics to research; thus we provide them with some great ideas in these Series Conclusions!

And now, having introduced and described our three-volume book series, we move to the (brief) Introduction to this present volume.

Robbie Davis-Floyd, Adjunct Professor, Department of Anthropology, Rice University, Houston, Fellow of the Society for Applied Anthropology, and Senior Advisor to the Council on Anthropology and Reproduction, is a well-known medical/reproductive anthropologist and international speaker and researcher in transformational models of childbirth, midwifery, obstetrics, and reproduction. Over the course of her long anthropological career, which began in the early 1980s, she has taught at four universities (University of Texas, Austin; Trinity University in San Antonio, Texas; Rice University, Houston; and Case Western Reserve University in Cleveland, Ohio, where she served for a year as Visiting Professor), has given more than 1,000 talks at universities and at birth, midwifery, and obstetric conferences around the world, and has received various grants and awards. She is author of 86 peer-reviewed journal articles and book chapters, and 24 encyclopedia entries, of *Birth as an American Rite of Passage* (1992, 2003, 2022) and of *Ways of Knowing about Birth* (2018); coauthor of *From Doctor to Healer: The Transformative Journey* (1998) and of *Ritual: What It Is, How It Works, and Why* (2022); and lead or coeditor of 17 volumes, the latest of which are *Birth in Eight Cultures* (2019), coedited with Melissa Cheyney; *Birthing Models on the Human Rights Frontier: Speaking Truth to Power* (2021), coedited with Betty-Anne Daviss; *Sustainable Birth in Disruptive Times*, lead-edited by Kim Gutschow and coedited with Betty-Anne Daviss (2021); and the solo-edited *Birthing Techno-Sapiens: Human-Technology Co-Evolution and the Future of Reproduction* (2021). In process are a collection on *Traditional Midwives: Cross-Cultural Perspectives*, to be coedited with Pakistani anthropologist Inayat Ali and Canadian social scientist and midwife Betty-Anne Daviss; and a textbook on the anthropology of reproduction, to be coauthored with Maya Unnithan and Marcia Inhorn. Email:davis-floyd@outlook.com.

Ashish Premkumar is an Assistant Professor of Obstetrics and Gynecology at the Pritzker School of Medicine at The University of Chicago and a doctoral candidate in the Department of Anthropology at The Graduate School at Northwestern University. He is a practicing maternal-fetal medicine subspecialist. His research focus is on the intersections of the social sciences and obstetric practices, particularly surrounding the issues of risk, stigma, and quality of health care during the perinatal opioid use disorder epidemic of the 21st century. E-mail: premkumara@bsd.uchicago.edu.

References

Ali I, Sadique S, Ali S, Davis-Floyd R. 2021. "Birthing Between the 'Traditional' and the 'Modern': Dai Practices and Childbearing Women's Choices during COVID-19 in Pakistan." *Frontiers in Sociology* 6: 622223.

American College of Obstetricians and Gynecologists (ACOG) 2019a. "ACOG Committee Opinion No. 766: Approaches to Limit Intervention during Labor and Birth." *Obstetrics & Gynecology* 133(2): 164–e173.

———. 2019b. "ACOG Committee Opinion No. 761: Cesarean Delivery on Maternal Request." American College of Obstetricians and Gynecologists. Retrieved 10 September 2022 from https://www.acog.org/-/media/project/acog/acogorg/clinical/files/committee-opinion/articles/2019/01/cesarean-delivery-on-maternal-request.pdf.

Arney WR. 1982. *Power and the Profession of Obstetrics*. Chicago: University of Chicago Press.

Barker-Benfield GJ. 2000. *The Horrors of the Half-Known Life: Male Attitudes toward Women and Sexuality in Nineteenth-Century America*. London: Routledge.

Belizán JM, Minckas N, McClure EM, et al. 2018. "An Approach to Identify a Minimum and Rational Proportion of Caesarean Sections in Resource-Poor Settings: A Global Network Study." *Lancet Global Health* 6(8): 894–e901.

Betran AP, Torloni MR, Zhang J, et al. 2015. "What Is the Optimal Rate of Caesarean Section at Population Level? A Systematic Review of Ecologic Studies." *Reproductive Health* 12(1): 57.

Boerma T, Ronsmans C, Melesse VY, et al. 2018. "Global Epidemiology of Use of and Disparities in Caesarean Sections." *Lancet* 392(10155): 1341–1348.

Bohren MA, Mehrtash H, Fawole B, et al. 2019. "How Women Are Treated during Facility-Based Childbirth in Four Countries: A Cross-Sectional Study with Labour Observations and Community-Based Surveys." *Lancet* 394(10210): 1750–1763.

Bridges KM. 2011. *Reproducing Race: An Ethnography of Pregnancy as a Site of Racialization.* Berkeley: University of California Press.

Casper MJ. 1998. *The Making of the Unborn Patient: A Social Anatomy of Fetal Surgery.* New Brunswick NJ: Rutgers University Press.

Cheyney M, Davis-Floyd R. 2020a. "Birth and the Big Bad Wolf: A Biocultural, Co-Evolutionary Perspective, Part 1." *International Journal of Childbirth* 9(4): 177–192.

———. 2020b. "Birth and the Big Bad Wolf: A Biocultural, Co-Evolutionary Perspective, Part 2." *International Journal of Childbirth* 10(2): 66–78.

———. 2021. "Birth and the Big Bad Wolf: Biocultural Evolution and Human Childbirth." In *Birthing Techno-Sapiens: Human-Technology Co-Evolution and the Future of Reproduction,* ed. Davis-Floyd R, 15–46. Abingdon, Oxon: Routledge.

Davis DA. 2018. "The Labor of Racism." Anthro{Dendum}, 7 May. https://anthrodendum.org/2018/05/07/the-labor-of-racism/.

Davis DA. 2019a. "Obstetric Racism: The Racial Politics of Pregnancy, Labor, and Birthing." *Medical Anthropology* 38(7): 560–573.

Davis DA. 2019b. *Reproductive Injustice: Racism, Pregnancy, and Premature Birth.* New York: New York University Press.

Davis-Floyd R. 2003. *Birth as an American Rite of Passage,* 2nd ed. Berkeley: University of California Press.

———. 2018a. "The Technocratic, Humanistic, and Holistic Paradigms of Birth and Health Care." In *Ways of Knowing about Birth: Mothers, Midwives, Medicine, and Birth Activism,* Davis-Floyd R and Colleagues, 3–44. Long Grove IL: Waveland Press.

———. 2018b. "The Rituals of Hospital Birth: Enacting and Transmitting the Technocratic Model." In *Ways of Knowing about Birth: Mothers, Midwives, Medicine, and Birth Activism,* Davis-Floyd R and Colleagues, 45–70. Long Grove IL: Waveland Press.

———. 2022. *Birth as an American Rite of Passage,* 3rd ed. Abingdon, Oxon: Routledge.

———. 2023. "Open and Closed Knowledge Systems, the 4 Stages of Cognition, and the Cultural Management of Birth." In *Cognition, Risk, and Responsibility in Obstetrics: Anthropological Analyses and Critiques of Obstetricians' Practices,* eds. Davis-Floyd R, Premkumar A, Chapter 1. New York: Berghahn Books.

Davis-Floyd R, Georges E. 2023. "The Paradigm Shifts of Humanistic and Holistic Obstetricians: The 'Good Guys and Girls' of Brazil." In *Obstetric Violence and Systemic Disparities: Can Obstetrics Be Humanized and Decolonized?* eds. Davis-Floyd R, Premkumar A, Chapter 9. New York: Berghahn Books.

Davis-Floyd R, Gutschow K, Schwartz DA. 2020. "Pregnancy, Birth, and the COVID-19 Pandemic in the United States." *Medical Anthropology* 39(5): 413–427.

Davis-Floyd R, Cheyney M, eds. 2019. *Birth in Eight Cultures.* Long Grove IL: Waveland Press.

Davis-Floyd R, Laughlin CD. 2022. *Ritual: What It Is, How It Works, and Why.* New York: Berghahn Books.

Davis-Floyd R, Matsuoka E, Horan H, Ruder B, Everson CL. 2018. "Daughter of Time: The Postmodern Midwife." In *Ways of Knowing about Birth: Mothers, Midwives, Medicine, and Birth Activism.* Davis-Floyd R and Colleagues, 221–264. Long Grove IL: Waveland Press.

Davis-Floyd R, Premkumar A, eds. 2023a. *Obstetricians Speak: On Training, Practice, Fear, and Transformation*. New York: Berghahn Books.

———. 2023b. *Cognition, Risk, and Responsibility in Obstetrics: Anthropological Analyses and Critiques of Obstetricians' Practices*. New York: Berghahn Books.

———. 2023c. *Obstetric Violence and Systemic Disparities: Can Obstetrics Be Humanized and Decolonized?* New York: Berghahn Books.

Davis-Floyd R, Sargent C. 1997. *Childbirth and Authoritative Knowledge: Cross-Cultural Perspectives*. Berkeley: University of California Press.

DeVries R, Benoit C, van Teijligen E, Wrede S, eds. 2001. *Birth by Design: Pregnancy, Maternity Care, and Midwifery in North America and Europe*. London: Routledge.

Dixon LZ, Smith-Oka V, El Kotni M. 2019. "Teaching about Childbirth in Mexico: Working across Birth Models." In *Birth in Eight Cultures*, ed. Davis-Floyd R, Cheyney M, 17–48. Long Grove IL: Waveland Press.

Gaines AD, Davis-Floyd R. 2003. "Biomedicine." In *Encyclopedia of Medical Anthropology: Health and Illness in the World's Cultures*, ed. Ember CR, Ember M, 95–109. Boston MA: Springer US.

Georges E. 2008. *Bodies of Knowledge: The Medicalization of Reproduction in Greece*. Nashville TN: Vanderbilt University Press.

———. 2023. "Becoming an Obstetrician in Greece: Medical Training, Informal Scripts, and the Routinization of Cesarean Birth." In *Cognition, Risk, and Responsibility in Obstetrics: Anthropological Analyses and Critiques of Obstetricians' Practices*, ed. Davis-Floyd R, Premkumar A, Chapter 3. New York: Berghahn Books.

Georges E, Daellenbach R. 2019. "Divergent Meanings and Practices of Childbirth in Greece and New Zealand." In *Birth in Eight Cultures*, eds. Davis-Floyd R, Cheyney M, 129–164. Long Grove IL: Waveland Press.

Ginsburg F, Rapp R. 1995. *Conceiving the New World Order: The Global Politics of Reproduction*. Berkeley: University of California Press.

Gribble KD, Bewley S, Bartick MC, et al. 2022. "Effective Communication about Pregnancy, Birth, Lactation, Breastfeeding and Newborn Care: The Importance of Sexed Language." *Frontier Global Women's Health*, 7 February. Retrieved 9 February 2022 from https://www.frontiersin.org/articles/10.3389/fgwh.2022.818856/full.

Gutschow K, Davis-Floyd R. 2021. "The Impacts of COVID-19 on US Maternity Care Practitioners: A Follow-Up Study." *Frontiers in Sociology* 6:655401: 1–18.

Jones R. 2009. "Teamwork: An Obstetrician, a Midwife, and a Doula in Brazil." In *Birth Models that Work*, ed. Davis-Floyd R, Barclay L, Daviss BA, Tritten J, 271–304. Berkeley: University of California Press.

Jordan B. (1978) 1993. *Birth in Four Cultures: A Cross-Cultural Investigation of Childbirth in Yucatan, Holland, Sweden, and the United States*. Long Grove IL: Waveland Press.

Kramer K. 2002. Class paper for a course at Southern Methodist University taught by Robbie Davis-Floyd, unpublished.

Krisberg K. 2019. "Programs Work from Within to Prevent Black Maternal Deaths: Workers Targeting Root Cause—Racism." *The Nation's Health* 49(6): 1–17.

Kuan CI. 2014. "Suffering Twice: The Gender Politics of Cesarean Sections in Taiwan." *Medical Anthropology Quarterly* 28(3): 399–418.

Lalonde A, Herschderfer K, Pascali Bonaro D, et al. 2019. "The International Childbirth Initiative: 12 Steps to Safe and Respectful MotherBaby–Family Maternity Care." *International Journal of Gynecology & Obstetrics* 146(1): 65–73.

Lewis R. 2020. "What to Expect When You're in the Latent (Early) Phase of Labor." *Healthline Parenthood*, 30 June. Retrieved 10 September 2022 from https://www.healthline.com/health/pregnancy/latent-phase-of-labor.

Liese K, Davis-Floyd R, Stewart K, Cheyney M. 2021. "Obstetric Iatrogenesis in the United States: The Spectrum of Unintentional Harm, Disrespect, Violence, and Abuse." *Anthropology & Medicine* 28(2): 188–204.

Liu S, Liston RM, Joseph KS, et al. 2007. "Maternal Mortality and Severe Morbidity Associated with Low-Risk Planned Cesarean Delivery versus Planned Vaginal Delivery at Term." *Canadian Medical Association Journal* 176(4): 455–460.

Lokugamage A. 2011. "Fear of Homebirth in Doctors and Obstetric Iatrogenesis." *International Journal of Childbirth* 1(4): 263–272.

Long D, Hunter C, van der Geest S. 2008. "When the Field Is a Ward or a Clinic: Hospital Ethnography." *Anthropology & Medicine* 15(2): 71–78.

Lukere V, Jolly M, eds. 2002. *Birthing in the Pacific: Beyond Tradition and Modernity?* Honolulu: University of Hawaii Press.

Mayo Clinic Staff. 2022. "Stages of Labor and Birth: Baby, it's time!" *Mayo Clinic*, January 13. Retrieved 10 September from https://www.mayoclinic.org/healthy-lifestyle/labor-and-delivery/in-depth/stages-of-labor/art-20046545.

McGregor DK. 1998. *From Midwives to Medicine: The Birth of American Gynecology*. New Brunswick NJ: Rutgers University Press, 1998.

McNabb D. 2023. "The Changing Face of Obstetric Practice in the US as the Percent of Women in the Specialty Has Grown." In *Obstetric Violence and Systemic Disparities: Can Obstetrics Be Humanized and Decolonized?* ed. Davis-Floyd R, Premkumar A, Chapter 11. New York: Berghahn Books.

Miller S, Abalos E, Chamillard M, et al. 2016. "Beyond Too Little, Too Late and Too Much, Too Soon: A Pathway towards Evidence-Based, Respectful Maternity Care Worldwide." *The Lancet* 388(10056): 2176–2192.

Murphy M. 2017. *The Economization of Life*. Durham NC: Duke University Press.

Murphy-Lawless J. 1998. *Reading Birth and Death: A History of Obstetric Thinking*. Cork: Cork University Press.

O'Driscoll K, Meagher D, Robson M. 2003. *Active Management of Labour: The Dublin Experience*. London: Mosby Elsevier.

Pérez D'Gregorio R. 2010. "Obstetric Violence: A New Legal Term Introduced in Venezuela." *International Journal of Gynecology & Obstetrics* 111(3): 201–202.

Ram K, Jolly M, eds. 1998. *Maternities and Modernities: Colonial and Postcolonial Experiences in Asia and the Pacific*. Cambridge: Cambridge University Press.

Reynolds PC. 1991. *Stealing Fire: The Mythology of the Technocracy*. Palo Alto CA: Iconic Anthropology Press.

Roberts DJ. 1999. *Killing the Black Body: Race, Reproduction, and the Meaning of Liberty*. New York: Vintage Books.

Sadler M, Santos MJDS, Ruiz-Berdún D, et al. 2016. "Moving Beyond Disrespect and Abuse: Addressing the Structural Dimensions of Obstetric Violence." *Reproductive Health Matters* 24(47): 47–55.

Scully D. 1980. *Men Who Control Women's Health: The Miseducation of Obstetrician Gynecologists.* Boston: Houghton-Mifflin.

Selin H, Stone PK, eds. 2009. *Childbirth across Cultures: Ideas and Practices of Pregnancy, Childbirth and the Postpartum.* New York: Springer.

Soliday E. 2012. *Childbirth in a Technocratic Age: The Documentation of Women's Expectations and Experiences.* Amherst NY: Cambria Press.

Smith-Oka V. 2021. *Becoming Gods: Medical Training in Mexican Hospitals.* New Brunswick NJ: Rutgers University Press.

Smith-Oka V, Dixon LZ. 2023. "On Risk and Responsibility: Contextualizing Practice among Mexican Obstetricians." In *Cognition, Risk, and Responsibility in Obstetrics: Anthropological Analyses and Critiques of Obstetricians' Practices*, ed. Davis-Floyd R, Premkumar A, Chapter 7. New York: Berghahn Books.

Thaddeus S, Maine D. 1994. "Too Far to Walk: Maternal Mortality in Context." *Social Science & Medicine* 38(8): 1091–1110.

Villar J, Carroli G, Zavaleta N, et al. 2007. "Maternal and Neonatal Individual Risks and Benefits Associated with Caesarean Delivery: Multicentre Prospective Study." *British Biomedical Journal* 335(7628): 1025.

Villar J, Valladares E, Wojdyla D, et al. 2006. "Caesarean Delivery Rates and Pregnancy Outcomes: The 2005 Who Global Survey on Maternal and Perinatal Health in Latin America." *The Lancet* 367(9525): 1819–1829.

WHO Statement on Caesarean Section Rates. 2015. *Reproductive Health Matters* 23(45): 149–150.

Williamson E, Matsuoka E. 2019. "Comparing Childbirth in Brazil and Japan: Social Hierarchies, Cultural Values, and the Meaning of Place." In *Birth in Eight Cultures*, eds. Davis-Floyd R, Cheyney M, 89–128. Long Grove IL: Waveland Press.

Wolf J. 2020. *Cesarean Section: An American History of Risk, Technology, and Consequence.* Baltimore MD: Johns Hopkins University Press.

INTRODUCTION TO VOLUME I
Obstetricians Speak

Robbie Davis-Floyd and Ashish Premkumar

For the first time in social science history, this coedited volume—with the exceptions of the preceding Series Overview, this Introduction, and the Conclusions—consists entirely of chapters written by obstetricians (obs) who have been much critiqued by others yet rarely have had the chance to speak for themselves in the social science literature. Some of its chapter authors are also studying to get their PhDs in medical anthropology or already have them; these authors describe what that means for their ability to autoethnographically self-reflect and self-analyze within the broader context of their cultures, countries, and professions, which in this volume include Hungary, Brazil, India, Turkey, Canada, Australia, and the United States.

In the Series Overview, we presented some theoretical constructs and frameworks that will be employed in all three volumes. These include Robbie Davis-Floyd's delineations of the technocratic, humanistic, and holistic paradigms of birth and health care, which are much used by the chapter authors in this volume, along with her descriptions of the "4 Stages of Cognition" and "Substage." Now we proceed to a summary of what you can expect to find as you read through these chapters.

Introducing the Chapters in This Volume

In Chapter 1, US obstetrician Scott Moses provides an autoethnographic account of becoming an abortion provider and the ethical dilemmas that entailed for him. While still in medical school, he was attracted to the field of obstetrics because of his fascination with life cycle events and their rituals. In his words, he was "drawn to the privilege of building a relationship with the patient and family during a time of significant and unique vulnerability and wonder," evoking Rabbi Abraham Joshua Heschel's term "radical amazement." He details his original uncertainty about becoming an abortion provider, his trajectory in moving from rabbinic candidate to women's health care provider—particularly in relation to pregnancy termination—and his extensive research on ethics. He describes his ultimate full commitment to providing a service that so many women need, precisely because of that need and because of his ability to provide it. He also addresses the implications of the Supreme Court's overturning of *Roe v Wade*, and of the recent Texas law that prohibits abortions in almost all cases.

The trope of abortion provision continues in Chapter 2, "Abortion, Professional Identity, and Generational Meaning Making among US Ob/Gyns" by medical anthropologists Rebecca Henderson and Chu J. Hsiao and obstetrician Jody Steinauer. These authors explore the meaning-making processes through which abortion provider interlocutors (who include coauthor Steinauer) have incorporated the provision of abortion as a key part of their professional identities and as an enactment of their core values. The authors show how the meaning of abortion provision has changed over time via the use of narratives from four ob/gyns of four different generations. The *Roe v Wade* generation of abortion providers tended to place primary focus on the lifesaving purposes of safe, doctor-provided abortions, framing them as medical necessities. Over the subsequent decades, abortion access for pregnant people and access to medical education about abortion steadily eroded in a politically fraught climate that generated the marginalization and stigmatization of abortion providers. Then, during the early 1990s, abortion provision became linked with values on feminism, advocacy, activism, and justice. Thus, subsequent generations have moved their meaning making around abortion to a primary focus on reproductive rights and reproductive justice. Like Scott Moses, these abortion providers consistently framed abortion as central to their professional identities as ob/gyns, describing their abortion work as affirming and as "expressing their most important professional values and obligations." They frequently engaged in political advocacy, seeing abortion as a means of addressing the "root causes" of injustice and as "mission-driven" medicine. The links that these interlocutors generated between abortion and ethical obligations also resonate with the ideas described by Moses in the preceding chapter.

In Chapter 3, series coeditor Ashish Premkumar autoethnographically describes his transformation from an obstetrician to a maternal-fetal medicine (MFM) subspecialist, also called a perinatologist. In the United States, becoming an ob/gyn requires four years of training after completion of medical school. To achieve subspeciality training in

MFM—the practice of taking care of pregnant people and fetuses with complex medical issues—one must undertake three additional years of training after residency. While anthropological inquiries into ob/gyn training have used ethnographic accounts to evaluate how obstetricians understand the body through surgery, or how risk is conceived of and enacted through obstetric practices, there has been a limited inquiry into the phenomenological and embodied experiences of undergoing training as a subspecialist, particularly the crafting of the body through procedures unique to the perinatologist—for example, performing maternal-fetal therapies and surgeries, and engaging with pregnant people in the construction and clinical management of maternal-fetal risk. By utilizing autoethnography, Premkumar seeks to shed light on how an MFM's viewpoint is maintained and (re)produced, and what the stakes are for both the burgeoning anthropology of obstetrics (as evidenced in our three volumes) and for wider theories of knowledge production, power, and the body.

In Chapter 4, "Cold Steel and Sunshine," Kathleen Hanlon-Lundberg, also an MFM specialist, provides both ethnographic and autoethnographic perspectives on two perinatal careers "from across the chasm" between biomedicine and anthropology. She compares her obstetric trajectory with that of her friend and colleague Emily: Kathleen worked in large tertiary hospitals, while Emily chose to open a private practice serving members of a small community—a practice that gives her great personal and professional satisfaction. Kathleen achieved her greatest satisfaction during the years when she worked at a humanistic hospital that fully integrated nurse-midwives and the midwifery model of care. Yet once she had children of her own, the long commute became unsustainable, and she moved to a large, nearby hospital where she experienced so much tragedy and grief that, after some years, she left obstetrics behind, eventually deciding to study anthropology to better understand the human condition. Throughout her chapter, Handlon-Lundberg emphasizes that the vast majority of obstetricians whom she knows are "caring, thoughtful, and dedicated to the health and well-being of the persons whom they serve." Yet the first American Anthropology Association meeting sessions on reproduction that she attended "centered on how the obstetricians of the world wrong and harm women. I was surprised, as this was certainly not representative of my experience. I was clearly out of my territory, surrounded by members of a hostile tribe that seemed determined to totalize and essentialize 'the other' using a plethora of multisyllabic words and liberal suffixes."

Let her words be an inspiration to all social scientists to avoid "totalizing" and "essentializing" the members of any groups we study. There should not be a "chasm" between biomedicine and anthropology, but rather a "plethora" of mutually rewarding interactions and fewer uses of "multisyllabic words and liberal suffixes"—of which we admit that we and our chapter authors are guilty of doing, as these days it seems that one cannot be an anthropologist without using plenty of those multisyllabic words and liberal suffixes.

In Chapter 5, US obstetrician Jesanna Cooper describes how she experienced "an awakening" after her difficulties with breastfeeding her first child, whose birth was highly medicalized. These difficulties led her to rethink her role as an obstetrician. Noting that "we obstetricians suffer from a flawed and dehumanizing maternity care system," she states that obs work in a professional setting of fear—fear of being wrong, of lawsuits, of professional ostracism, of being bullied, of disappointing their patients and themselves. They also fear the consequences of not meeting standards set by courts, hospital governance bodies, governments, and insurance companies, and of not being able to support their families financially and emotionally. Cooper explains the traumas of her own years of residency in terms of the "Dementor's Kiss" described in the Harry Potter book series, and how she graduated from residency as "a shell of her former self." Bullying, fatigue, and fear had extinguished her intellectual curiosity, joy, and love of service. Then she had an awakening. She said, "I remembered who I was. I realized that my position in the medicalized maternity care system gave me a platform for change. I could partner with midwives and doulas. I could create a culture where our team approaches patients with understanding, compassion, and respect." Her chapter goes on to describe the resulting changes she made to her practice, the tolls her paradigm shift has taken on her mental, emotional, and physical health, and, paradoxically, the successes and personal satisfaction this paradigm shift has given her. Yet ultimately, those tolls proved too much for her to bear, so, as she explains in her chapter, she sold her clinic in 2021, and is now officially retired.

In Chapter 6, Rosana Fontes, a Brazilian obstetrician, also describes the repercussions of a similar paradigm shift from Stage 1 technocratic to Stage 4 humanistic practice (for explanations of these terms, see the Series Overview, this volume) in both her professional and personal lives. Fed up with the "blind obedience" required by the technocratic approach, which excludes and punishes those who don't conform, Fontes and her like-minded partners conceived and founded the Mátria Clinic, where "deeply humanistic" (again, see the Series Overview) practitioners responsibly attended over 1,000 deliveries in the Paraíba Valley, São Paulo, Brazil, in a multi-professional team. In her chapter, Fontes provides the excellent statistical results associated with this Stage 4 humanized care, and notes that including midwives generated this clinic's success.

Fontes demonstrates that pregnant women attended at the Mátria Clinic were more satisfied with their labor processes because their choices were respected. The workload and responsibility normally entirely deposited in the obstetrician, Fontes, were reduced, along with her stress levels. The implementation of multidisciplinary group prenatal care also contributed to success in this model, as did the fact that clinic practitioners followed the WHO recommendations to ensure maternal and child safety. Fontes demonstrates that, even within a country where the cesarean rate is very high (56%), it is remarkable to see that adaptation to this humanistic model is easy to perform, low cost, and entirely possible. Yet eventually, tired of the persecutions she experienced from other doctors, and in an effort to achieve a better work/life balance and in hopes of having a family, Rosana sold the Mátria Clinic despite the strong objections of the staff, and today attends only a few births per month—those referred to her by the midwives with whom she still works.

The trope of the repercussions of a paradigm shift, this time to entirely holistic practice, is continued in Chapter 7 by former Brazilian obstetrician Ricardo Jones, who told us that he found his chapter both "emotionally challenging and psychologically cathartic" to write. He details his paradigm shift to Stage 4 holistic obstetric practice and his reasons for making it, and briefly describes his 34 years of attending both home and hospital births with his midwife and doula team. Jones then proceeds to the major focus of his chapter—the heavy prices he paid for practicing outside the Stage 1, fundamentalist, and often fanatical technocratic silo in the forms of bullyings and persecutions by the obstetric establishment in his city of Porto Alegre in the far South of Brazil and the ways in which he managed to withstand these. Jones concludes with an account of how the obstetric establishment finally managed to take away his license over a neonatal death that he did his best to avoid, only to be defeated in his efforts by NICU doctors who failed to give the baby the proper antibiotics in time to save his life. With this chapter, Jones hopes to call attention to the persecutions as experienced by himself and by many other holistic obstetricians and midwives like him, and to offer his own efforts to withstand these as a pathway for others who are presently experiencing the same types of persecution, in what many call "the global witch hunt."

By far the most famous obstetric practitioner who experienced the effects of that "witch hunt" is Hungarian obstetrician and midwife Ágnes Geréb. Coauthored with her friend and colleague Katalin Fábián, in Chapter 8, "Hungarian Birth Models Seen through the Prism of Prison: The Journey of Ágnes Geréb," Ágnes (Agi) describes her transformation from working as an ob/gyn for 17 years to becoming a certified midwife, her efforts to re-establish home birth in her country, the love and support she received from her homebirth clients, the trumped-up malpractice accusations against her, and her resultant 77-day imprisonment and years of house arrest. Agi's official prison term was for two years, but, due to the flood of letters and petitions the Hungarian President received from multiple national and international organizations and thousands of individuals, he granted her an early release, followed by house arrest for an additional three years and two months, lasting until February 2014. She was additionally prohibited from practicing for ten years; she was 67 at the time. Agi is now an international heroine and inspiration to the birth humanization movement, and we are proud to include her chapter in this volume!

In Chapter 9, "Adopting the Midwifery Model of Care in India," obstetrician Evita Fernandez describes how, in its 63rd year of existence, the Fernandez Hospital in Hyderabad, India, launched an in-house two-year Professional Midwifery Education and Training (PMET) program. At the time, the word "midwife" (*dai*) was perceived as referring to traditional midwives/traditional birth attendants (TBAs), who are very much disparaged as "illiterate" and "ignorant" among biomedical personnel and the middle and upper classes of this country. Prior to Fernandez's work, India did not have a dedicated cadre for professional midwifery care. As Fernandez shows, the challenges faced in introducing professional nurse-midwives as accountable and trustworthy healthcare professionals and colleagues into a strongly biomedically led maternity hospital were enormous. Evita, who played a major part in initiating this change, describes that with growing numbers of nurses trained in midwifery, there has been a visible change in childbirth practices. Women receiving midwifery care endorse their services with positive feedback. The obstetricians also began to appreciate midwifery care and new working relationships between obs and midwives were established.

Fernandez also explains that the government of India had been battling with an unacceptably high cesarean birth (CB) rate. National consultation on the causes and determinants of the high CB rate in 2016 suggested midwifery care as a vital option to help decrease unnecessary interventions, including CBs. The government of Telangana State, with the highest CB rates in the country, decided to pilot its first midwifery training program with a cohort of 30 registered nurses. The success of this program led the Government of India to launch the *Guidelines on Midwifery Services* in India and to establish 14 national midwifery educator training institutes to help scale up midwifery training to meet India's enormous needs. Evita's chapter tells the story of this journey, which she describes as "the start of a revolution."

In Chapter 10, Turkish obstetrician Hakan Çoker first describes his 19 years as a "classic" obstetrician whose main concern was a healthy mother and baby at the end of the birth. Yet after sneaking into a childbirth education class in Turkey out of sheer curiosity, and later attending childbirth classes in multiple countries, "my perception of birth irreversibly changed." He cocreated a birthing team called "Birth with No Regret," which consists of an obstetrician, a midwife who also acts as a doula, and a birth psychotherapist, who importantly helps both the practitioners and the families they attend process their emotions before, during, and after the birth. Hakan and his team organize childbirth classes for families, childbirth educators, and doulas, "so that we can grow the concept of humanistic births everywhere"—a much-needed process, as in Turkey, the cesarean rate is 58%, with many routine interventions. Hakan has become a widely known advocate for humanistic births and humanistic birth teams, yet there were heavy prices to pay in the form of attacks by other obs, as he describes in his chapter. Importantly, his responses to those attacks were neither defensive nor argumentative; rather, he took each attack as an opportunity to further explain the benefits of evidence-based, humanistic care. This respectful approach led to some of the obs who attacked him secretly attending his childbirth education classes and eventually adopting his model of "Birth with No Regret."

In Chapter 11, Australian obstetrician Andrew Bisits explains that in Australia, Canada, New Zealand, and the United States over the past decades, there has been a near-complete disappearance of vaginal breech birth as a legitimate option for women with babies in the breech position at term, as obs in those countries are no longer trained in breech delivery techniques. Other countries in Scandinavia and Europe have maintained vaginal breech birth as a supported and responsible option for such women. In his chapter, Bisits describes how his interest in breech births developed and what he has learned about vaginal breech deliveries over time, with the aim of informing, teaching, and giving confidence to all obstetricians and midwives so that they can be safe breech birth practitioners as well.

In Chapter 12, US ob Marco Gianotti describes how he mixes modalities in his "traditionalist," technocratic obstetric practice, and the ideology and rationales that underlie that practice. He notes that, although biomedical obstetric practice became much more trying during the coronavirus pandemic, he still found it possible to integrate more humanistic and holistic measures into care plans for patients seeking such a balance. Gianotti demonstrates the difficulties of incorporating more holistic practices into traditional biomedicine and how they depend on a particular physician's practice style and philosophy, relating back to how the physician was trained and to personal beliefs. Gianotti believes that the practice of obstetrics presents a particular opportunity to incorporate home deliveries, the support of doulas, and holistic modalities.

In Chapter 13, world-renowned obstetrician André Lalonde takes us to the global stage by describing his career trajectory as it developed over 40 years to address respectful maternity care and promote physiologic childbirth. From the introduction of humanistic changes as Chief of Maternity Services in a community hospital to teaching residents at McGill University, André questioned the "paternalistic practices" of obstetrics that gave childbearers few choices. Having made major humanistic changes in labor and delivery practices in these places, he then served as President of the Society of Obstetricians and Gynecologists of Canada for 21 years, during which he helped to draft many guidelines that addressed women's major concerns. Also during that time, he served on the Executive Board of the International Federation of Gynecology and Obstetrics (FIGO) and as Chair of FIGO's Safe Motherhood and Newborn Committee. As he describes in his chapter, André's work on this international committee led to the development of important international policies and guidelines and to the launch of the *International Childbirth Initiative* (ICI): *12 Steps to Safe and Respectful MotherBaby-Family Maternity Care*. The ICI Principles and 12 Steps are now being implemented in multiple birth facilities and practices around the world (see Robbie's bio below); André lists all of them in his chapter.

Having completed our brief Introduction to this volume, we now turn to its chapters, in which, as our book title states, "obstetricians speak."

Robbie Davis-Floyd, Adjunct Professor, Department of Anthropology, Rice University, Houston, Fellow of the Society for Applied Anthropology, and Senior Advisor to the Council on Anthropology and Reproduction is a cultural/medical/reproductive anthropologist interested in transformational models of maternity care and an international speaker. She is also a Board member of the International MotherBaby Childbirth Organization (IMBCO), in which capacity she helped to wordsmith the *International Childbirth Initiative: 12 Steps to Safe and Respectful MotherBaby-Family Maternity Care* (found at www.icichildbirth.org). Researchers are needed to study the barriers to and the effects of ICI implementation. If you are interested, please contact Robbie at davis-floyd@outlook.com.

Ashish Premkumar is an Assistant Professor of Obstetrics and Gynecology at the Pritzker School of Medicine at The University of Chicago and a doctoral candidate in the Department of Anthropology at The Graduate School at Northwestern University. He is a practicing maternal-fetal medicine subspecialist. His research focus is on the intersections of the social sciences and obstetric practices, particularly surrounding the issues of risk, stigma, and quality of health care during the perinatal opioid use disorder epidemic of the 21st century. E-mail: premkumara@bsd.uchicago.edu.

CHAPTER 1

On Becoming an Abortion Provider in the United States
An Autoethnographic Account

Scott Moses

Introduction

After many generations of silence about abortions and abortion provision, the past few decades have seen a relative abundance of literature on these topics. Most relevant articles and books engage the topic by celebrating and prioritizing the principle of autonomy above all other ethical constructs. This is true whether the authors are advocating for the pregnant patient's ability to abort a fetus or, in stark contrast, focusing on the personhood of the fetus as irrefutable. I am not an expert in anthropology, philosophy, religion, or law, although I am interested in all of these disciplines. Nor am I considered an abortion expert in my field because I have not completed a Family Planning Fellowship.[1] In fact, performing abortions constitutes only a small portion of my clinical practice. However, I have participated in, and performed, many hundreds over the past 30 years. I write this chapter in part because I believe myself to be, like many obstetrician/gynecologists in the United States, someone who lives in the realm of the lifecycle with patients and struggles with the impossibly complicated dilemma of abortion. For some patients, pregnancy signifies the quintessential manifestation of love and optimism about the future, while for others, pregnancy poses a devastating predicament. In my 30 years as an obstetrician, I have been struck by the fluidity within which many patients and providers vacillate in contemplating the options and implications of those choices. I humbly write this chapter describing my trajectory through reproductive health care using abortion as the lens. I write as a generalist ob/gyn who has always worked in university medical centers, as a graduate of a religious seminary, as a father, and as a male gynecologist inspired by the feminist movement.

My Career Trajectory

In some ways, this chapter grew out of a talk I gave to small groups of medical students several times a year over two decades. After finishing my formal ethics training during Fellowship,[2] I started to teach in the first-year ethics course at Northwestern University Medical School in 1997. I was surprised that the course, while excellent, did not address abortion at all. When asked, the course director described the failure of past discussions. She felt that the sessions on abortion inevitably resulted in an argument between the two opposing positions. Nevertheless, I was committed to working the issue into the formal curriculum. After being transformed by my own studies with this course director, who was one of the pioneers in the field of "narrative ethics" (Hunter 1991), I developed a talk designed to begin to understand the fragility and vulnerability of the patient going through the process. I did this through use of patients' narratives, and also through modeling the precariousness of being an abortion provider, including how I decided to participate in this particular lifecycle event of these patients, and often their families. The talk became exponentially better, and more well-received, when it incorporated my dear friend and colleague, who described how and why she decided not to provide abortions. Thereby, the students were exposed to two attendings who worked together and liked and respected each other.[3] Both of us were active members of religious communities, and we had arrived at very different conclusions about abortion provision. Modeling the ability to learn from those with different worldviews paved the way to allow the respect and humility the topic required.

While I believe that my training was perfect to prepare me for a career in clinical medicine, it was not the most common trajectory. The fact that my father was orphaned in Nazi Germany and escaped to France, later establishing a life with foster parents in Chicago, contributed greatly to my choice to become a doctor. I was far from the only first-generation Jewish American child to make a life as a physician. Yet my path was a bit circuitous. As an undergraduate, I was privileged to study simultaneously at both Columbia University, where I was pre-med, and the Jewish Theological Seminary, where I was "pre-rabbi." I received two undergraduate degrees, one in biology and the other in

Jewish philosophy. I felt very lucky to be able to weave the two disciplines and cultures of study. Physician and rabbi both felt like worthy paths of service.

During my undergraduate coursework, I took a variety of classes in philosophy, including a class on Jewish medical ethics. I even wrote a paper on Jewish views on abortion.[4] I remember contemplating the topic as a textual puzzle, hunting for clues in the Talmud and in commentaries to discern rabbinic perspectives. That abstract approach stands in stark contrast to the often painful, agonizing, real-life dilemmas that my patients and I face.

Upon graduating from college, I realized that I would have to choose one discipline to the exclusion of the other. I took a year to decide whether a life in medicine or the rabbinate would be the best fit and most fulfilling. During that year, I worked in a clinical research lab while writing a thesis on the great 12th-century rabbi, philosopher, and physician, Maimonides—the iconic Jewish leader of the Medieval Era who embodied the synthesis between the theological and scientific worlds. I am not completely certain what ultimately pushed me to clinical rather than pastoral care, but by the end of the year I had firmly decided on medicine.

Later, like all US medical students, I took a first-year Medical Ethics course. While many of my colleagues considered the class a distraction from the rigorous science curriculum, I found it fascinating. Throughout medical school, ethics served as a frame for me to integrate subjects like biochemistry and anatomy. Ethics and the medical humanities created lenses through which to view my study of the "hard sciences."

My fourth year of medical school was an extraordinary time. I was reminded of reading van Gennep and Turner—the anthropological experts on rites of passage—as I experienced the elation of the completion of medical school, only to be thrust into the humility of assuming medical care for other human beings, armed solely with the sparse clinical knowledge of a new resident house officer. This estrangement from the life of a lay person and integration into the new world of the professional healer encouraged me to truly appreciate the power and precariousness of liminality—of being "betwixt and between" (Turner 1969). Arnold Van Gennep's description in *The Rites of Passage* (1960) of the phases of "separation, transition, and integration" gave me words and concepts that helpfully elucidated my trajectory through biomedical education and my transformation into professionalism.

When I started medical school, I assumed that I would become a pediatrician, but found that I loved the energy and drama of surgery, particularly the rituals of the operating room. As a young provider, surgery challenged my self-confidence and sense of preparedness in ways the more "cognitive fields" did not. One couldn't talk around the problem, eventually homing in on a plan of care. Surgery requires precision and action. To my surprise, psychiatry also mesmerized me; it struck me that psychiatry was the foundation of clinical medicine. The daunting task of earning access to the thoughts and fears of another human being with the goal of helping to alleviate pain seemed to merge my two seemingly incongruous academic backgrounds. Again, I had a difficult time deciding on my next career step. Choosing a field of biomedicine in which to specialize forced me to become more aware of my own strengths and weaknesses. I painfully acknowledged to myself that I really didn't like taking care of sick people. I wasn't very good at it, and honestly, it frightened me. I was awed by and even jealous of my colleagues who had the competence and dedication to care for patients as their health declined and death became a reality. After completing four extremely trying years in medical school, admitting that the care of the very ill was not my skill set was difficult.

Choosing My Ultimate Career Path

Obstetrics inspired me as the field that most dramatically fostered the care of patients on the upswing of life. As I forged my career path, perhaps I was trying to incorporate my experiences in seminary, where I witnessed clergy being granted the awesome task of stepping in during the most intense aspects of human experience. Likewise, I became energized by the privilege and opportunity of sharing in a patient's lifecycle events. The opportunity to attend the birth of a baby felt impossibly thrilling; that a patient would allow me to participate and a family would welcome me into the scene to me epitomized the privilege of care. These factors ultimately led me to only submit ob/gyn programs to the match for residency,[5] after initially applying and interviewing in three fields: ob/gyn, pediatrics, and psychiatry.

I matched into a large, private, university hospital program, which was far more academic and formal than my prior public medical school. I was one of eight residents chosen per year in a hospital that, at the time, provided services for more than 5,000 births per year. We received significant training in low- and high-risk obstetrics, gynecology, gynecologic oncology, infertility, and urogynecology. There was also one rotation in the third year of residency during which abortions were performed. Today, 25 years later, this hospital has a Family Planning Fellowship incorporating several attending physicians, but at that time, there was only one attending who was responsible for performing the second trimester pregnancy termination procedures. A few others in the department performed abortions in the early second trimester, and many faculty and private attendings did first trimester abortions.

The doctor who ran that abortion rotation was extremely competent. She had been trained as a perinatologist but practiced as a generalist obstetrician and abortion provider. Counseling and performing first trimester abortions were part of the rotation, but the transformative experiences involved caring for the families who had a second trimester loss or a fetus with a structural or genetic deviation. Most devastatingly, a teen or a victim of sexual assault would occasionally come to the clinic for an abortion. During the rotation, we never really discussed the ethics of abortion, nor do I remember anyone ever asking me about my emotional response to performing them. The focus was on the technical skills and on emotional support for the patient.

I was aware that I could have opted out of performing abortions if I so chose. Most years, at least one resident chose not to participate in the family planning/abortion rotation for moral or religious reasons. My sense was that these residents were neither discriminated against for removing themselves nor glorified for forgoing this portion of the curriculum according to their beliefs.[6] It wasn't really discussed amongst the residents, other than "so-and-so does not do abortions." I did not have a difficult time deciding to participate in abortion care when my turn came for the family planning rotation. I never wanted to be in a position where a patient presented to the emergency department bleeding heavily, and I didn't have the skills to perform a dilation and curettage or fetal extraction to save her life. I viewed residency as a gift that allowed me to be exposed to all possible clinical experiences under supervision, to prepare me for what I would face when alone as a graduate. What I was not prepared for was how much this rotation would affect me.

Learning to Listen and Finding Balance

The office appointments both before and after abortions were raw, intense, and emotionally draining. During my prior three years of residency, I had gained a basic proficiency in talking to patients; however, during my time with the population in the family planning clinic, I often had no words. Crucially, I learned how to listen with the intention of *caring* rather than *curing*—the role I had previously been far more comfortable inhabiting. For the first time in my training, I profoundly appreciated the aspect of my job that required and deserved another kind of competence. It demanded being wholly present, making eye contact, and often, simply holding a hand. Meeting with these patients and their partners challenged and humbled me as the most intense and intimate embodiments of the patient-physician relationship I had yet experienced. I was reminded of the time when my mentor at the seminary called me into his office to discuss my conundrum of choosing a future career. He told me that "sometimes you can serve people better as a doctor than a rabbi." I believe that he was trying to give me permission to transition away from the safety and assuredness of religious education, while also kindly making it clear that I was not truly suited for a life in the clergy. Yet in assisting patients with abortions, I had found the balance of clinical and pastoral care that I had sought in my earlier life.

Initially, while still unaccustomed to and uncomfortable with the sadness, anger, and vulnerability of this patient population, I found the procedures themselves to be technically challenging, even (shamefully) satisfying. This was a clinical scenario where I could identify a "problem" and solve it through treatment in a matter of minutes. Somehow, at that time in my development, I unquestioningly lived with the cognitive dissonance between the emotional complexity of this lifecycle event and the relative simplicity of the surgical treatment. Thinking about abortion procedurally, rather than as an integrated part of a patient's life, was a defense against contemplating the ethical complexities.

During my months in training focused on abortion, I found myself thinking about this population around the clock. I had vivid, difficult dreams. I yearned to speak about the experiences of caring for these patients and their families, but lacked the language to do so. Abortion was not the kind of topic one spoke about at social gatherings, other than in the most theoretical manner. I didn't know how to integrate the experience into my life. The fact that my wife was pregnant with twins at that time made the decisions my patients faced seem impossible to fathom, while also painfully close.

Emotional Responses to Performing Abortions

One of my closest friends in medical school and residency had a profound impact on my emotional responses to participating in abortions. While she was on the abortion rotation, which I had already completed, I noticed that she was more withdrawn and quieter than usual. When I asked about her mood, she urgently brought me into a room to talk, and asked if I had a hard time sleeping after I did the procedures. She asked if the muscles in my hand ever cramped while doing second trimester terminations from the simple strain and force necessary to grasp the fetus during the extraction. Both of us started to cry when she asked whether my mouth ever started to water when struggling to reach the fetal skull with the forceps used to collapse and remove the largest part of the fetus. I replied that I had also experienced these reactions on multiple occasions, and that I, too, was scared and confused about my reactions.

Beyond that short conversation with her, I was never provided with the opportunity to share and process these experiences. I still am unsure if my mouth watering was a response of nausea or the single-minded focus required for the surgery, but the memory of my own physiologic reaction associated with second trimester abortions still unsettles me 30 years later. I knew that I had developed an important skill that was too often unavailable in this country. Still, I was perplexed by my visceral response to the physical dismemberment of the fetus required while doing the procedure—a response that left me feeling both quintessentially humane and inhumane at the same time.

Facing Loss

One of the most surprising and powerful realizations of my time in the family planning clinic was that almost all of the patients understood and interpreted their experience as a loss, regardless of whether the fetus had a heartbeat or not, and also regardless of the motivation for the abortion. Sometimes the loss was of possibilities and the fantasy of parenting, or in cases of fetal anomalies, parenting a child without anatomic or genetic challenges. Sometimes it was the sense of loss one feels when forced to select the best choice available instead of the perfect one. While each situation was different, the emotional response of loss was ubiquitous for patients. My clinical experiences alerted me to see the distinction between miscarriage and abortion as relatively insignificant. In both clinical scenarios, I felt pride in my ability to help a person in need and sadness about the need to do so, regardless of the indication for the surgery. I did not expect that sadness to be so similar, whether for a chosen pregnancy termination or assisting with a dead fetus.

When the time came during residency to do the required research project, I was drawn back to the population undergoing the terminations of their pregnancies. I investigated psychological responses to second trimester terminations by surgery or induction of labor. Patients were contacted throughout the six months after their experience and filled out a variety of psychological evaluations. Most crucially, I personally called each of the patients to ask questions about the process. Every conversation was emotionally challenging, but I will never forget the woman who described the harrowing experience of returning to work after her loss. She had brought a card with the footprints of her dead child to work and placed it on her desk.[7] Unimaginably, someone mocked her, and she fled her office in tears, later attempting suicide. She ultimately landed in the hospital to receive mental health services. Through speaking with her, my inexperience and lack of training to care for her mental health needs became clear, as did the hospital's lack of a mental health professional appropriately trained to handle the profound impacts these experiences had on patients and families. I wrote a proposal to create a perinatal grief position in our hospital. After three attempts and failures to fund the project, the hospital finally added the position to its budget.

Studying Ethics

After completing my residency in obstetrics and gynecology, I realized that I missed the humanities, so I looked around for places to continue to work in the areas that I had found so enriching while in the seminary. Over the next two years, I enrolled in two different ethics programs, one focusing on clinical ethics and one more dedicated to the medical humanities. I learned how to assist in an ethics consultation in the hospital. I also studied great thinkers in philosophy, sociology, anthropology, religion, and literature, attempting to gain some grasp of the textual canons of ethics and medical humanities. I had the privilege of taking a year of healthcare law taught by an incredible educator, and I studied weekly with a brilliant and kind Jesuit priest, exploring St. Thomas Aquinas' masterpiece *Summa Theologica* (which he worked on from 1265 until his death in 1274), in addition to other Catholic texts. During these two years, I read everything I could find on reproductive ethics and gained a deeper appreciation of perspectives on abortion held by a wide range of religious, ethnic, and subcultural communities.

The Emotional Impacts of Performing Abortions and My Definitive Moment of Choice

Still, I was not aware of the significance of the distinction between the intellectual exploration of the field and the emotional impacts of actual patient care until I started my clinical practice as a general ob/gyn in the same large university hospital in which I had done my residency. I was a young provider eager to build a patient base. After practicing for a couple of months, I looked at my schedule for the day and saw the name of a patient labeled as "New OB." I had just started to see newly pregnant patients and relished the opportunity to care for and get to know these pregnant people throughout this transformative process. After initial introductions and a review of her medical history, this patient started to speak about her relationship history and also started to cry. She told me that she had been divorced for several years and had a teenage daughter. She had recently begun her first significant relationship after her divorce, and there had been a condom failure during intercourse. She did not say the word, but it was clear that she was in my office to discuss having an abortion. I am embarrassed to say that after five years in seminary, four years in medical school, four years in a residency in obstetrics and gynecology, and Fellowships in both clinical and reproductive medical ethics, I did not know if I would perform abortions in my own clinical practice. I did know that I supported the choice of a patient to have an abortion, and that I was competent to perform the procedure, but I hadn't yet faced the reality of what it would mean to perform one without a senior provider responsible not only for the surgical competence, but also responsible for the choice to perform it. I hadn't realized the extent to which I had deferred the ethical questions as a trainee.

I excused myself for a moment and stood in the hallway. As described, I worked in a hospital that had a family planning program. The city also had several high-quality abortion clinics. Additionally, the doctor with whom I had joined in practice performed abortions, and I could have easily scheduled the procedure with him. However, during my few moments of discomfort standing in the hall, I realized that I was connected to the patient as her doctor, and that I needed to help her through whatever lifecycle events were ahead. In fact, I later understood this realization as an acknowledgment and a synthesis of both my medical and religious oaths. Guided by a sense of the patient's need and vulnerability, my ambivalence, confusion, and fear melted into a more confident and calm appreciation of my responsibility. I felt that I had not only the permission to perform the abortion, but also the obligation to do so. Ultimately, I did the termination and felt comfortable with my choice. I believed that I had provided both capable and supportive care during a particularly stressful period for another human being.

A Patient's Ethical Challenge

As my practice grew and I saw more newly pregnant patients, I subsequently performed several other terminations, eventually seeing a patient who came in explicitly for an abortion. Often patients would book an appointment giving "counseling" or "family planning" as the reason for the visit. This was my first patient who simply stated that her goal was to terminate her pregnancy. I was caught off guard. Did I require any other information? Did I deserve any other information? By this point, I had heard many patients describe tumultuous lives, including stories about difficult relationships and financial struggles. Sometimes there were other children whose needs would have to be sacrificed if an additional child were added to the family. This patient told me that she just didn't want a baby. I was again thrust into what I imagined to be a new ethical challenge. It occurred to me that I had significant empathy for prior patients for whom I had terminated a pregnancy, and that I was judging this patient because I didn't think that her reason was good enough, or that she didn't feel, or wasn't expressing, sufficient remorse or pain to satisfy my threshold for "a good reason." I was troubled as I wrestled with whether or not I could participate in her abortion. I had started to feel comfortable with my identity as an abortion provider and was now confused by the question of whether I had limitations on this role. Deciding on parameters based on gestational age or personal hardship struck me as motivated by science or by compassion. This patient helped me realize that deciding which abortions were and were not permissible needed to be about the patient, not about me.

Ultimately, I grew to understand my performance of abortions as originating in the responsibility dictated by the patient-physician relationship. My judgement of that patient was unfair and inappropriate. I could not and should not be the arbiter of what "a good reason" was to terminate a pregnancy. At some level, the medical oath that I took,[8] and perhaps even more substantively, the religious oath that is the scaffolding of my medical ethics, led me to the understanding that I had the knowledge of how to perform this procedure and, because I held this knowledge, I was obligated to assist those who needed or even simply wanted an abortion, all in the safest, most respectful way possible.

In *Life's Work: A Moral Argument for Choice*, Dr. Willie Parker (2017) poignantly describes his life's journey to becoming an abortion provider. While Dr. Parker and I come from very different religions and theological beliefs, I was moved by his synthesis of religion and medicine. His use of the word *conversion* to becoming an abortion provider resonates deeply as I think about my own experiences. There is power in reclaiming traditional language in new ways. I am particularly empathetic with the ways in which theology informs his medical actions, while still rigorously avoiding judgment or proselytizing. Parker (2017:53) stated:

He loved you in your brokenness . . . He didn't need you to be perfect. That was the miracle. That same understanding informs my approach with my patients. As they feel compelled to explain themselves, to rationalize their abortion decision, they often feel the need to invent a narrative that makes them appear virtuous, or that "cleans up" the details of their circumstances, in order to evoke my compassion. When I sense this, I tell them of my understanding (though I keep God out of it): "Your need makes you worthy. You are fine the way you are."

Using a religious lens to guide my practice while preserving and celebrating the autonomy and humanity of the patient can be a tightrope walk. Dr. Parker has been a role model in helping me to keep my balance.

More recently, *You're the Only One I've Told: The Stories Behind Abortion* by Dr. Meera Shah (2020) helped me fine-tune my thinking on the matter. I share her understanding of narrative as a powerful mode of communication. Her ability to practice without judgment of the patient also challenged me to confront the ways in which I may not fit into the classic mold of the community of abortion providers, which surprised me, given that I share the politics of the majority of this group. Of course, I am not really certain about what this group of professionals think and feel about the abortions that they perform. Publicly disclosing and revealing the narratives of abortion providers has a relatively short history; much remains to be discussed and processed. Shah (2020:12) wrote, "We can simultaneously believe that there is a potential life growing inside a uterus *and* trust the person carrying the pregnancy to do what is right for them in their own lives." This sentence cogently articulates my own understanding. However, earlier in Shah's book, where she contributed her own narrative as an abortion provider in the form of an introduction to the narratives of the patients, she wrote: "I never, ever, ask anyone *why* someone makes the decision they make, whether that is to continue a pregnancy, have an abortion, or pursue adoption . . . . I give my patients the most information I can provide and support them in whatever they decide. I don't decide *with or for* them" (Shah 2020: 12). I am not certain whether that sentence caught my attention because I agree with her and I fall short of this lofty goal, or maybe because I see the process differently. I certainly don't decide *for* a patient, but I had a more difficult time understanding the word *with*. As I mentioned, I no longer probe to understand the inner motivations of the patient (although, to be honest, I am drawn to do just that). This is consistent with Dr. Shah's position, but her model doesn't seem to account for the transformation of the surgeon by the event.

Shared Decision-Making?

I do not mean to imply that this is some sort of shared decision-making model, as in the case where I recommend a cesarean birth to a patient who strongly desires a vaginal birth. I don't believe that the decision to have a child or not is equivalent to deciding between vaginal or abdominal delivery, and I understand and accept that there are people for whom these are enormous outcome differences and others for whom these are negligible. In the healthcare community, at least in the United States, there has been an historic shift from paternalism to autonomy, progressing to the more fashionable, and I believe appropriate, concept of today: "shared decision making" (see Veatch 1972). I will never know what it is like to be this patient and yet I have a certain expertise that informs my recommendations. Together we are challenged to come up with a plan of care. I struggle with the ways in which the "abortion conversation" is or is not similar to other counseling situations. How does the fact that women and other pregnant people are often unseen and unheard in society, especially regarding health care and, even more significantly, regarding reproductive choice, change the way we counsel about abortion? It seems to me that, particularly among abortion providers, nuance is a luxury that is too threatening to be tolerated. Given the constant attacks on reproductive rights (see the Epilogue to this chapter), it is rare to hear an abortion provider say privately, much less publicly, that it is sometimes difficult to perform abortions, or even to perform one specific abortion that was uniquely fraught.

I think there is something to be learned from the construct of "shared decision-making" as it applies to the field of abortion ethics. As in the case of birth, I do not claim that the person performing the abortion is as profoundly impacted by the choice as the patient who has it done. However, the fact that the process should be patient-centered does not preclude the possibility of a significant impact on the doctor. As I think back to my emotional responses to Dr. Shah's and Dr. Parker's words, I wish to be the person who is distinct from the decision of the patient. My task should be service. I know how to do a safe abortion, and I am the facilitator of that task.

Responses to Loss

The problem is that I often do not experience abortion in that way. Just as I am exhilarated by the privilege of assisting in the birth of a child, I am affected by the reality that the fetus I extract from the uterus will not become a child. Surprising even to myself, my emotional response is similar whether I remove a live fetus during an abortion or a dead fetus after a miscarriage. In both cases, these losses are complex and difficult. They are sometimes sad, and sometimes only less sad than the alternatives, and I strongly believe that the decision as to whether or not to continue the pregnancy should be up to the patient. But I am changed as well. I wish to explore how the doctor is transformed during the process of caring for the patient. Both patient and provider (as well as the nurse, scrub tech, anesthesiologist, and many other people involved in the experience) have distinct yet interconnected narratives that warrant further investigation.

Dr. Lisa Harris has written powerfully about this subject; she is the academic/clinician in the field doing some of the most important work facing the complexities of these issues with real attention to nuance. Her piece in the *New England Journal of Medicine* (Harris 2012) is a fierce yet vulnerable article that I require all ob/gyn residents to read when I teach about abortion. In another of her articles, "Second Trimester Abortion Provision: Breaking the Silence and Changing the Discourse" (Harris 2008), she brilliantly addresses the possible pain and subtlety of the in-between, never wavering from the mission of providing care to those in need (see also Martin et al. 2017; Czarnecki et al. 2019), asking:

> How do abortions providers determine how late in pregnancy they will provide abortion services? . . . personal and psychological aspects, visceral responses to the fetus and fetal parts in later gestations, feeling that second trimester abortion is violent, and ethical concerns with second trimester abortions. Providers may censor themselves with respect to these issues, fearing that honest acknowledgements of difficult aspects may be dangerous to the pro-choice movement. (Harris 2008:74)

What should be or can be the methods of addressing these complex feelings for me or any abortion provider?[9] I am drawn to the increase in narratives published about patients' experiences and emotional responses to having an abortion, whether written by doctors about the patients they care for or written by the patients themselves. Narratives of providers and those associated with the procedures have also become available (see Wicklund 2008). Most frequently, abortion providers reference "patient autonomy" as the foundation of any rationale for abortion. I share the importance of that perspective, but it feels incomplete, satisfying the intellectual but not fully the emotional aspects of the experience. This model fails to open up space for those involved to express pain and sadness.

I am very familiar with the formidable resources, media, and sophisticated organizations dedicated to prohibiting abortion, and I am also deeply empathetic with the desire to refute the ever-present restrictions and intolerance of the patient's right to choose. However, we need a way to discuss the topic with more subtlety, in the public forum as well as in academic medicine. My experience as a clinician has shown me that many patients are yearning for an outlet to grieve and mourn their loss. Whether a miscarriage, abortion, or loss of any kind, I attempt to help them find ways to mark their unique event. The loss of a pregnancy is most common, but the patient may face a new diagnosis of cancer or the death of a parent, among many other potential tragedies. How can the patient mourn authentically and personally, be it through religious or secular expression? I have talked about baptism and burial services. I have facilitated patients going to the Mikvah—a Jewish tradition of ritual immersion in water[10]) as a method of creating a distinction between the loss and the possibility of a future child or after the completion of chemotherapy. I have had patients start to write poetry and begin to paint as responses to loss. Once, I had a patient who had suffered her second miscarriage in a row; she responded by cloistering herself in her home. Eventually, she described the feeling of becoming tired of her own sadness and isolation, and she walked into a food shelter in her neighborhood—one that she had passed hundreds of times before. She spent the day volunteering at the shelter, serving meals in memory of her fetus and mourning the loss of the opportunity to parent that child. Another woman I cared for early in my career had delivered two healthy children in the past. She came in because she had been bleeding at six weeks gestation. After I confirmed that she had a miscarriage, she was devastated. I was not expecting the depth and profound nature of her grief and mourning. I witnessed how her loss telescoped onto other sad or difficult life experiences.

Over the years, I have found that I too need a ritual to mark the events of loss—a way to express my own pain as well as the patient's. I would be disingenuous if I said that I am constantly searching for a way to ritualize every medical event I encounter. In fact, some abortions feel merely procedural, or worse. Often while performing an abortion, I may be thinking about how many patients are upstairs in labor or simply ruminating over one of the many daily distractions of life. These distractions lead me to feel less proud of the ways in which I am participating in patient care. The words of Rabbi Shai Held (2013:30) are powerful: "One of the crucial tasks . . . is to struggle against the anesthetizing effects of our over-familiarization with life and reality, and to instill in us a sense of perpetual surprise, a willingness to encounter the world again and again as if for the first time."

I liken this challenge to my experiences in synagogue. I rarely have a spiritual encounter when I attend synagogue, but I do go with the desire to be changed by my attendance. In fact, I am not sure if I could continue to go to synagogue if I believed it impossible to be moved by my participation. As Abraham Joshua Heschel, one of the great modern Jewish theologians and activists, wrote, "To pray is to take notice of the wonder, to regain the sense of the mystery that animates all beings . . . Prayer is our humble answer to the inconceivable surprise of living" (1977:341). Shouldn't I want to be affected by sharing a lifecycle event with a patient, especially one as significant as abortion? I wish to emphasize that I have no judgment about how patients or other abortion providers find significance. In fact, I completely respect the position that rejects the need for any act at all to mark the event. Further, I am sympathetic to those who believe it is inappropriate that I insert myself so dramatically in the story at all.

Marking the Event: My Personal Rituals

I do know that when I perform an abortion, I need to mark the event—or more precisely, I desire to feel the need to mark the event. Throughout my adult life, I have become accustomed to establishing time through rituals. I use the period prior to the termination while I scrub—ritually cleanse—to think about the event. Scrubbing becomes one of the pivoting behaviors transforming me into someone different from who I am in my daily life. I wrestle with the implications of the upcoming task, just as I struggle with how to view my role in the narrative. Is it better to transform into a technician? Would I, as a patient, want a practitioner to be thinking about the emotional and ethical implications while operating? In contrast, should the abortion be treated just like the removal of an ovarian cyst?

There is a seldom-mentioned component of surgical termination that only abortion providers fully understand. After the surgery, one of the final tasks is to open and inspect the suction canister to ensure that the embryo or fetus has, in fact, been evacuated. In later gestation abortions, it is expected to actually account for the fetal parts. After fulfilling this medical ritual many times, it becomes fairly routine—the spell only broken when demonstrating the process to inexperienced students. Seeing the process through their eyes has often been jarring to me.

Over the years, I have sought to provide some sort of appropriate acknowledgment of the abortion, particularly during this surreal task of counting fetal body parts. I desired a personal religious response to the medical ritual of pregnancy termination. I have never spoken about this with anyone until writing this chapter. After caring for a patient in a particularly challenging social situation, I tried saying the phrase used in the traditional Jewish community when one hears of a death—*Baruch Dayan HaEmet*—"Blessed is the true Judge."[11] Initially, this blessing helped me to pay attention to the seriousness of the act on my part, maybe even helped me to obtain an element of closure. Creating a ritual for myself as the surgeon also served to ground my own feelings as distinct from the patient's feelings about choice and loss. Perhaps, by uttering these words, I was also defusing the complex ethical challenges of providing abortions. I am, after all, not the "true Judge." I am merely the one allowed to perform the task, given my training.

Saying these three simple words brought me back to an experience I witnessed while on sabbatical in Israel, where the Termination Committee absorbs the responsibility of deciding whether a desired abortion is permissible or forbidden. The Committee consists of social workers and physicians who make the decision as to the appropriateness of the abortion. The individual physicians providing abortions seemed to be liberated from the ethical dilemmas because a separate group decided on the permissibility. In 2019, *The Jerusalem Post* reported that 99.4% of Israeli patients seeking abortions were granted permission: "We don't have doctors here who would say 'This is against my belief. I am not going to give you this'" (Sharon Orshalimy, quoted in Kavaler 2021).

This is in contrast to the situation in the United States, where the majority of obstetricians do not perform abortions. One large study (Stulberg et al. 2011) showed that only 14% of practicing US obstetricians perform abortions. Eight years after that study was published, another study (Grossman et al. 2019) demonstrated that approximately 24% of obstetricians were participating in abortions. The authors suggest that barriers to performing abortions include the hospital institution or hiring body, which often make the decision for the provider. Others have decided not to provide abortions due to deference to their staff or to difficulty finding support to assist with the procedures. The unique requirements associated with prescribing Mifepristone for medical abortions are also seen as significant barriers to abortion provision (Boonstra 2013).[12] I have heard from many providers that they don't feel sufficiently skilled to perform second trimester terminations, but I am confident that their unease stems more from the ethical issues than from the technical requirements.[13]

I have stopped reciting *Baruch Dayan HaEmet*. Uttering these few words, even under my breath, never felt completely appropriate or respectful. I am all in favor of adapting traditional language to new situations, but I ultimately couldn't justify using the quintessential prayer of humility at the exact moment when I purposefully engaged in such an emotionally and physically powerful act. I have not yet found a better replacement to mark the act and my participation in it. In retrospect, I can see that the lectures I gave to medical students functioned as the most significant healing rituals for my encounters with abortion. I always felt energized by the responses of the next generation of doctors and their interest and concern while engaging with this challenging topic. Inevitably, a few students would linger to talk after class to ask more personal questions related to their lives as well as to mine. Mostly, they wanted to show support, and standing in a group, even silently, struck me as a strong, powerful, and nourishing expression of their solidarity.

Cross-Cultural Perspectives

Over the years, I thought I might be comforted by learning how a wider range of communities understand the nature of the fetus, and ultimately how abortion may fit into the larger worldview. In what ways do other religions and cultures mourn a fetus? While I still do not have adequate language, or ritual, or prayer to help me with the task, I increasingly consider that I may be looking too hard. Can any religion or culture provide meaningful insight into how one is to mourn this common, yet under-discussed, lifecycle event of miscarriage and abortion for both patient and provider? I sought understanding by exploring the foundations of my own Jewish tradition. I was surprised when I learned of the practice of *Milah*—ritual circumcision—performed on a child born dead but with visible male genitalia. Most understand this unusual circumcision to be performed to ensure that this child would be identifiably Jewish when the resurrection of the dead occurs during the Messianic Era (Talmud, Sanhedrin, 110b; see also Steinsaltz 2012).

The Catholic Church also struggled with the nature of the fetus. I was fascinated by the passages in the *Summa Theologica* where Aquinas discusses when the soul is imparted, as seen through the embryological progression from plant to animal to cognizant human (Aquinas Question 64). While certainly not normative, during the Middle Ages there were even examples of in utero baptism in the Catholic church to address the problem of the fetus/child remaining in limbo without the sacrament of baptism (Pope Benedict XIV).[14] The long and prolific history of the Hindu textual tradition includes many rituals surrounding death, burial, and grieving, but they are too complex to respectfully address here. I was most perplexed when I learned that in the Hindu religion, adults are cremated, but when a fetus or young child dies, the tradition is to bury that individual, offering yet another perspective into the unique status of the fetus (Paraskara's *Grihyasutra*[15]). The Japanese ritual of *Mizuko Kuyo* (a memorial service for a dead child/fetus, literally "Water Child") started in the 1950s and became more common in the 1960s. The practice of *Mizuko Kuyo* has now been described in many articles and books in English, and has definitely had an impact on mourning loss even outside of Japan. "The main focus is on children who died very young or were stillborn (*shizan*), miscarried (*ryuzan*), or aborted (*ninshin chuzetzu*)" (Smith 2013:7). Until this practice, these "children" had been left out of the usual Japanese Buddhist funeral and memorial services for the dead. Because the question of whether a fetus is a child is not generally debated in Japan, the term *mizuko* can be translated as "dead," "lost," or in another reading of *mizuko* as "unseen child." I was particularly moved because the Japanese tradition doesn't make any significant distinction between miscarriage and abortion, seeing both simply as loss (Smith 2013:7).

Ultimately, the language of Heschel (1945:156) speaks to me, comforts me, and inspires me most of all:

> Prayer is no panacea, no substitute for action. It is, rather, like a beam thrown from a flashlight before us into the darkness. It is in this light that we who grope, stumble, and climb, discover where we stand, what surrounds us, and the course which we should choose. Prayer makes visible the right and reveals the false. In its radiance we behold the worth of our efforts, the range of our hopes, and the meaning of our deeds.

For me, the humility of meditative prayer "makes visible the right." At this point in my life and in my career, I indeed have "discovered where I stand," and performing abortions firmly gives "meaning to my deeds" because I feel better participating than not, and because I now understand that it is the right thing for me to do.

Epilogue

This chapter was written several months prior to June 24, 2022, when the Supreme Court overturned Roe v. Wade—the 1973 decision affirming the constitutional right to abortion. By overturning Roe, the Supreme Court placed the legal status of abortion and abortion provision in the hands of the individual states. As I write the final edits on this chapter in early November, 2022, there are 26 states that have banned or plan to ban abortion through a variety of legislative actions. The laws and the interpretations of these new laws are in constant and dramatic flux. Perhaps the most striking legislation during this tumultuous past year is Texas Senate Bill 8 (2021), also known as the "Texas Heartbeat Act." SB8 was passed and allowed to stand by the Supreme Court in the months leading to the fall of Roe. It was initially thought to be an extreme version of what a state may legislate. However, post Roe, SB8 has proven to be an inspiration for several other states with the agenda of significantly curtailing or eliminating abortions altogether. Starting on September 1, 2021, the law prohibited abortion after fetal cardiac activity, which outlaws approximately 85% of all abortions in Texas. The ban would still stand in cases of rape or incest, but an exception exists for life-threatening risks to the mother. Further, the law allows for civil suits not only against the abortion provider, but also against all who assist the patient in obtaining the abortion (Texas Heartbeat Act 2021). The most novel aspect of the law is that the state is not to be its enforcer. Rather, private citizens are allowed, and financially incentivized, to sue abortion providers and anyone who assists in the process.

Although Illinois—the state in which I practice—was not impacted by the federal legal decision, we have seen a significant increase in requests for abortions at my institution. I was told by our Family Planning team that there is now a two-to-three week wait for first trimester abortions, and that approximately one-third of the patients presenting are coming from states that have either already made abortion illegal or have legislation pending, making the patient concerned about legal action. These numbers were informally confirmed by a colleague who directs another abortion facility in the city. Many people I speak with in reproductive medicine have told me that there are more patients asking about permanent sterilization and the possibility of long term contraception out of fear of losing contraception availability and/or insurance coverage. The university has expanded clinical services in family planning. I have been in several meetings addressing the legal complexity and fluidity of the current situation with the agenda to diminish the anxieties of abortion providers. Often providers describe fears of losing a medical license, or worse, facing a prison sentence.

Personally, I have investigated how I may be of some service to patients requiring care. I am bombarded with opportunities for fundraising and social and political action. For now, these expressions are motivating and powerful on both the local and national levels. Unfortunately, as a healthcare provider who performs direct care, I am even more vexed by the vulnerability of the patient in need of service as well as by the increasing vulnerability of the community of abortion providers serving these patients.

Scott Moses is a faculty member at the Pritzker School of Medicine, University of Chicago, in both the Department of Obstetrics and Gynecology and the Maclean Center for Clinical Medical Ethics. Previously, he served on the clinical faculty in Obstetrics and Gynecology and in the Department of Bioethics and Medical Humanities at Northwestern University Feinberg School of Medicine. He was active in medical education both clinically and as the Director of Ethics Education for the Department of Ob/Gyn, where he established a Medical Humanities curriculum for residents incorporating ethics, philosophy, literature, art, religion, and ritual studies.

Notes

1. Family Planning Fellowships started in 1991 at the University of California San Francisco. Today, there are 28 institutions with accredited programs providing clinical training and research support for post residency ob/gyn with the objective of providing leaders in the fields of complex contraception and abortion.
2. Currently, many universities offer a Master's degree in Medical Ethics. When I finished residency, advanced ethics and humanities training consisted of two-year programs offered by a handful of major biomedical centers. The term "Fellowship" attempted to place the academic discipline of ethics firmly in the biomedical model, similar to gynecologic oncology or maternal-fetal medicine.
3. The term "attending" refers to the physician who has completed training. Prior to practicing biomedicine autonomously in the United States, one has to finish medical school and residency. The first year of residency is sometimes called "internship."
4. There is no monolithic view on abortion in the Jewish tradition, but analysis of traditional sources suggests that abortion in the first 40 days would generally be permissible. From that point until labor, abortion is not only permissible but obligatory if the pregnancy puts the life of the mother in jeopardy. Otherwise, abortion would generally be forbidden. There is debate among the diverse Jewish communities as to how much mental health should be considered a threat to the mother's life. For further discussion, see Rosner and Bleich (1980) and Dorff (1999).
5. During the fourth year of medical school, students apply to their field of choice within the different biomedical disciplines. The specific programs decide on which candidates to interview, and ultimately both the student and program submit rank lists. The entire country uses a central computer system to "match" the student with the program maximizing the students' preferences with those of the hospital.
6. Please see Dr. Lisa Harris's excellent article "Recognizing Conscience in Abortion Provision" (2012), in which she describes how both abortion providers and those who choose not to provide abortions can be informed by conscience.
7. "Child" was the patient's word and bears no reflection on whether a fetus is a child by scientific or religious definition, but rather reflects her sense of the relationship.

8. A variety of oaths are used in US biomedical schools. Many schools have students recite the oath when they first receive their white coat, some when starting clinical medicine, and all upon graduation. The "Oath of Geneva" (1948), the "Hippocratic Oath" (originally 5th century BCE), and the "Physician's Oath" by Markus Hertz of Berlin (1790) are each used in US medical schools. For more information on medical oaths, see Miles 2005.
9. It should be mentioned that having an emotional response is not unique to performing abortions, of course. I have attended term deliveries that have made me sad because I was concerned about the difficult life that child might be starting, just as I have felt joy in the opportunity to help a patient in need by terminating her pregnancy.
10. See Davis-Floyd's (2023) chapter in Volume II of this series for descriptions of the roles of ritual in reducing stress, and note that in that chapter, she defines "rituals" as "patterned, repetitive, and symbolic enactments of cultural—or individual—values and beliefs." See also the Series Overview, this volume, for a description of that chapter.
11. It should be stated that *Baruch Dayan HaEmet* is traditionally only recited after hearing about the death of one that lived through the neonatal period, although there is much diversity of rituals among Jewish communities and individuals.
12. Mifepristone, also known as RU-486, is an anti-progesterone oral medication used to cause an abortion. The FDA has approved its use up to 70 days from the last menstrual period. The FDA requires the healthcare provider to register to prescribe RU-486, and both the patient and the provider must sign an "agreement form" prior to dispensing the drug. Also, the pill can only be dispensed in a clinic, a hospital, or a medical office.
13. First trimester abortions are performed with a suction curette removing the fetus and placenta. After approximately 14–16 weeks gestation, the cervix is often readied for the surgery with medications such as Misoprostol or Laminaria sticks, which slowly help to dilate the cervix to prevent cervical trauma during dilation and extraction of the fetus and placenta. Depending on the size of the fetus, the uterus, and cervical dilation, extraction forceps are used to empty the uterus.
14. Pope Benedict served as Pope 1740–1758. He spoke of the need for "conditional Baptism," even if an instrument is required for the Baptismal waters to reach the fetus.
15. This information comes from a conversation with Professor Charles Preston, University of Chicago. Paraskara's *Grihyasutra* describes rituals of the home and is dated to the last centuries BCE. Its first volume has been translated into English (Oldenburg and Max 2016).

References

Aquinas T. 1997. *Summa Theologica: A Concise Translation*. Chicago IL: Thomas More Publishing Reprint.

Boonstra H. 2013. "Medication Abortion Restrictions Burden Women and Providers and Threaten US Trend toward Very Early Abortion." *Guttmacher Institute Policy Review* 16(1): 18–23.

Czarnecki D, Anspach R, DeVries R, et al. 2019. "Conscience Reconsidered: The

Moral Work of Navigating Participation in Abortion Care on Labor and Delivery." *Social Science and Medicine* 232: 181–189.

Davis-Floyd R. 2023. "Open and Closed Knowledge Systems, the 4 Stages of Cognition, and the Obstetric Management of Birth." In *Cognition, Risk, and Responsibility in Obstetrics: Anthropological Analyses and Critiques of Obstetricians' Practices*, ed. Davis-Floyd R, Premkumar A., Chapter 1. New York: Berghahn Books.

Dorff E. 1999. *Matters of Life and Death: A Jewish Approach to Modern Medical Ethics*. Philadelphia PA: Jewish Publication Society.

Grossman D, Grindlay K, Altshuler A, et al. 2019. "Induced Abortion Provision among a National Sample of Obstetrician-Gynecologists." *Obstetrics & Gynecology* 33(3): 477–483.

Harris L. 2008. "Second Trimester Abortion Provision: Breaking the Silence and Changing the Discourse." *Reproductive Health Matters* 16(31 Suppl): S74–81.

———. 2012. "Recognizing Conscience in Abortion." *New England Journal of Medicine* 367: 981–983.

Held S. 2015. *Abraham Joshua Heschel: The Call of Transcendence*. Bloomington: Indiana University Press.

Heschel AJ. 1945. "Prayer." *Review of Religion* 9(2): 153–168.

———. 1977. *Moral Audacity and Spiritual Grandeur*. New York: Farrar, Straus and Giroux.

Hunter KM. 1991. *Doctor's Stories: The Narrative Structure of Medical Knowledge*. Princeton NJ: Princeton University Press.

Kavaler T. 2021. "Israel's Abortion Rate Continues 32-Year Decline." *Jerusalem Post*, Jan 5.

Martin L, Hassinger J, Debbink D, et al. 2017. "Dangertalk: Voices of Abortion Providers." *Social Science and Medicine* 184: 75–83.

Miles S. 2005. *The Hippocratic Oath and the Ethics of Medicine*. Oxford: Oxford University Press.

New York Times. 2022. "Tracking the States Where Abortion is Now Banned." October 13.

Oldenburg M, Max F. 2016. *The Grihya-Sutras, Rules of Vedic Domestic Ceremonies Volume 1*. New York: Palala Press.

Parker W. 2017. *Life's Work: A Moral Argument for Choice*. New York: Atria Books.

Rosner F, Bleich JD. 1980. *Jewish Bioethics*. New York: Hebrew Publishing Company.

Shah M. 2020. *You're the Only One I've Told: The Stories behind Abortion*. Chicago IL: Chicago Review Press.

Smith B. 2013. *Narratives of Sorrow and Dignity*. New York: Oxford Press.

Steinsatz A. 2012. *Talmud Bavli with Commentary*. Jerusalem: Koren Publishing.

Stulberg D, Dude A, Dahlquist I, et al. 2011. "Abortion Provision among Practicing Obstetrician-Gynecologists." *Obstetrics and Gynecology* 1118(3): 609–614.

Texas Heartbeat Act. 2021. Texas Senate Bill 8. Austin TX: Texas Legislature.

Turner V. 1969. *The Ritual Process*. New York: Penguin Books.

Van Gennep A. 1960. *The Rites of Passage*. Chicago IL: University of Chicago Press.

Veatch RM. 1972. "Models for Ethical Medicine in a Revolutionary Age: What Physician-Patient Relationship Roles Foster the Most Ethical Relationship?" *The Hastings Center Report* 2(3): 5–7.

Wickland S. 2008. *This Common Secret: My Journey as an Abortion Doctor*. New York: Public Affairs.

CHAPTER 2

Abortion, Professional Identity, and Generational Meaning Making among US Ob/Gyns

Rebecca Henderson, Chu J. Hsiao, and Jody Steinauer

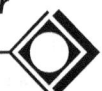

Introduction: Professional Identity and Meaning Making

Providing abortions has long been framed as "dirty work" (Ward 2021)—a fraught and often stigmatized practice that obstetrician/gynecologists (ob/gyns) may choose to include in their care provision. While multiple studies have sought to understand the impacts of political changes, stigmatization, and fear on the abortion workforce (Harris et al. 2011; Martin et al. 2014; Britton et al. 2017), fewer studies have situated the abortion workforce within the context of professional identity and meaning-making work. In this chapter, we follow Anuradha Kumar's (2013) call for scholarship that moves abortion work beyond a stigmatization framework, and Elisa Andaya and Joanna Mishtal's (2016) call for renewed anthropological attention to abortion in the United States in the face of new and vigorous anti-choice movements. The June 2022 Supreme Court decision overturning Roe v. Wade, leaving the legality of abortion to the states, has further heightened the urgency for scholarship on abortion care.

We argue that abortion comprises an integral part of the professional identity of physicians who choose to provide this service, as indicated in the preceding chapter by abortion provider Scott Moses. Rather than either experiencing abortion as stigmatized work that ostracizes them from their professional community or as a tangential or mundane part of practice, ob/gyns who perform abortions describe abortion as meaningful precisely because the practice resonates directly with their value-based physician identities. Moreover, we argue that the resonance of abortion for ob/gyn professional identity is not static, but rather socially and historically situated, altering in response to political forces and changes to physician professional identity over time. Herein, we trace these shifts through narratives drawn from semi-structured interviews with ob/gyns who provide abortions. We relate the meaning-making practices of these physicians both to abortion politics and to shifting notions of meaning in biomedicine. Through these narratives, we demonstrate that abortion has transformed from being a small component of the ob/gyn physician identity to constituting the anchoring foundation of ob/gyn physician identity for the abortion providers we interviewed. The politicized nature of abortion work, and the marginalization of abortion work by restrictive legislation, have led to the increased centralization of abortion in the professional identities of the ob/gyns who provide them. Instead of framing their identities as marginalized, the ob/gyn abortion providers we interviewed frame abortion as an affirmation of their core ob/gyn physician values and identities. While descriptions of "abortion as professional identity" have remained rooted in the values-based language of physician professional identity, the particular values emphasized have shifted. Rather than being concerned solely with preventing physical harm to individual patients, providers are increasingly embracing values such as advocacy and justice. Over time, providing abortions has been less frequently framed as meeting an urgent public health need and increasingly viewed as part of a larger identity of activism, outreach to vulnerable communities, human rights, and social justice.

Professional Identity, Biomedicine, and Abortion Provision

Institutionalized occupations, especially those in which personal values and beliefs are closely entwined with work and institutional order, often produce deep professional identities (Barbour and Lammers 2015). Professional identity is of vital importance in understanding how individuals enact and draw meaning from their work (Zikic and Richardson 2015). The study of professional identity provides a means for examining the intersection of institutional authority with individual values, allowing for an investigation of how work and work environments are made meaningful (Alvesson and Willmott 2002). Professional identity is therefore a concept in which personal values, motivations, and identities are entangled with external power structures, where values, beliefs, and attitudes may contribute to a sense of shared belonging (Ibarra 1999; Britton et al. 2017).

Physicians are expected to conform to the norms, values, and ideals of their profession, and developing a professional identity is an explicit part of biomedical school curricula (Cruess and Cruess 2006). Defined in biomedicine as "the integration of personal values, morals, and attributes with the norms of the profession," professional identity among biomedical physicians is deeply entangled with meaning making in medical work (Wilson et al. 2013). Learning and teaching professional identity, termed "Professional Identity Formation" (PIF), is considered a key part of biomedical professional education (Wald 2015). PIF is often framed around a shared set of professional values, which, in one framework, include attitudes, personal characteristics, duties, habits, relationships, and perceptions (Holden et al. 2015). Within this particular "professional identity" framework, becoming a physician involves not simply developing competency in doctoring but also reorienting oneself toward a collective set of personal moral and ethical commitments. Despite the emphasis on PIF in biomedical education, literature on the stability or transformation of professional identity among mature physicians, rather than learners, is scarce. Much of the literature seems to presume that professional identity, once formed through a generic and appropriate medical education, remains stable throughout practice and across different types of practitioners. Additionally, relatively few studies have attempted to understand how differences in biomedical practice may impact professional identity among physicians.

In this chapter, we seek to understand the self-conceptions of professional identity in a particular group of practitioners: ob/gyns who incorporate abortion into their professional practices. Much of the current research on abortion providers has focused on the impacts of stigma and restrictive laws on experiences and quality of life (see, for example, Martin et al. 2014), suggesting that stigmatization may likewise affect how ob/gyn abortion providers view their identities as physicians. In North Carolina, Laura E Britton and colleagues (2017) found that new abortion restrictions increased negative characterizations of abortion providers and made abortion care more complicated and difficult. Despite these negative characterizations, abortion providers' senses of professional identity, including their motivations to provide abortions, their pride in their work, and their values and beliefs remained strong.

Shifting and Generational Identities

We recognize that physician professional identities, like all identities, can change over time (Jarvis-Selinger et al. 2019). We further acknowledge that identities are intersectional, and that professional identity is informed by diverse identifications and experiences, including those of race, ethnicity, gender, sexuality, and others (Atewologun, Sealy, and Vinnicombe 2016). In this chapter, informed by themes emerging from our interview data, we have chosen to focus on how professional identity for abortion providers has changed over time. Several studies have identified generational divides within conceptions of physician professional identity (e.g., Hoonpongsimanont et al. 2018); for ob/gyns, the growth of subspecialities, as well as new technologies such as laparoscopic surgical techniques, have caused a reexamination and redefinition of meaning and sense of professional self (Zetka 2011, 2020).

Particularly for a politically charged practice like abortion, we argue that the relationship between professional identity and abortion has been in constant flux as both the medical and political landscapes evolved over the past several decades. The place of abortion in the professional identity of ob/gyns is therefore historically situated. Sociologist Carole Joffe and her colleagues have traced the history of the relationship between physicians and feminists in the fight for abortion legality through *Roe v. Wade*,[1] describing the situation as an "uneasy alliance" (Joffe, Weitz, and Stacey 2004: 775). Physicians' firsthand experiences with patients directly harmed by the criminalization of abortion forced the mobilization of a generation of committed physicians in the late 1960s and early 1970s, despite a fundamental disjuncture with feminist movements working toward the same goal. While physicians tended to medicalize and professionalize abortion to legitimize stigmatized abortion services, feminists framed physicians as having a more limited, technical role in abortion care. Physicians' framing of abortion transitioned from this early disjunctive alliance into a period of marginalization. The nearly nonexistent training pathways after *Roe v. Wade* was passed in 1973 resulted in a severe decline in the number of abortion providers in the 1980s and early 1990s. This situation culminated in a resurgence of abortion as a central issue for some physicians in the early 1990s, in which abortion providers viewed themselves as more firmly allied with the interests of a feminist movement that had since bureaucratized and become less radical (Joffe, Weitz, and Stacey 2004).

To illustrate the shifting roles of abortion care within ob/gyn professional identities over time, we have structured this chapter around four narratives from a larger study of semi-structured interviews conducted by the first author, Rebecca Henderson, then an MD-PhD candidate. Henderson conducted 34 telephone interviews between 2018 and 2019 with US abortion providers (Table 2.1).

Table 2.1. Demographic characteristics of participating abortion care providers, N=34. © Rebecca Henderson

Provider region		Specialty		Gender	
Midwest	6	Family medicine	11	Male	6
Northeast	6	Ob/gyn	21	Female	28
West Coast	8	Emergency medicine	2		
Southeast	7				
Southwest	7				

Each narrative presented below represents the voice of a physician who trained and matured their professional identity during a different time period. We begin with an ob/gyn who trained in the early 1980s, and follow with the narrative of one of our coauthors, Dr. Jody Steinauer, who trained in the early 1990s. We then share the story of an ob/gyn who finished training in 2005, and end with a 2019 medical student. All narratives have been partly fictionalized; names, dates, places, and specific experiences have been altered to protect the anonymity of participants, with the exception of coauthor Steinauer. While each narrative presented is based on the story of a specific interlocutor, quotations and themes presented are drawn from the larger sample of 34 interviews.

"This *Is* Ob-Gyn"

When Dr. William Barnes began medical school in 1980, he rarely encountered or thought about abortion care. He did not remember abortion ever being discussed in his medical school curriculum, and first encountered abortion care after beginning an ob/gyn residency in the southwestern United States. He described walking into a residency program in which all ob/gyn practitioners routinely performed second trimester abortions several days a week. "It was just assumed I would participate in this care," he said. While he was assured that he did not have to initiate the termination himself, "the attitude was that 'we're going to expect you to help us take care of patients who have had a termination, and if you don't, well there's the door and you can leave.'" According to Dr. Barnes, "it was rare that ob/gyns would take the stance that 'I'm not participating in this.'"

Abortion was taken for granted by Dr. Barnes and his co-residents as a natural part of ob/gyn work. "I mean, this was the mid-1980s," he said:

Roe v. Wade was 10 years old. Everybody who did ob/gyn remembered the dark times of septic abortion and horrible outcomes, and I just thought "This *is* ob/gyn—this is what I signed up to do. This is part of the practice. This feels great. Let's take care of them." I didn't have to do any soul searching, I didn't have any moral qualms. I mean, it was just an accepted part of ob/gyn practice.

His mentors described abortion as vitally important and lifesaving work, frequently reminding trainees of the consequences of a pre-Roe world: "Anybody who practiced prior to *Roe v. Wade* was thankful that women weren't going to be dying from the complications of unsafe abortions."

Then in the mid-1980s, hospital leadership changed, and fewer abortions were performed at the hospital where Dr. Barnes worked. "I didn't really realize at the time, but I came to understand that was the beginning of the political embattlement," he described. "Our new boss didn't really want to do it, didn't think that it was necessary for residents to participate in that care. So, we stopped doing them for a couple of years, except for fetal malformations and for people with cancer." When he joined a southwestern clinical practice after finishing training, abortion care was increasingly rare, and abortion training opportunities for residents dwindled through the early 1990s. Abortions, discouraged by hospital administrators, were left to the discretion of individual providers, who frequently opted not to perform them.

Dr. Barnes continued, "So then, in the late 1990s, that's when all the trouble started." First, an ob/gyn in private practice in a nearby city was harassed by an anti-choice group. "They sent his picture to all of his patients with the word 'murderer' scratched across it and claims that he worked in a practice killing babies." The mailing frightened the administrators of local hospitals, who worried that they would likewise be targeted if they allowed their physicians to perform abortions. According to Dr. Barnes, "The climate for ob/gyns became much more hostile." At the same time, the state passed its first legislation restricting abortions, preventing hospitals from receiving certain kinds of reimbursement if they performed abortions. In response, Dr. Barnes's practice made all ob/gyns sign an agreement in which they certified that they would not perform abortions. "That was the first time in my career when I was forced to say I wouldn't do them anymore. I had to keep my job. I mean, we weren't really doing them at that point anyway, but it just felt wrong having to sign that piece of paper, and I was annoyed by that."

Dr. Barnes's narrative follows the historical trajectory outlined by Joffe, Weitz, and Stacey (2004). The generation of ob/gyns who practiced prior to *Roe v. Wade* viewed abortion as a vital service that protected patient's lives. Gradually, through the 1980s, as the issue was increasingly politicized, conservative hospital administrations distanced themselves from abortion. Abortion practice and abortion training programs were eroded by this loss of administrative support. Abortion practice and training were completely cut off in many large facilities as ob/gyns became the targets of destructive, and sometimes violent, political actions throughout the 1990s, and restrictive laws made it more difficult to continue to provide abortions. Dr. Barnes's reaction reflects the centrality of abortion in his identity as an ob/gyn: "I remember thinking, this feels wrong, this feels un-American and awful, and we should argue about it because it's the right thing to do—to argue about it. We're supposed to be training students, and this is wrong." At the same time, he felt powerless in the face of institutional policy.

In the late 2000s, Dr. Barnes experienced a major shift in perspective. As he moved up within his own organizational hierarchy, he felt increasingly empowered to engage in the politics surrounding abortion. He reached out to abortion provider communities that had grown nationally and interacted with the new generation of ob/gyns who provided abortion care as a central part of their practices. Dr. Barnes described his prior views of abortion-only providers: "Abortion providers that I had known in the past who were strictly abortion providers were not the world's most reputable people. Some of them were ok people, but they've lost their ability to practice in the normal world [of ob/gyn] for a variety of reasons." His view of abortion-only providers as marginal figures unqualified to be "normal" ob/gyns changed as a result of interacting with the new generation of ob/gyns who considered abortion and abortion advocacy central to their work. "I met all these wonderful young women who were doing this work and were passionate about it and so committed, and were putting themselves, their careers, their families, on the line. It inspired me to keep working really hard on the advocacy side of it." Dr. Barnes eventually left his position to take on a full-time role oriented around abortion practice and advocacy. At the time of our interview, Dr. Barnes spent 75–85% of his time engaged in clinical work, primarily abortion, with the remaining time spent on administrative and advocacy responsibilities.

In explaining his commitment to abortion, Dr. Barnes related his work directly to his identity as a physician, particularly to his professional responsibility to provide direct patient care: "Well, what being a doctor means to me is, we take care of people who are in trouble, and provide them with the health care they need as best we can. Abortion is health care . . . it's no different than giving insulin to a diabetic." With these words, Dr. Barnes frames abortion as an unexceptional physician service, albeit one with an urgent need, inextricable from his identity as an ob/gyn: "It was a part of the world of ob/gyn when I started doing ob/gyn, and I hope it's always going to be a part of the world of ob/gyn." As an older white male physician practicing in the conservative environment of the US southwest, Dr. Barnes utilized his status, seniority, and identity as a respected member of his professional community to legitimize his work as an abortion provider:

> I have two business cards I carry with me. One says my real job, but I'm also a leader of my state's association of ob/gyns. So I just hand them that card if I'm in a conservative office, and I use it to remind them, "This is what ob/gyns think." There is unanimity between all ob/gyns that we ought to be fighting for abortion.

In his advocacy, Dr. Barnes sought to bring abortion practice back into alignment with his professional identity as an ob/gyn.

"We Felt Like We Had to Do Something"

Coauthor Dr. Jody Steinauer entered medical school in the early 1990s with a deep commitment to what was then termed "women's health" and a theoretical desire to perform abortions as a part of her eventual practice. She had prior experience working in a feminist health center, and a childhood during which abortion was openly discussed and framed as a deeply important human right. Feminism and an activist commitment to women's health were already part of her personal identity and her conception of physician identity: "I thought that you could provide medical care as an activist. Abortion fit into this idea that as a physician I could be an advocate for patients . . . I wasn't sure I would be an ob/gyn yet, but I knew for sure that I was going to be an activist around abortion care."

Abortion was scarcely mentioned in the medical school she attended, and the few mentions were highly charged, stigmatized moments. Speaking of one such moment, Dr. Steinauer says: "It was so fascinating—I could palpably feel discomfort in the lecture hall of students. When he [the professor] said the word 'abortion' and talked about it, people were uncomfortable. And I remember thinking, 'That's a problem, that people are so freaked out.' And I was so excited that he brought it up." Far from Dr. Barnes' first encounter with abortion, which occurred much later in training and was framed as a natural part of being an ob/

gyn, Dr. Steinauer's early encounters distanced and alienated abortion from normal clinical practice. Abortion care continued to be stigmatized throughout Dr. Steinauer's first years of medical school. A major turning point came when an anti-choice group disseminated a pamphlet to all student members of the American Medical Association that ridiculed abortion providers. Entitled "Bottom Feeders," the pamphlet was "like, 20 pages long with a lot of really offensive jokes about abortionists." Almost simultaneously, Dr. David Gunn, an ob/gyn providing abortions in Florida, was shot and killed outside of his practice. "The mailing plus his murder just totally upset us, and we felt like we had to do something."

Still a medical student, Dr. Steinauer was galvanized by the increasing politicization of abortion care and organized educational talks and advocacy events: "We made all these little flyers that we hung around the school, like 'Do you think you could provide abortions?' . . . We had a panel of abortion providers, with family physicians and ob/gyns . . . So from that moment on, from like June of my first year, I would say I was talking about abortion nonstop." Steinauer reacted against the anti-choice political activists and the increasing alienation of abortion providers by acting from within the biomedical establishment. "It was not super easy—my flyers would disappear off the walls—so students were pretty uncomfortable with the attention to abortion." Abortion was already a core component of Steinauer's sense of self as a future activist physician, and she worked to integrate this aspect of her identity with those of her classmates and the biomedical establishment.

Dr. Steinauer spent her first summer in medical school working with the National Abortion Federation (NAF) to engage students in abortion training; she said:

> NAF and ACOG [American College of Obstetricians and Gynecologists] were concerned that the number of abortion providers was declining . . . all of these physicians who had been doing abortions because of the morbidity and mortality of the pre-Roe era—they were really motivated to make sure people get safe abortion care, but now that it was the '90s, a lot of them were near retirement and [very few] ob/gyn programs had abortion training.

Dr. Steinauer began her bioeducation during the early 1990s—the period in which Dr. Barnes noted the withdrawal of ob/gyns from the abortion workforce and the gradual marginalization of abortion care in his practice. Increasingly, Steinauer connected with medical students around the country who shared her core value of physicians as activists committed to increasing abortion training. That summer, this group of activist medical students formed a new national organization, Medical Students for Choice, which Dr. Steinauer spent a year away from medical school to cultivate.

When she returned to medical school, Dr. Steinauer was still undecided on ob/gyn as a biomedical specialty and had yet to experience providing abortion care firsthand. Despite this lack of experience, abortion had already formed a core part of her burgeoning professional identity:

> I was like, "Okay, I really hope I like a specialty in which I can easily do abortions"... When I went into my first [abortion procedure], I thought, "Oh my God, what if I really don't want to do this? This is going to be a huge identity crisis for me"... And then I watched my mentor do it, and thought to myself, "I would love to be able to provide this safely for women."

After deciding on ob/gyn, Dr. Steinauer sought out residency training programs that provided high-quality training in abortion, actively mentioning her desire for this training during the interview process. "Just by asking about it, it really changed how ob/gyn program directors thought of training. I mean it was a requirement at that point, but they still weren't advertising it." Unlike Dr. Barnes, who had encountered abortion in residency as an unremarkable aspect of his professional ob/gyn identity, Dr. Steinauer's commitment to abortion as a core part of her physician identity preceded and superseded her identity as an ob/gyn. In the process of becoming a biomedical provider, Dr. Steinauer sought to re-legitimize abortion as the predominating part of her new ob/gyn identity through returning abortion to mainstream discussions in training programs.

Eventually, Dr. Steinauer completed both an ob/gyn residency program and a Family Planning Fellowship, building an academic career: "I would say the bigger part of my identity is now being an educator about abortion, so, not only do I do abortions, but if I train people to provide abortion, that will have a bigger impact." Despite the fact that she currently provides a broad variety of care as an ob/gyn, Dr. Steinauer reflected "If you said to me, 'You can only do one thing in all of your future life related to clinical care,' I would 100% do abortion care." Dr. Steinauer related this deep commitment to abortion to the early place of advocacy in her professional physician identity: "I think it comes back to my identity as an activist. If I don't do abortion, that means there's one less person providing this care people need, and it's such a stigmatized area of medicine, it's so politicized... I would not be doing the right thing if I didn't do it anymore."

Dr. Steinauer also noted that her motivations for performing abortions differed from the motivations of the earlier generation of abortion providers she encountered as a student. Echoing the findings of Joffe, Weitz, and Stacey (2004), Steinauer described a movement away from framing abortion as a "public health" and "patient safety" issue toward a more feminist agenda:

> We would interact with lots of people who had done abortions before Roe or had just started providing right after Roe had overturned the abortion law and had seen people dying and suffering from unsafe abortion. And they were coming to this from an urgent public health mindset, like "We have to do this or people will die." And we also had [younger] mentors coming at it from more of a feminist place, like saying "This is a right that we should have, and it's really satisfying work, and if you can do it, you should do it"... I could see my generation was feeling much less aligned with the public health message. I mean we knew that people had died, but that wasn't really our primary motivation.

Steinauer also reflected on how her early framework for abortion as meaningful work differed from that of subsequent trainees she encountered, both through Medical Students for Choice and through teaching at her academic center:

> The first re-framing [that I encountered in my students] was about disparities and barriers to access, and that brought in race, class, and socioeconomics. And then, on social and structural determinants of health, then expansion to LGBTQ care and abortion within a bigger framework. It has sort of grown so that abortion is just one piece of the puzzle, and all those things are really interconnected.

While initially Medical Students for Choice was built around abortion advocacy and activism, these activist values have since expanded beyond abortion, as Steinauer explains:

> For example, back then, it was "Women, women, women. Women's rights, women's access." I think feminism can be inclusive, but of course the feminism that I learned back in the '80s was not inclusive of people other than those who identified as women. Now there's more of a justice frame, more holistic ... people who are activists around abortion are more likely to also be thinking about people's rights and the various people who are excluded from care. Like the

importance of providing trans care, providing high-quality care for people who are pregnant with substance use disorders, providing high-quality care for people with few resources, and engaging the community as partners in care ... The new framework is about reproductive justice, and I think it's bigger than reproductive justice.

From a small group of medical students who felt drawn to abortion through activism as a core part of physician professional identity, Dr. Steinauer now sees a community of physicians for whom activism, advocacy, equity, and justice are fundamental physician values, inextricable from each other and from the meaning of biomedical work.

"If I Can Politically Participate, I've Helped So Many More Women"

Dr. Kelly DeLaurentis, like Dr. Steinauer, entered medicine as a feminist knowing that she wanted a career that allowed her to empower women through health care. DeLaurentis said:

> It was pretty obvious to me that women face certain hurdles just because of the XX chromosome. And males have all this privilege assigned to them just because of the Y chromosome. So I wanted to go into medicine and to take care of women and try to address that disparity at least as much as I could in my own practice of medicine.

As with Dr. Steinauer, Dr. DeLaurentis too found that abortion was stigmatized within the biomedical school establishment. While abortion was not mentioned in her medical school curricula in the early 2000s in the southern United States, she connected with a larger community of abortion providers through organizations like Planned Parenthood and Medical Students for Choice. Dr. DeLaurentis described having to feign ignorance with a faculty mentor who provided abortions at Planned Parenthood. "I was not allowed to acknowledge her role at Planned Parenthood at the university or really that I knew her in any capacity other than as a medical student at the university."

As Dr. DeLaurentis's sense of professional identity as an ob/gyn matured around the importance of abortion, she began to see pregnancy as a nexus of social forces, a point of intervention in reshaping larger injustices:

> It became really clear to me that if a person cannot control their fertility, the socioeconomic, physical, mental, sort of consequences

of that are so profound that that's what I really wanted to focus on . . . If you have a child when you are not ready or don't have the financial resources, or physically you're not in the best health, these are things that have very downstream consequences. They don't allow you the same possibilities as far as future things like completing school and your education, getting jobs, moving forward in your career—those kinds of things.

Abortion provided a means of medically intervening in a patient's life in an expansive manner that could also improve social factors such as the patient's socioeconomic status, education, or career. In contrast to Dr. Barnes, who framed abortion in terms of prevention of physical harm, "just like giving insulin to a diabetic," Dr. DeLaurentis sought to address more than her patients' physical bodies; she sought to expand care for their social and economic lives.

After medical school, DeLaurentis chose a residency program based on the availability of abortion training, and subsequently pursued a Family Planning Fellowship. After her Fellowship, she became faculty at the university hospital where she had studied. At the time of the interview, Dr. DeLaurentis had left her academic position to pursue full-time work as an abortion provider:

> You know, recently I gave up my obstetrics practice and went full-time to Planned Parenthood, partly because there's just not a lot of other people willing to do the work and there's a lot of need, and there sure are a lot of people who will deliver babies and help you get pregnant and there are providers willing to do that.

Dr. DeLaurentis, like Dr. Steinauer, considered abortion to be the central bedrock of her identity as an ob/gyn and physician. Both of these doctors were willing to sacrifice other aspects of their work as ob/gyns to fill the need for abortion care in their communities. This need played a key role in forming DeLaurentis's professional identity as a physician:

> We take the oath about our patients' autonomy, you know, all of our ethical principles—there's nowhere in there that says, "As a physician, I should be dictating care because of my own personal beliefs" . . . You know, there's so many easy ways to help people that are not so supported by society . . . providing ob care, for instance. That's just ok. Like, that's not a struggle, and there are a lot of people out

there doing that work. I feel there's such a need on the other side of the coin that there's not enough people doing this work.

In contrast to obstetric care, which is "just ok," abortion care—an area with an urgent unmet health care need—provided Dr. DeLaurentis with the sense that she was most fully enacting her professional values.

For DeLaurentis, there was an additional component to her abortion work: the imperative to be politically active. She saw the need to advocate not only at the patient level or even within the medical establishment but also within larger social and political systems:

> If we want to remove the stigma from abortion, we have to talk about it, and that has to be *providers* talking about it . . . the more we fly under the radar and keep quiet about it and let the other side say whatever they want, the stigma is never going to go away when it really, to my mind, it is just a basic human right to control your fertility. So, if I want to change things, then I have to be out there, which is why I've done some extra training to become an advocate . . . . I have chosen legislative advocacy . . . . If I can politically participate, I've helped so many more women.

Dr. DeLaurentis felt that *all* physicians, not just abortion providers, had the responsibility to be politically active on behalf of their patients, and that this responsibility extended beyond abortion: "I think it's definitely physicians' responsibility and role to advocate on a larger scale for a justice-oriented healthcare system that really [places] the patient [at] the forefront of how we provide care, and this is how I am choosing to enact myself in that role." DeLaurentis acknowledged that her identity as an abortion provider had fundamentally changed, and even superseded, other aspects of her ob/gyn identity. She described how abortion has changed her ob/gyn professional identity:

> I feel like my goals are still the same, but I'm no longer willing to be that person that's providing [without challenging the status quo] in my practice. . . . [ob/gyn] is comprehensive care, we do what the patient needs, but unfortunately, politically, everybody's all in your exam room and shaming women . . . And so to stop that, I think you have to come out of that ideal practice model where you're just providing comprehensive care, whatever that is—abortion and prenatal care. You have to come out of that role and be an advocate for your patients, and there's risk involved with that, of course. You know,

historically, I think that's a big reason why abortion providers have been quiet are the risks involved, the stigma, and there's always that rare chance you could be killed.

For Dr. DeLaurentis, her devotion to providing abortion care despite the risks expanded her professional obligation from providing comprehensive reproductive health care within the confines of her practice to public-facing political advocacy. Her core professional identity had only been strengthened by her abortion work: "Before I am a man or a woman or a Jew or a Christian or white or Black or green, I am a physician. It is my heart and my soul. It is more than a career. It is part of my identity, and being an abortion provider has always been part of it, but because it's needed now to be loud, I'm happy to be loud about it."

"All the Abortion Stuff, All the Queer Stuff, and All the Trans Stuff"

Maggie Henrique was still in her first year of medical school at the time of our interview, yet she was already taking time away from her studies to attend a weekend-long Abortion Training Institute hosted by Medical Students for Choice. Abortion was the key reason she wanted to become a doctor: "I'm here because my ultimate goal is to become a second- and third-trimester abortion provider. This is the goal I settled on. That's why I decided to go to medical school. I had this very singular focus." Her drive to become an abortion provider began during her senior year of high school when she started learning about and advocating for reproductive health. Throughout college, she considered other career paths, but after taking on an organizer role in response to anti-choice activism targeting Planned Parenthood, Maggie realized that advocacy work would ultimately be unsatisfying: "I really came to terms with the grinding pace of policy and community organizing work, and I felt like if I was going to do that work long term, I would lose my mind because there was so much work to get to even the smallest of wins. So I was like, 'I need something more immediately gratifying than this.'"

Maggie did not consider a career in biomedicine until her senior year in college, after completing her thesis on disparities in abortion care:

> The abortion stories we see in the media are like, a middle-class white woman who goes to get an abortion and it's liberating for her. But I wanted to reflect that the majority of people who get

abortions are women of color. We are completely overlooking queer and trans people who get abortions. Their stories are not being told.

After graduating, Maggie worked for a national organization promoting access to abortion care while she applied to medical school. It was a job that she loved despite long hours and low pay.

Since starting medical school, Maggie has shadowed an abortion provider at her university whom she met through Medical Students for Choice. While abortion has only been brought up a few times in her first six months of medical school, she feels that her interest is generally supported by her colleagues and faculty. As the President of her school's chapter of Medical Students for Choice, as well as for the school's LGBTQ health group, "I talk about all the abortion stuff, all the queer stuff, and all the trans stuff." Maggie's drive toward abortion care is framed in the language of reproductive justice, and she reflects critically about power dynamics within biomedicine and the pro-choice movement:

> Broadly speaking about the reproductive health rights justice community, it is a lot of white women. What does [reproductive justice] mean when all the people in power are white women? The communities we're predominately working with, who have historically been negatively impacted by our movement, are Women of Color, particularly Black women. And we really do push queer and trans people off to the side and then bring them in when it's convenient to talk about . . . The language of the pro-choice movement is very [white] women-centric.

Maggie's goal to provide second- and third-trimester abortions means that she is already certain about becoming an ob/gyn. She already recognizes that the intense need for abortion providers, especially for later procedures, means that abortion may end up supplanting most of the other responsibilities of an ob/gyn. She wonders:

> Am I okay with only doing one procedure for the rest of my life? And so that's kind of hard, in that once I finish residency, I won't be able to do any of the other things that come with obstetrics and gynecological care . . . I'm going to have to go through all the training and become board certified and do all of the things, and only do one thing.

At the same time, though, when asked how abortion fits into her sense of herself as a future physician and her developing professional identity, Maggie immediately replied: "I think that it's just part and parcel of being an ob/gyn for me. I feel like those two things are completely inseparable."

Conclusion: Abortion Care and Physician Values

The meaning of abortion to the professional identities of ob/gyns who choose to provide it has, in many ways, radically shifted over the past four decades. In the wake of *Roe v. Wade*, abortion care was framed as a medical necessity, a service that all ob/gyns should provide as a part of their normal scope of practice. Ob/gyns who experienced pre-Roe practice knew that abortion saved the lives of patients, and framed its place within their practices as one of a number of necessary medical services to keep their patients healthy. However, over the subsequent decades, as access to abortion was steadily eroded and an increasingly fraught political climate pushed hospitals and practitioners to gradually step away from abortion care, abortion became increasingly marginal to ob/gyn work and stigmatized within biomedical education.

As anti-choice activism and political violence directed at abortion providers surged in the early 1990s, the framing of abortion began to shift. Framed at first in feminist terms, abortion care became linked with a new set of values, in which physician identity is inextricable from advocacy, activism, and justice. According to our interlocutors, younger generations of abortion providers see abortion as a core part of their identities as both ob/gyns and physicians because it gives them the opportunity to express these values. Increasingly, they feel that physicians have responsibilities not just to care for the patient in front of them, but also to change society socially and politically. Pregnancy has become a potential site of intervention into social and economic aspects of the lives of patients, and abortion a means of addressing the "root causes" of injustice. Increasingly, these younger ob/gyns feel that as physicians, they have social and political roles framed around rights and justice—roles that extend their obligations beyond abortion or feminism and toward historically marginalized communities.

The abortion providers interviewed for this project acknowledged the various ways in which they experienced stigma and marginalization from professional communities, yet they consistently framed abortion as central to their professional identities as ob/gyns. Instead of drawing them away from their "core" selves as physicians and ob/gyns, abortion work was consistently described as affirming and as expressing their most important professional values and obligations. This sense of abortion as the key practice of meaning and identity led the interlocutors to feel comfortable "giving up" other aspects of the care that they had been trained to provide as ob/gyns. These abortion providers feel that political advocacy and activism are core to their professional identities as ob/gyns and physicians, even if this means having inadequate time for other aspects of the specialty. Increasingly, they recognized abortion as central to practice and identity early in their physician careers, and their careers are increasingly framed around abortion as "mission-driven" medicine. The links that these interlocutors drew between abortions and ethical obligations, and the importance of personal narratives to abortion provision as a career path, also resonate with the ideas described by Moses in the preceding chapter in this volume.

The links that these interlocutors drew between abortions and ethical obligations, and the importance of personal narratives to abortion provision as a career path, also resonate with the ideas described by Moses. The orientation of physician identity toward advocacy is not confined to abortion providers, who may form the vanguard of what is undoubtedly a larger trend in biomedicine. In 1995, the idea that physicians should initiate actions on behalf of their communities was proposed as an opportunity for change and growth in the biomedical profession (Boelen 1995). Over subsequent decades, major medical organizations have included advocacy as a core competency, including the American Medical Association and the American College of Obstetricians and Gynecologists. A 2006 national survey of practicing physicians in the United States found that 90% of the physicians surveyed rated community participation and advocacy as "very important" (Gruen, Russell, and Blumenthal 2006). This importance has also been noted in countries outside of the United States. For example, in her anthropological examination of biomedical education in Malawi, Claire Wendland (2004) noted that young physicians felt a strong drive toward political activism as a part of their physician identities. Encountering systematic inequities that crippled the delivery of appropriate care, they identified the root causes of disease as lying both in their patients' bodies and in the larger dysfunctional health and political systems preventing them from solving straightforward health problems.

In 2012, US biomedical educators were considering the inclusion of advocacy as a core part of undergraduate medical education (Croft et al. 2012). By 2017, a survey of US ob/gyn residents found that 95% of those surveyed thought that political advocacy was important to the field of ob/gyn, and 90% felt that formal training in advocacy should be integrated into their residency training (Hall, Quinlan, and Gerber 2017). Organizations that guide biomedical education curricular content also consider advocacy core competencies. For example, the Association of Professors of Obstetrics and Gynecology, which publishes reproductive health educational objectives for US medical schools, includes in its recommendations that all medical students should be able to "describe the public health impact of the legal status of abortion, and discuss how health policy and advocacy, as well as social and environmental factors, impact access to abortion" (2019:56). As advocacy and political involvement have become more clearly integrated into the core of biomedical professional identity, abortion provision has been increasingly framed as a way of expressing this value.

James R. Zetka (2011) identified key shifts in ob/gyn professional identities related to increasing specialization. Zetka notes that specialization within biomedicine often arises as a result of preexisting divisions of medical work, and that new specialties most often arise in areas "that others have no interest in, and when their programs dovetail with the programs of the dominant elites" (2011:838). The centrality of abortion provision to the professional identities of some ob/gyns may be related to the placing of abortion as a specialist skill and to the development of Fellowships such as the Complex Family Planning Fellowship, accredited in 2020 (Schreiber and Madden 2021). The increasingly siloed nature of abortion care, and the politically motivated sidelining of abortion from the mainstream of ob/gyn practice, may contribute to the centrality of abortion to physician identity and to the framing of abortion as a specialist skill.

Through four narratives from four different generations of ob/gyns, we have demonstrated that abortion is core to the identities of the abortion-providing interlocutors, and that the specific values underlying these identities have shifted over time. Gradually, as our interviews have shown, the orientations of abortion providers, and physicians more broadly, have evolved toward political advocacy as a core professional responsibility and value. The narratives provided above suggest a further evolution among abortion providers to core values of equity, human rights, and social justice. We suspect that these core values reflect an evolution in the values of physicians overall, which will grow as the newest generation of physicians responds to the inequities magnified through the COVID-19 pandemic, the Black Lives Matter movement, the LGBTQQA1+ movement, and the movement for reproductive justice.

As restrictions to access to safe abortion care multiply following the overturn of Roe v. Wade, the professional identities of abortion providers may likewise continue to shift. Perhaps the increasing scarcity of safe abortion services will make more visible the consequences of lack of safe access and the vitality of abortion training, and it will again be framed as a "public health" necessity, as it was for older, pre-Roe v. Wade physicians. This may cause abortion provision to be once again seen as a core part of ob/gyn identity, rather than one which is specialized or optional. Alternatively, as the overturn of Roe v. Wade leaves the decision to individual states, abortion and abortion training may become more politicized and fragmented as they are confined to regions where abortion is legal. This politicization may further the sense of abortion care as a political calling, and may also further the need for ob/gyns who see abortion care at the center of their professional identities. Physicians training in states where abortion is illegal may either see abortion as critical and challenge the law, encourage their institutions to expand indications for legal abortion care, and/or leave the state to practice. Or they may see abortion as unnecessary and even inappropriate to their practices, increasing the marginalization of abortion care within the identities of practicing ob-gyns.

Rebecca Henderson received her PhD in Medical Anthropology from the University of Florida in 2022. She is currently completing her medical degree. Her interests include reproductive health, cancer, and precarity, and models in healthcare.

Chu J. Hsiao is an MD/PhD candidate at the University of Florida in Biological Anthropology. She studies how sociocultural experiences become biologically embodied using biocultural approaches. Her research interests include reproductive health, developmental origins of health and disease, and health disparities.

Jody Steinauer is a Professor of Obstetrics, Gynecology and Reproductive Sciences at the University of California, San Francisco, based at San Francisco General Hospital (SFGH). She directs the Bixby Center of Global Reproductive Health and the Kenneth J. Ryan Residency Training Program in Family Planning. Dr. Steinauer teaches and provides clinical care at SFGH, and her academic areas are family planning education and teaching learners to provide patient-centered care.

Note

1. "*Roe v. Wade* was a landmark legal decision issued on January 22, 1973, in which the U.S. Supreme Court struck down a Texas statute banning abortion, effectively legalizing the procedure across the United States. The court held that a woman's right to an abortion was implicit in the right to privacy protected

by the 14th Amendment to the Constitution. Prior to *Roe v. Wade*, abortion had been illegal throughout much of the country since the late 19th century." (Quoted from Roe v. Wade: Decision, Summary & Background—HISTORY)

References

Alvesson M, Willmott H. 2002. "Identity Regulation as Organizational Control: Producing the Appropriate Individual." *Journal of Management Studies* 39(5): 619–644.

Andaya E, Mishtal J. 2016. "The Erosion of Rights to Abortion Care in the United States: A Call for a Renewed Anthropological Engagement with the Politics of Abortion." *Medical Anthropology Quarterly* 31(1): 40–59.

Association of Professors of Gynecology and Obstetrics. 2019. *APGO Medical Student Educational Objectives*, 11th ed. Crofton MD: Association of Professors of Gynecology and Obstetrics.

Atewologun D, Sealy R, Vinnicombe S. 2016. "Revealing Intersectional Dynamics in Organizations: Introducing 'Intersectional Identity Work.'" *Gender, Work & Organization* 23(3): 223–247.

Barbour JB, Lammers JC. 2015. "Measuring Professional Identity: A Review of the Literature and a Multilevel Confirmatory Factor Analysis of Professional Identity Constructs." *Journal of Professions and Organization* 2(1): 38–60.

Britton LE, Mercier RJ, Buchbinder M, Bryant AG. 2017. "Abortion Providers, Professional Identity, and Restrictive Laws: A Qualitative Study." *Health Care for Women International* 38(3): 222–237.

Boelen C. 1995. "Prospects for Change in Medical Education in the Twenty-First Century." *Academic Medicine* 70(7): S21–31.

Croft D, Jay SJ, Meslin EM, Gaffney MM, Odell JD. 2012. "Perspective: Is It Time for Advocacy Training in Medical Education?" *Academic Medicine* 87(9): 1165–1170.

Cruess RL, Cruess SR. 2006. "Teaching Professionalism: General Principles." *Medical Teacher* 28(3): 205–208.

Gruen RL, Campbell EG, Blumenthal D. 2006. "Public Roles of US Physicians: Community Participation, Political Involvement, and Collective Advocacy." *Journal of the American Medical Association* 296(20): 2467–2475.

Hall E, Quinlan M, Gerber S. 2017. "Attitudes and Self-Reported Competencies in Advocacy among OB/GYN Residents [25I]." *Obstetrics & Gynecology* 129(5): 99S.

Harris LH, Debbink M, Martin L, Hassinger J. 2011. "Dynamics of Stigma in Abortion Work: Findings from a Pilot Study of the Providers Share Workshop." *Social Science & Medicine* 73(7): 1062–1070.

Holden MD, Buck E, Luk J, et al. 2015. "Professional Identity Formation: Creating a Longitudinal Framework through TIME (Transformation in Medical Education)." *Academic Medicine* 90(6): 761–767.

Hoonpongsimanont W, Sahota PK, Chen Y, et al. 2018. "Physician Professionalism: Definition from a Generation Perspective." *International Journal of Medical Education* 9: 246–252.

Ibarra H. 1999. "Provisional Selves: Experimenting with Image and Identity in Professional Adaptation." *Administrative Science Quarterly* 44(4): 764–791.

Jarvis-Selinger S, MacNeil KA, Costello GRL, et al. 2019. "Understanding Professional Identity Formation in Early Clerkship: A Novel Framework." *Academic Medicine* 94(10): 1574–1580.

Joffe CE, Weitz TA, Stacey CL. 2004. "Uneasy Allies: Pro-Choice Physicians, Feminist Health Activists, and the Struggle for Abortion Rights." *Sociology of Health & Illness* 26(6): 775–796.

Kumar A. 2013. "Everything Is Not Abortion Stigma." *Women's Health Issues* 23(6): e329–331.

Martin LA, Debbink M, Hassinger J, et al. 2014. "Abortion Providers, Stigma and Professional Quality of Life." *Contraception* 90(6): 581–587.

Schreiber CA, Madden T. 2021. "Complex Family Planning: A Newly Accredited, Landmark Fellowship." *Contraception* 103(1): 1–2.

Wald HS. 2015. "Professional Identity (Trans)Formation in Medical Education: Reflection, Relationship, Resilience." *Academic Medicine* 90(6): 701–706.

Ward KM. 2021. "Dirty Work and Intimacy: Creating an Abortion Worker." *Journal of Health and Social Behavior* 62(4): 512–525.

Wendland CL. 2010. *A Heart for the Work: Journeys through an African Medical School.* Chicago IL: University of Chicago Press.

Wilson I, Cowin LS, Johnson M, Young H. 2013. "Professional Identity in Medical Students: Pedagogical Challenges to Medical Education." *Teaching and Learning in Medicine* 25(4): 369–373.

Zetka JR. 2011. "Establishing Specialty Jurisdictions in Medicine: The Case of American Obstetrics and Gynaecology." *Sociology of Health & Illness* 33(6): 837–852.

———. 2020. "Innovation, Professional Identity, and Generational Divides in Medicine: The Case of Gynecologic Laparoscopy in the USA." *Social Science & Medicine* 266: 113350.

Zikic J, Richardson J. 2015. "What Happens When You Can't Be Who You Are: Professional Identity at the Institutional Periphery." *Human Relations* 69(1): 139–168.

CHAPTER 3

My Transformation from an Obstetrician to a Maternal-Fetal Medicine Subspecialist
Autoethnographic Thoughts on Situated Knowledges and Habitus

Ashish Premkumar

In this chapter, I describe my development as a maternal-fetal medicine (MFM) subspecialist/perinatologist through the lens of my training of residents in obstetrics and gynecology in MFM-related procedures, understood from my simultaneous positionality as a medical anthropologist. According to the Society for Maternal-Fetal Medicine (2021), an MFM "treats two patients at the same time"—the pregnant person and the fetus.[1] More specifically, an "MFM" (a commonly used shorthand for "maternal-fetal medicine subspecialist") either acts as a consultant (i.e., guides a consulting midwife or obstetrician in clinical decision-making), or as the primary obstetrician in a situation of pregnancy complications that could increase the likelihood of morbidity or mortality for the pregnant person, the fetus, or both. In this chapter, I intend to not only describe my own positionality as an MFM specialist and my reflections on that positionality, but also to provide, through vignettes, some understandings of what MFMs do that other ob/gyns don't, and of how we teach others.

Regarding training, in the United States, an MFM must complete four years of residency in obstetrics, followed by a three-year Fellowship in MFM.[2] The seven years between graduating from medical school and becoming an attending MFM are filled with hours spent in outpatient clinics, ultrasound units, operating rooms (ORs), lecture halls, and global conferences to sculpt one's thought process and practice in line with current evidence-based data and opinions regarding optimal treatment of the pregnant person and also to internalize biomedicine's "hidden curriculum,"[3] which often consists of non-evidence-based biomedical traditions.[4] My focus within this chapter is to consider: (1) How my knowledge base as an MFM/anthropologist developed in tandem with engagement with biomedical and anthropological perspectives; and (2) How I embody this knowledge base within my surgical and procedural practices, and how this embodiment positions me in relationship with the pregnant people whom I had the privilege of caring for throughout my training.

Through two clinical vignettes concerning Melanie, a pregnant woman whose twins were affected with twin-to-twin transfusion syndrome (TTTS),[5] I draw on Donna Haraway's (1988) concept of situated knowledges, as well as on insights from Pierre Bourdieu and his interlocutors (Farquhar 2005; Prentice 2005, 2007, 2012; Wacquant 2004, 2005; Pitts-Taylor 2015) focused on "habitus" (Bourdieu 1977, 1997), to argue that the crafting of an MFM configures a physician in a specific affective orientation with a pregnant person, particularly in the creation of a medical subject (i.e., a fetus) with a diagnosable pathology and need for medical intervention (Weir 2006). By utilizing autoethnography, I hope to shed light on how an MFM's "view from somewhere" (Haraway 1988) is maintained and (re)produced, and what the stakes are for both the anthropology of obstetrics and obstetricians—a field that Robbie Davis-Floyd and I intend to officially create with this three-volume book series—and for wider theories of knowledge production, power, and the body.

Reflections on My Training in MFM

My desire to train as an MFM sprang from a long-standing interest in working with pregnant people who, due to medical issues affecting themselves and/or their fetuses, were deemed too high risk for non-MFM obstetricians to treat. I also felt deeply drawn toward reproductive health in general because of its strong sociopolitical bent toward healthcare equity, especially as relates to issues around reproductive choice (Paul and Norton 2016; Ross and Solinger 2017) and, particular to MFM, to reductions in morbidity and mortality (D'Alton 2010). These aims are primarily achieved through clinical training in complex obstetric procedures, management of critically ill pregnant people and their fetuses, and research methodologies aimed at describing and intervening to prevent adverse health outcomes (see below). I had cultivated this interest since

I was a medical student and was particularly struck by one key event when I was on a clinical rotation on a labor and delivery ward in South Africa.

Miriam and My Decision to Become an MFM

I first met Miriam in the obstetrical triage bay, her bony frame tenting up the rough hospital bedsheets, her face barely mustering a grin. An ambulance had brought her six hours from her rural home to our public hospital in East London, the largest city in the poorest district of South Africa, for complaints of abdominal pain and vaginal bleeding. She told us that she was in her mid-30s, HIV positive, and pregnant. After finding absent fetal heart tones, indicative of a fetal demise, she gave birth silently, looking away as her child was taken to the pathology lab for further testing. Given that I was still a medical student, I had never seen such suffering; I felt overwhelmed being with Miriam during her most vulnerable of moments, giving birth to a child already dead in a cold hospital room. I came in early the next day to speak with her, only to have my resident inform me that she had died overnight. The resident attributed her death to AIDS-related malnutrition and cardiorespiratory collapse—words that sounded woefully inadequate to me. I could not find an explanation for what had happened, and it gnawed at me—medically, philosophically, and most importantly, morally.

I became drawn to obstetrics and gynecology, and particularly to MFM as a modality to combat everyday inequalities in the lives of the people I had come to see and know. In particular, by focusing my scope of practice among highly marginalized populations who suffer from medical conditions that lead to higher risk of adverse pregnancy outcomes and early maternal mortality, I felt that my clinical work could help to improve the lives of vulnerable people (Farmer 2010). Furthermore, as someone who also hoped to practice at the intersection of MFM and family planning, being able to counsel and provide options for contraception and abortion became my way of helping to enact reproductive justice (Ross and Solinger 2017; and see the two preceding chapters in this volume). Finally, by trying to treat each person who came to see me with dignity, kindness, and respect—regardless of intersectional forms of inequity—I sought to improve the highly disempowering experiences that mark most engagements with biomedical care (Washington 2006; Davis 2019).

The process to train as an MFM is long. In addition to the pedagogical, clinical, and surgical training that MFMs undergo as residents in obstetrics and gynecology, the additional three years spent during the Fellowship are filled with acquiring skills that may be inconsistently taught or not taught at all during ob/gyn residency, such as: the clinical management of critically ill pregnant people; maternal-fetal therapy; prenatal diagnosis of congenital and genetic anomalies; family planning techniques that include initiation of contraception in medically complex people; complex obstetric surgeries, such as cesarean hysterectomies; and research methodologies, culminating in a thesis prior to graduation.[6] Throughout the hundreds of hours spent on labor and delivery wards, the antepartum wards, and in classrooms—both learning from professors and teaching medical students and residents about MFM—I began to become the doctor that people would come to for research advice, the one called into the OR for a difficult birth, the one whose phone would ring at odd hours of the night with a physician on the other end of the line, panicked or concerned about a sick pregnant person, looking to me for guidance and support. In short, training as a Fellow in MFM cultivated my positionality as a consultant who could aid other reproductive health practitioners during particularly dangerous moments in pregnancy and birth. (As an MFM friend of my coeditor Robbie once put it, "Everybody relaxes when they see me coming, because they know that I will know what to do.")

It is from these positions as a subspecialist and consultant, and as a medical anthropologist, that I now engage my critical theoretical lens toward the pedagogy surrounding the clinical decision-making aimed at improving pregnant people's health and health care. Thus, I turn to my experiences with Melanie during my Fellowship, in order to elucidate the particularities of knowledge production and affect—understood as the emotional atmosphere engendered during a clinical encounter—within procedural and surgical encounters during a high-risk pregnancy.

Vignette 1: Amnioreduction at the Bedside

I met Melanie at a busy, quaternary urban hospital on the day she was admitted to the antepartum service for management of TTTS,[7] a complication unique to monochorionic gestations (twins that share a placenta). Due to the sharing of blood vessels between each twin via the placenta, there is a possibility for imbalanced blood flow between high-pressure arteries and low-pressure veins. In TTTS, blood flow has shunted from one twin (the "donor twin") to the other twin (the "recipient twin"). This pathophysiology can lead to reduced amniotic fluid in the donor twin and excess amniotic fluid in the recipient twin. Depending on the severity of the TTTS, if left untreated, it can lead to stillbirth for one or both twins; among liveborn neonates who are affected with TTTS in utero, there is a higher likelihood of adverse neurodevelopmental outcomes and cardiac dysfunction (Society for Maternal-Fetal Medicine and Simpson 2013; Hecher et al. 2018).

Melanie had initially come to our care center on referral from her obstetrician, several hundred miles away, to assess whether she would be a candidate for maternal-fetal surgery to treat TTTS. Based on the degree of TTTS affecting Melanie's twins, the recommended course of action would have been a fetoscopic laser obliteration of the intertwin blood vessels with subsequent removal of the excess amniotic fluid surrounding the recipient twin (Senat et al. 2004; Slaghekke et al. 2014). This is performed by placing a special kind of fetoscope—a slender, fiberoptic instrument with a camera at its tip and ports for inserting surgical instruments at its hub—percutaneously through the maternal abdomen, uterus, and into the recipient twin's amniotic sac. By visualizing the intertwin blood vessels via the camera installed in the fetoscope—and subsequently projected onto a television screen in an operating room—the surgeon can introduce a laser fiber into the surgical tool port of the fetoscope to ablate ("turn off") the vascular connections and thus stop the blood flow imbalances that lead to TTTS.

When Melanie had presented to the maternal-fetal care center attached to our hospital in the early part of her third trimester of pregnancy, she was complaining of worsening contractions, which had started the day before. Given the concern for preterm labor—which can be associated with TTTS—she was sent to labor and delivery for further evaluation, where she was found to be in early labor. Due to the technical limitations of being able to perform fetoscopy during labor and the high risk of complications associated with fetoscopy, such as iatrogenic rupture of the amniotic membranes, our maternal-fetal surgical care team decided to avoid fetoscopy. Over the course of the next half day, Melanie's contractions reduced and, for the time being, it seemed that her labor had subsided. After a team discussion, we recommended an amnioreduction—the placement of a long needle under ultrasound guidance through the maternal abdomen, uterus, and into the amniotic sac of the recipient twin. A large glass evacuated container is attached to the needle hub via plastic tubing, which, through negative pressure, will remove excess amniotic fluid from around the recipient twin (Moise et al. 2005).

When I met Melanie for the first time, I was prepared to counsel her about an amnioreduction. My attending—Dr. Williams, a senior MFM attending physician who had been practicing for more than 20 years—

and one of our junior residents in obstetrics and gynecology, Pearl, were also in the room. In addition to seeking to save the life of the recipient twin, the goal of the procedure was to allow me to "proctor" or guide the junior resident through the amnioreduction, with Dr. Williams, the MFM attending, supervising the procedure.

We asked Melanie to lie flat on her back before we began the procedure. After cleaning her pregnant abdomen with soap, we placed a series of towels in a square formation around her abdomen to create a sterile space in which to perform the amnioreduction. I then placed an ultrasound probe over her abdomen to view the twins. Immediately, we could see a sea of black on the ultrasound screen, consistent with the known excess amniotic fluid around the recipient twin. We could also see the recipient twin lying on the lower portion of the screen as a bundle of bright lines moving intermittently on the screen, the fetal heartbeat easily visualized as a rapid sequence of flickers, like an eye blinking open and closed. "There's the recipient twin, swimming at the bottom of the ocean!"[8] Dr. Williams exclaimed, whispering within earshot of myself and Pearl, softly enough so that Melanie, who was awake during the procedure—for which we used an injectable local anesthetic—could not hear.[9] After finding a good area to place the needle, I whispered into Pearl's ear the tricks I had picked up throughout my training: using one's finger to gently poke the skin of the abdomen near the ultrasound probe in order to visualize the dimpling and relaxation of the skin on the ultrasound screen indicating the position and course of the needle; making sure to keep the probe as close to the needle as possible in order to visualize it continuously with the ultrasound; and moving one's hands in tandem—if one is to reposition the needle to point closer toward the head, the ultrasound probe, usually held in the opposite hand, should move with it. "Move slowly, with small changes in the position of your hands," I added, thinking back to the times I had trained in amniocentesis and had moved my hand holding the needle so quickly that I lost sight of my needle tip, which can be particularly dangerous as the needle may unintentionally pierce other structures (such as the umbilical cord or the intertwin amniotic membrane) and cause complications. I had learned from my own mistakes, and thus was able to transmit that learning to Pearl to keep her from making the same ones.

I handed the local anesthetic to Pearl and watched on the ultrasound screen as the needle went into Melanie's skin. As the fluid entered the tissue lying just beneath her skin, you could see a brief expansion of gray on the ultrasound screen, emanating from the hyperechoic,[10] bright area where we could easily see the needle tip. Pearl was then handed the amnioreduction needle; as she introduced it along the same track that the anesthetic had created, I could see it approaching the anterior wall of the uterus. I would adjust her hand ever so slightly to keep the needle directly in line with the ultrasound probe so that we could track the bright, hyperechoic line representing the needle through the ultrasound screen. Trying not to speak too loudly, I whispered, quickly, "Now, jab like you're throwing a dart!" On the screen, I could see a brief jiggle, and then a bright line within a sea of darkness—the needle now inserted into the amniotic sac of the recipient twin. We quickly attached tubing from the needle hub to the evacuated container and began to perform the amnioreduction.

The time that it takes to perform an amnioreduction can vary but, given the degree of fluid and the narrow caliber of the tubing between the needle and the container, this one took almost ten minutes to complete. During this time, there is not much to do other than stand still and try, as much as possible, not to move the needle. Every minute or two, we would move the ultrasound probe slightly to evaluate the fetal heartrates to ensure that both twins were alive. It is during these moments—usually filled with silence—that one or both senior physicians in a room will sometimes start to quietly talk, pointing out things that would be useful for this junior resident physician to know and things that the patient would want to understand. It was during one of these moments, as we could see the recipient twin moving away from the "bottom of the ocean" and higher up on the screen as excess amniotic fluid was being removed, that Dr. Williams was able to point out the fetus for Melanie to see. "And there's your baby, you can see how the fluid is decreasing," she said, pointing to the now-smaller black, hypoechoic space surrounding the recipient twin.[11] Two liters of fluid later, now with an ultrasound demonstrating a relatively normal amount of fluid surrounding the recipient twin, Pearl removed the needle from Melanie's abdomen.

Thinking about the Medical Subject: A View from Somewhere

My description of showing Pearl how to do an amnioreduction highlights a particular form of pedagogy classic to medical training (i.e., the often-mentioned maxim "see one, do one, teach one"[12]), but that also reinforced my transition from an obstetrician to an MFM as I proctored Pearl: namely, a highly specified focus on the fetus—or, in this case, fetuses. Here, I hearken to Donna Haraway's (1988) concept of "situated knowledge," which emphasizes that knowledge itself, and the means of acquiring knowledge, are always partial, never universal. She reached this conclusion by dissecting universal theories, historically proposed by

Enlightenment thinkers who did not themselves acknowledge the racist, classist, and misogynistic roots from which their theories arose. As Haraway put it: "I am arguing for a view from a body, always a complex, contradictory, structuring, and structured body, versus the view from above, from nowhere, from simplicity" (1988: 589). Haraway's emphasis on the locality of knowledge acquisition and making vis-à-vis the body is critical for my exegesis of Pearl's first amnioreduction. Principally, Haraway acknowledges the contingencies associated with a partial perspective from a corporeal perspective (e.g., the bodily capacity to see or not to see[13]). It is this emphasis on the body that interests me in terms of how knowledge production and acquisition are occurring simultaneously during an amnioreduction. The act of putting a needle into Melanie's uterus to remove excess amniotic fluid—itself based on visual findings from an ultrasound—emphasizes a particular form of objective knowledge—that is, there is a condition called TTTS, which our team has diagnosed, that can be treated with an amnioreduction; the amnioreduction also highlights the production of a given subject(s) that is intimately connected with the act of amnioreduction: Melanie's fetuses.

I argue that by employing the situated knowledge around TTTS and proctoring Pearl through the amnioreduction, we were bringing Melanie's fetuses from static ultrasound findings into tangible medical subjects who were the recipients of medical treatment. I theorize the transition in our minds of Melanie's fetuses from abstract ultrasonographic pictures to medical subjects by hearkening to Lorna Weir's (2006) use of the term "threshold"—namely the shift from one temporal and ontological moment to another during the window of pregnancy. The creation and maintenance of the threshold of the medical subject, I further posit, is a job that is key to being an MFM, and one that is unique to this specialty. It is the role of an MFM to perform prenatal diagnoses of fetal conditions and to recommend treatments based on the severity of the disease process; these care foci are much different than those of obstetricians, who primarily focus on the prenatal, birth, and postpartum care of childbearing people.

Yet in serving the fetus, the MFM's creation and maintenance of the threshold of the medical subject bring up concerns about the erasure of the pregnant person. The very nature of the amnioreduction—centered around an ultrasound depiction of Melanie's fetuses, with limited attention focused on Melanie—highlights where the theoretical concept of the medical subject meets the embodied act of intervening upon the mother for fetal benefit. Melanie's amnioreduction as I have narrated it was notably bereft of Melanie herself: the erasure, however temporary, of the pregnant person during a procedure aimed at improving fetal health has important consequences for how I want to proceed in my analysis. My narrative depicts a common problem that MFMs face: namely, the moments in which a care team must work on a pregnant woman to care for her fetus, not for her; this, at face value, contradicts the holistic ideological assumption that mother and baby are one, and that what is good for the mother is good for the baby (Davis-Floyd [1992] 2003, 2022). Yet, ontologically, this tenet of holism is not actually contradicted in Melanie's case, as her own best interests are served when her twin fetuses are rendered healthy, as our team attempted to do in performing the amnioreduction.

Vignette 2: An Emergent Cesarean Birth, a Death

The first amnioreduction was successful; repeat ultrasounds of Melanie's twin fetuses demonstrated a normalization in the fluid around both twins, with evidence of fluid in both twin's bladders. This latter finding was a sign that the severity of the TTTS was reducing, which, overall, was reassuring. However, over the course of the next two weeks, these ultrasound findings would increase in severity, and Melanie would undergo further amnioreductions to try to treat the TTTS.

I started on an evening shift with another one of my attending physicians, Dr. Molina—a junior faculty MFM who had been intermittently caring for Melanie alongside me. At the beginning of our shift, we were informed that today's ultrasound bore a poor prognosis: despite the multiple amnioreductions, one of the twins had progressed in the severity of TTTS and had developed a life-threatening condition called "hydrops fetalis."[14] Given the inability of conservative measures to appropriately treat the TTTS affecting Melanie's twins, and the high risk of mortality of one or both of her twins, we recommended proceeding with delivery. Since the twin closest to Melanie's cervix was not in the vertex (head down) position, but rather was breech, and given the high likelihood that the twin affected with hydrops fetalis would undergo intrapartum asphyxia, we recommended a cesarean birth.[15]

I remember walking into Melanie's room prior to the cesarean. She was already dressed in one of the light green hospital gowns we had the patients wear prior to moving to the OR. When I had first met her for her first amnioreduction, and in subsequent meetings in the clinic, she was cheerful, talking about her other children, her life in the Great Plains prior to moving to the Midwest, and her hopes that, despite the odds, the amnioreductions would work and she would be able to meet and raise both of her twins. Now we had to tell her that, despite our interventions, we were unable to successfully treat the TTTS. Furthermore, given the fact that we were going to proceed with delivery at a very early gestational age, there was a high likelihood of the neonatal death of the twin affected with hydrops fetalis. Prior to going into Melanie's room, Dr. Molina had told me, "If she wants a hope of holding her kid before it dies, we need to proceed with delivery." Melanie began to cry when we discussed this possibility, her husband looking down at the floor, trying to comfort her with a hand over her shoulder.

Julia, one of the senior residents in obstetrics and gynecology, and I, alongside Dr. Molina, performed the cesarean. As opposed to an emergency cesarean birth, for which a pregnant person may be placed under general anesthesia unless she already has an epidural (which happens in only around 7% of cesarean births) our anesthesiology team was able to place an epidural, allowing Melanie to be awake for the births of her children. The operating room was packed full of people—along with Melanie's husband, our usual anesthesiology team, nursing staff, and a surgical technician in the room, we also had two neonatal resuscitation teams made up of multiple people to care for both twins. My team tried to keep the noise down to a minimum so that we could focus on the surgery and alert the other teams regarding any complications. Once we had delivered the first twin and handed the baby to the neonatology team, we could hear an initial cry coming from the resuscitation table; I could hear Melanie and her husband also start to cry. One of the neonatologists announced that the child was doing well, which provided some measure of relief to all of us. We then proceeded with delivery of the twin affected with hydrops fetalis. After delivery, the newborn looked puffy and swollen, and was not moving as vigorously as the first twin. We handed the infant to the neonatologist for resuscitation.

I have become attuned, particularly as an MFM, to listen for how a given neonatal resuscitation is going. As the Fellow physician in this operation, my goal was to assist and supervise Julia through the cesarean birth, as I have done for many other residents; therefore, showing residents how to improve the dexterity of their surgical instrumentation, knot tying, and dissection abilities becomes a rote skill, one that requires little thought unless issues like hemorrhage or untoward organ injury occur. Thereby, my attention can be freed up in a way that is not the same as when I was training as an ob/gyn. During Melanie's birth, after delivery of the twin affected with hydrops fetalis, all I could hear as I listened was the near-silence surrounding a code event during which cardiopulmonary resuscitation is being administered—the soft hiss of bag mask ventilation, the muffled sounds of the neonatology team trying to place appropriate lines to administer medications and perform chest compressions, Melanie whispering to her husband, "What's going on?," the anesthesiologist trying to comfort Melanie: "The doctors are trying to do all they can for your little one."

It was after we had finished the surgery—after Melanie and her husband had the opportunity to see Colin, the firstborn twin, in an incubator moving to the neonatal intensive care unit—that the neonatology team had brought over Caleb, the twin affected with hydrops fetalis, swaddled in a white blanket, a blue beanie covering his head. After speaking with Melanie, the lead neonatologist came to me, Julia, and Dr. Molina and said, "The family has opted for comfort [palliative] care." Melanie had already been moved off the surgical table onto a stretcher; she was sitting upright, holding Caleb and crying. Her husband, dressed in a white pullover "bunny" suit, was also crying. "Don't worry, Caleb, it'll be ok," Melanie kept saying, cuddling Caleb. I could not find the strength to look at Melanie or her husband during this incredibly intimate moment in a cold OR, surrounded by the anesthesiologist, Melanie's nurse, and her MFM team. It felt eerie, almost disembodying, to be in the midst of a family openly grieving the death of their child—as if I had mistakenly chimed into a conversation not meant for me. Having been so involved with Melanie and her pregnancy, it would almost seem that I should also be involved with Caleb's passing. However, in moments like these, I have usually been able to excuse myself from the room so the family can grieve privately. Yet because this was occurring in an OR, it did not feel like the right place to leave Melanie—she should be back in her own private room, not in a cold space meant for surgery. Reflecting back on this moment, I realize that we should have moved Melanie and her family out of the OR and into a private room, but that did not occur to us at the time. So we stood in the OR with her for almost half an hour, frozen while she and her husband continued to mourn the loss of Caleb, before she handed Caleb to her nurse, and we wheeled Melanie to her room.

Thinking about Affect in the OR

These two vignettes about my time spent with Melanie and her twins, training a resident physician in amnioreduction, and helping to perform a cesarean birth with the ultimate death of Caleb, bring up critical questions for how I, as an MFM specialist, think about situated knowledge and the body—particularly the bodies of physicians in relationship to medical subjects (such as Melanie and her fetuses). Discussions of the body as it pertains to clinical practice have largely been confined to two bodies of literature: (1) Those that analyze the crafting of the "medical gaze," a term used by Michel Foucault (1978:108) to signify how physicians use their knowledge to objectively observe the patient and look for telling signs in order to properly diagnose and treat whatever illness is ailing the patient, seeing patients not as individuals but as problems to be solved (see also Good 1994; Davenport 2000); and (2) Those that elucidate the pedagogy of surgical training, both within the realm of medical hierarchy (see e.g., Cassell 1991, 1998; Bosk [1979] 2003) and in the cultivation of surgical practice (e.g., Prentice 2005, 2007, 2012). For the purposes of this chapter, I am focusing on the latter issue as it relates to the creation of medical subjects, and how, through employing situated knowledges in training residents in MFM-related procedures (e.g., amnioreduction and a cesarean birth with difficult consequences), affect—the emotional atmosphere engendered during a clinical encounter—is cultivated.

I also employ Pierre Bourdieu's (1977, 1997) concept of habitus. For Bourdieu, the term "habitus" refers to the physical embodiment of cultural capital, and to the collective entity by which and into which dominant social and cultural conditions are established and reproduced. In Bourdieu's words (1977:86), habitus refers to "a subjective but not individual system of internalised structures, schemes of perception, conception, and action common to all members of the same group or class"; in simpler terms, habitus can be seen as a cognitive space where group perceptions live, a space that they inhabit. The parameters of that space will be determined by the cultural capital of its inhabitants. Bourdieu (1997:141) further described the modalities of reproducing habitus, focusing on the effects of bodily practices: "We learn bodily. The social order inscribes itself in bodies through this permanent confrontation, which may be more or less dramatic but is always largely marked by affectivity [emotionality], and, more precisely, by affective transactions with the environment."

Anthropologists such as Rachel Prentice (2005, 2012) have hearkened to Bourdieu's theory of habitus within obstetrical and gynecological practice to describe the minute ways in which surgical methods are taught and how they are valued and crafted within modern biomedical hierarchies. I build upon Prentice's work on surgical training by focusing on how affect is created in the midst of MFM procedures. While affective/emotional work is part and parcel of clinical work, the ability to effectively produce and maintain a particular affective environment—one that emphasizes quietness, allowing simultaneously for the potential for calm to a patient, yet able to effectively allow for communication and coordination of multiple medical care teams—during difficult, and often traumatizing, situations is a hallmark of transitioning from an obstetrician/gynecologist to an MFM.

From taking Pearl through her first amnioreduction to training Julia in a complex cesarean birth, I am acutely aware of how training resident physicians in cases involving MFM brings about questions focused on the body: how to improve Pearl's evaluation of her needle placement in the amniotic sac of the recipient twin and her bodily coordination with the ultrasound probe and monitor; how to swiftly guide Julia through a cesarean birth by concomitantly focusing on the performance of her incision, knot tying, and handling of the surgical needle. Yet there are particular affects that become reproduced, whether consciously or unconsciously, that define the atmosphere within the space of a given procedure: the emphasis on silence, whether in the midst of an amnioreduction or the performance of cardiopulmonary resuscitation on a critically ill newborn; the ability to successfully juggle performing a surgical procedure and being aware of other teams working simultaneously; the moments in which it is deemed socially acceptable to offer insight into how a given medical procedure is proceeding; and the feeling of intrusiveness while a family grieves the loss of their son in an cold operating room filled with strangers.

While I have previously touched on the situated knowledges that are used to guide interventions, such as the amnioreduction, it is also important to note that situated knowledges are additionally employed to promote particular affective atmospheres. Hearkening to the silences that arose during Melanie's amnioreduction and subsequent cesarean birth, as well as to Dr. Williams's comments about the success of the amnioreduction, I can say that the opportunities to vocalize findings, or not, are things that are socially and experientially taught during medical training. For example, teaching medical students and other trainees when it is appropriate to ask questions or discuss the progress of a given surgical case and when it is not, is often fraught with tension. Within modern biomedical pedagogy, it is expected that medical students can ask questions and receive effective guidance on how medical decisions are made. Yet within the realm of surgery, the timing of these questions is critical, as physicians may be unable to explain their thought processes during a given situation due to the critical nature of the task at hand—for example, it is inappropriate for a medical student to ask an attending physician why a newly postpartum woman is being moved to the OR while she is hemorrhaging and is showing dangerous signs of hemodynamic instability, such as a high heart rate and/or low blood pressure.

These highly affective moments are (re)produced through relations with bodies and medical interventions through the construction of medical subjects, technologies, and surgeries. They center the body as "an object *and* means of inquiry" (Wacquant 2005:465, italics mine), and emphasize how the pedagogical training that I helped to perform as an MFM fellow with obstetrics and gynecology residents helped to mold my particular transition from being an obstetrician to being an MFM. For to become a teacher in this way is to accept that you are an ultimate authoritative figure, and that what you teach will be passed on, so it had better be right. Becoming an MFM generated a transition in my position in the obstetric hierarchy with which I had to come to terms—as in US President Truman's famous phrase,"The buck stops here." The sense of responsibility that this competence generates feels to me to be as large as the competence I had to develop to reach this habitus. I often feel the weight of this responsibility as an MFM in ways that I did not as an obstetrician.

Coda

Melanie's relationship with me and our MFM team brought up issues focused on the development of an obstetrician into an MFM: the creation of medical subjects through an understanding of situated knowledges, as well as how affective environments are produced during complex procedures, understood via habitus—that cognitive space where group perceptions live. These arenas of thought are not necessarily unique to MFM praxis, but, given the sociopolitical, economic, racial, gendered, and ableist underpinnings surrounding reproductive health and childbirth, are critical to consider.

I reached out to Melanie almost a year and a half later to see how things were going with Colin, her living child. She sent me a picture of a chubby toddler, smiling during a morning drop-off at a local daycare. "Would never know he had a rough start!" she said.

Ashish Premkumar is an Assistant Professor of Obstetrics and Gynecology at the Pritzker School of Medicine at The University of Chicago and a doctoral candidate in the Department of Anthropology at The Graduate School at Northwestern University. He is a practicing maternal-fetal medicine subspecialist. His research focus is on the intersections of the social sciences and obstetric practices, particularly surrounding the issues of risk, stigma, and quality of health care during the perinatal opioid use disorder epidemic of the 21st century. E-mail: premkumara@bsd.uchicago.edu.

Notes

1. For a further discussion of the historical creation of the fetal patient, particularly through maternal-fetal interventions (e.g., in-utero treatment of particular medical conditions), please see Casper (1998). For bioethical quandaries associated with the creation of the fetal patient, particularly the false separation of the fetus from the pregnant person, please see Lyerly, Little, and Faden (2008); Premkumar and Gates (2016); Davis-Floyd (2022).
2. MFMs may go on to complete additional training in other subfields, such as clinical genetics, maternal-fetal surgery, family planning, global health, or critical care. They may, like me, pursue additional research training or advanced degrees during and/or after fellowship (e.g., Masters in Public Health; Masters in Clinical Science and Investigation; PhD in Medical Anthropology—the path I chose).
3. As opposed to residents or fellow physicians who are in the midst of (sub) specialty training, an "attending" physician has completed all of the necessary training to practice independently. The vast majority of attending physicians in obstetrics and gynecology have passed a series of written and oral examinations administered by the American Board of Obstetrics and Gynecology.
4. For critiques of evidence-based medicine practices, see Timmermans and Berg (2003); Timmermans and Mauck (2005); Armstrong (2007).
5. Permission was sought from the individuals who are depicted in the vignettes, and all names have been changed to ensure confidentiality.
6. For example, my thesis evaluated the most cost-effective strategy for management of opioid use disorder during pregnancy. For further information, see Premkumar et al. (2019).
7. Hospitals are designated based on different levels of care, depending on the types of perinatal health care services they provide. The lower the level of designation, the fewer complex perinatal care services a given center may provide. For further information regarding hospital designations, see Kilpatrick et al. (2019).
8. In the setting of marked polyhydramnios, it is common to see the fetus at the bottom of the ultrasound screen; this does not necessarily define the presentation of the twins (i.e., it does not state which twin is presenting, that is, closest to the cervix), but rather defines where the fetus is in relationship to the abdominal wall (anterior) and the maternal spine (posterior).
9. For analyses of the moral and political work performed through medical technologies utilized to visualize fetuses, such as ultrasound, please see Petchesky (1987); Zechmeister (2001); Ivry (2009).
10. When describing ultrasonographic features using gray-scale ultrasound (i.e., black-and-white ultrasound pictures), MFMs and radiologists will normatively describe them as hyperechoic (bright-appearing) or hypoechoic (dark-appearing).
11. Often, obstetricians will vacillate between using "fetus" or "baby" to discuss ultrasound findings. As a rule of thumb during my training, we would mirror the language that the patient would use (e.g., if the patient said, "Oh, look at the baby on the screen!" the MFM would use the term "baby" to describe any ultrasound findings).

12. This phrase, common to the unofficial curriculum within biomedical training, emphasizes the need for a clinician-in-training to observe procedures, do them, and then guide others through the procedure.
13. "There are lessons that I learned in part walking with my dogs and wondering how the world looks without a fovea and very few retinal cells for color vision but with a huge neural processing and sensory area for smells" (Haraway 1988:583).
14. "Hydrops fetalis" refers to collections of fluid in at least two areas of the body where fluid normally does not collect to a significant degree (e.g., scalp edema, pericardial effusion) (Society for Maternal-Fetal Medicine [SMFM] et al. 2015). Etiologies for hydrops fetalis are numerous, though in the setting of TTTS, this can demonstrate failure of the heart to pump appropriately. Hydrops fetalis in the setting of TTTS portends a poor prognosis with a high likelihood of fetal demise (Society for Maternal-Fetal Medicine [SMFM] and Simpson 2013).
15. The method of delivery (i.e., planned vaginal or planned cesarean birth) for twin gestations is the subject of discussion. The Twin Birth Study, a multicenter randomized controlled trial, showed that, among the most common types of twins (i.e., twins that either have two placentas and two amniotic sacs or one placenta and two amniotic sacs), there was no difference in perinatal outcomes based on mode of delivery (Barrett et al. 2013). However, inclusion criteria for the trial included twins between 32 weeks 0 days and 38 weeks 6 days gestation, with the presenting twin (i.e., the twin closest to the maternal cervix) in vertex (i.e., head down) presentation. In places like France, supporting a vaginal birth in the setting of the presenting twin in non-vertex presentation has been described (Korb et al. 2020).

References

Armstrong D. 2007. "Professionalism, Indeterminancy, and the EBM Project." *BioSocieties* 2: 73–84.

Barrett JFR, Hannah ME, Hutton EK, et al. 2013. "A Randomized Trial of Planned Cesarean or Vaginal Delivery for Twin Pregnancy." *New England Journal of Medicine* 369(14): 1295–1305.

Bosk CL. (1979) 2003. *Forgive and Remember: Managing Medical Failure*, 2nd ed. Chicago: University of Chicago Press.

Bourdieu P. 1977. *Outline of a Theory of Practice* (R. Nice, Trans.) Cambridge: Cambridge University Press.

Bourdieu P. 1997. *Pascalian Meditations*. Stanford, CA: Stanford University Press.

Casper MJ. 1998. *The Making of the Unborn Patient: A Social Anatomy of Fetal Surgery*. Piscataway, NJ: Rutgers University Press.

Cassell J. 1991. *Expected Miracles: Surgeons at Work*. Philadelphia, PA: Temple University Press.

Cassell J. 1998. *The Woman in the Surgeon's Body*. Cambridge, MA: Harvard University Press.

D'Alton ME. 2010. "Where Is the 'M' in Maternal–Fetal Medicine?" *Obstetrics & Gynecology* 116(6): 1401–1404.

Davenport BA. 2000. "Witnessing and the Medical Gaze: How Medical Students Learn to See at a Free Clinic for the Homeless." *Medical Anthropology Quarterly* 14(3): 310–327.

Davis D-A. 2019. *Reproductive Injustice: Racism, Pregnancy, and Premature Birth.* New York: NYU Press.

Davis-Floyd R. (1992) 2003. *Birth as an American Rite of Passage*, 2nd edn. Berkeley: University of California Press.

———. 2022. *Birth as an American Rite of Passage*, 3rd edn. Abingdon, Oxon: Routledge.

Farmer PE. 2010. *Partner to the Poor: A Paul Farmer Reader*, ed. Sussey H. Berkeley: University of California Press.

Farquhar J. 2005. "Whose Bodies?" *Qualitative Sociology* 28(2): 191–196.

Foucault M. 1978. *Discipline and Punish: The Birth of the Prison.* New York: Pantheon Books.

Good B. 1994. *Medicine, Rationality, and Experience: An Anthropological Perspective.* New York: Cambridge University Press.

Haraway D. 1988. "Situated Knowledges: The Science Question in Feminism and the Privilege of Partial Perspective." *Feminist Studies* 14(3): 575–599.

Hecher K, Gardiner HM, Diemert A, Bartmann P. 2018. "Long-term Outcomes for Monochorionic Twins after Laser Therapy in Twin-to-Twin Transfusion Syndrome." *The Lancet Child & Adolescent Health* 2(7): 525–535.

Ivry T. 2009. "The Ultrasonic Picture Show and the Politics of Threatened Life." *Medical Anthropology Quarterly* 23(3): 189–211.

Kilpatrick SJ, Menard MK, Zahn CM, Callaghan WM. 2019. "Obstetric Care Consensus #9: Levels of Maternal Care." *Obstetrics & Gynecology* 134: e41–55.

Korb D, Goffinet F, Bretelle F, et al. 2020. "First Twin in Breech Presentation and Neonatal Mortality and Morbidity According to Planned Mode of Delivery." *Obstetrics & Gynecology* 135(5): 1015–1023.

Lyerly AD, Little MO, Faden RR. 2008. "A Critique of the 'Fetus as Patient.'" *American Journal of Bioethics* 8(7): 42–46.

Moise KJ, Jr., Dorman K, Lamvu G, et al. 2005. "A Randomized Trial of Amnioreduction versus Septostomy in the Treatment of Twin-Twin Transfusion Syndrome." *American Journal of Obstetrics & Gynecology* 193(3 Pt 1): 701–707.

Paul M, Norton ME. 2016. "Ensuring Access to Safe, Legal Abortion in an Increasingly Complex Regulatory Environment." *Obstetrics & Gynecology* 128(1): 171–175.

Petchesky RP. 1987. "Fetal Images: The Power of Visual Culture in the Politics of Reproduction." *Feminist Studies* 13(2): 263–292.

Pitts-Taylor V. 2015. "A Feminist Carnal Sociology?: Embodiment in Sociology, Feminism, and Naturalized Philosophy." *Qualitative Sociology* 38(1): 19–25.

Premkumar A, Gates E. 2016. "Rethinking the Bioethics of Pregnancy: Time for a New Perspective?" *Obstetrics & Gynecology* 128(2): 396–399.

Premkumar A, Grobman WA, Terplan M, Miller ES. 2019. "Methadone, Buprenorphine, or Detoxification for Management of Perinatal Opioid Use Disorder: A Cost-Effectiveness Analysis." *Obstetrics & Gynecology* 134(5): 921–931.

Prentice R. 2005. "The Anatomy of a Surgical Simulation: The Mutual Articulation of Bodies in and through the Machine." *Social Studies of Science* 35(6): 837–866.

Prentice R. 2007. "Drilling Surgeons: The Social Lessons of Embodied Surgical Learning." *Science, Technology, & Human Values* 32(5): 534–553.

Prentice R. 2012. *Bodies in Formation: An Ethnography of Anatomy and Surgery Education.* Durham, NC: Duke University Press.

Ross LJ, Solinger R. 2017. *Reproductive Justice: An Introduction.* Berkeley: University of California Press.

Senat M-V, Deprest J, Boulvain M, et al. 2004. "Endoscopic Laser Surgery versus Serial Amnioreduction for Severe Twin-to-Twin Transfusion Syndrome." *New England Journal of Medicine* 351(2): 136–144.

Slaghekke F, Lopriore E, Lewi L, et al. 2014. "Fetoscopic Laser Coagulation of the Vascular Equator versus Selective Coagulation for Twin-to-Twin Transfusion Syndrome: An Open-Label Randomised Controlled Trial." *Lancet* 383(9935): 2144–2151.

Society for Maternal-Fetal Medicine (SMFM). 2021. "High-Risk Pregnancy Information." *SMFM.* Retrieved 14 September 2022 from https://www.highriskpregnancyinfo.org.

Society for Maternal-Fetal Medicine (SMFM), Norton ME, Chauhan SP, Dashe JS. 2015. "Society for Maternal-Fetal Medicine (SMFM) Clinical Guideline #7: Nonimmune Hydrops Fetalis." *American Journal of Obstetrics & Gynecology* 212(2): 127–139.

Society for Maternal-Fetal Medicine (SMFM), Simpson LL. 2013. "Twin-Twin Transfusion Syndrome." *American Journal of Obstetrics & Gynecology* 208(1): 3–18.

Timmermans S, Berg M. 2003. *The Gold Standard: The Challenge of Evidence-based Medicine and Standardization in Health Care.* Philadelphia, PA: Temple University Press.

Timmermans S, Mauck A. 2005. "The Promises and Pitfalls of Evidence-Based Medicine." *Health Affairs* 24(1): 18–28.

Wacquant L. 2004. *Body and Soul: Notebooks of an Apprentice Boxer.* New York: Oxford University Press.

Wacquant L. 2005. "Carnal Connections: On Embodiment, Apprenticeship, and Membership." *Qualitative Sociology* 28(4): 445–474.

Washington HA. 2006. *Medical Apartheid: The Dark History of Medical Experimentation on Black Americans from Colonial Times to the Present.* New York: Doubleday.

Weir L. 2006. *Pregnancy, Risk and Biopolitics: On the Threshold of the Living Subject.* London: Taylor & Francis.

Zechmeister I. 2001. "Foetal Images: The Power of Visual Technology in Antenatal Care and the Implications for Women's Reproductive Freedom." *Health Care Analysis* 9(4): 387–400.

CHAPTER 4

Cold Steel and Sunshine

Ethnographic and Autoethnographic Perspectives on Two Obstetric Careers in the United States from across the Chasm

Kathleen M. Hanlon-Lundberg

Introduction

The training of an obstetrician is long and arduous; most enter the field because they enjoy the work that they do and are committed to the patients and families whom they serve. Standardized educational guidelines for basic training and post-graduate continuing medical education encourage practitioners to remain abreast of current practice. As with any group of people, obstetricians are not a homogeneous entity; they are individuals with unique backgrounds, interests, aptitudes, and experiences. Every obstetrician has witnessed the wonder of new life many times over; each has participated in cases complicated by tragedy and death. Largely maligned in reproductive anthropological literature as callous—if not brutal—self-serving effectors of the over-medicalization of childbirth, most obstetricians I know and have worked with are devoted to providing respectful, individualized care to their patients—the women and families whom they often get to know well in the course of many encounters over years. As a perinatologist who is also trained in anthropology, I have experienced both obstetrician and reproductive anthropologist perspectives.

In this chapter, I share reflections from two women from along their paths as they became physicians and obstetricians and on their medical practices. Through these stories of premedical and medical training, and later, of obstetric practice, I hope to illustrate the embodied, sustained devotion to providing high quality, sensitive care—often at great personal cost—that is typical of obstetric practitioners. In some ways, the paths of these two individuals were parallel. They are of the same age cohort, are now middle-aged women, originate from middle-class European American families, and live in the midwestern United States. After medical school, their paths diverged. Emily (a pseudonym) trained in a community-based residency program and practiced general obstetrics and gynecology in a small town. As the other obstetrician described herein, I trained at a large, urban public hospital, specialized in perinatal medicine, practiced in academic, tertiary hospitals, and then left active practice and studied anthropology. These stories are drawn from open-ended interviews conducted with Emily, and from my own retrospective, autoethnographic accounts. Herein I refer to persons seeking health care as "patients," in keeping with medical tradition, acutely aware of the justifiable problematization of this term.

Identifying Aptitude, Early Mentors

As a child, science and social studies were my favorite subjects. I was intrigued by life's creative adaptations to change, radiating in form and function across time. My interest in science was encouraged by engaged elementary and secondary school teachers. I had not been exposed to many options in applied or academic biology, so medicine was an obvious choice. I enjoyed and excelled at tasks requiring manual dexterity: knitting, beading, playing piano, and especially sewing. My father was a hospital administrator who advised that if I wanted to go into a medical field, "be a doctor, not a nurse. You want to be the one giving the orders, not taking them." I often recalled these words. However well meant, this advice did not consider the differentially gendered sex role stressors and work/life tradeoffs between the medical and nursing professions. It was a time and place when some young girls were told that they could do anything—they could have a challenging and successful career *and* a happy family. Born during the Depression and educated on the GI Bill, my father did not envision the collaborative practices among providers of all levels and patients that would replace earlier, hierarchical healthcare models. He did not anticipate the far-reaching structural changes in health care that have included corporate delivery systems, increased control by insurance companies, and the rising influence of the pharmaceutical industry, including direct-to-consumer marketing. Perhaps most importantly, the rapid development of the internet and the widespread use of smartphones has democratized information access, increased transparency, and fostered the notion that individuals should and must control their own care as responsible consumers.

In high school, I worked as a medical assistant, then known as a "nurses' aide," at an assisted care facility, then known as a "nursing home." No training was necessary, only a stated desire to become a nurse or a doctor. At the age of 16, this was my initial exposure to the workings of a healthcare facility. It was also my introduction to the care of debilitated persons, most of whom were confused, often non-verbal, sometimes aggressive, and who occasionally exhibited strange behaviors such as crying uncontrollably, getting fully dressed atop a full set of clothing, or smearing feces on themselves and their surroundings. I cared for a woman whose husband arrived every day to have lunch and to spoon feed his silent, immobile wife. He repeatedly showed me the worn picture from his wallet of the World War II fighter pilot he had been, his arm around the waist of "his Mina," a dark-haired beauty in a flowered dress. I followed the obituaries from my hometown for years.

Likewise, Emily showed an aptitude for science and math from an early age. Through accelerated high school courses, she found that memorization and keeping track of information came easily to her, prompting her to consider the challenge of studying medicine. Emily had a female pediatrician who exposed her to the possibility of becoming a doctor. Not all were supportive of women entering medicine in the 1970s–1980s. Emily's high school guidance counselor, who had four daughters himself, advised that "women should never become physicians because they can't have a family and practice medicine. I thought 'big middle finger to you! That's what I'm going to do.' I took it up as a challenge." Emily gravitated toward a surgical specialty, in part because she too enjoyed sewing, inspired by an excellent high school teacher. Stitching with a machine and sewing by hand "helps you think three-dimensionally"—skills that Emily honed. During high school, Emily applied for a job at her local hospital and was offered a position as a phlebotomist based on her expressed interest in studying medicine. "Don't I need a little more education to go and stick people with needles?" she asked her interviewer. Emily did not get the job, and worked at a Taco Bell instead.

Premedical Undergraduate Experience: Learning to Care for Persons and Bodies

At university, I quickly realized that I needed to study hard to earn the grades that would allow admittance into medical school. And study I did. I also worked as a home health aide for a woman with advancing multiple sclerosis and her husband, who had neurologic sequelae of past alcoholism. Five evenings a week, I rode my bike to their home, joining them for dinner and helping with various tasks as they verbally sparred, expressing the frustrations of a long yet unhappy marriage compounded by declining physical and mental health. I also worked as a nurses' aide on a hospital rehabilitation unit, caring for people recovering from motor vehicle accidents, strokes, complex orthopedic problems, and suffering from a variety of other maladies. One patient, periodically admitted to the unit for weeks on end, was a young woman with congenital absence of lymphatics producing immobilizing leg edema. Another was a teen who contracted primary genital herpes after her first sexual encounter, requiring in-patient pain control. I measured and recorded vitals, changed bedding, adjusted bodies and pillows. I fed, toileted, bathed, and dressed. I cleaned up all manner of messes and performed whatever chores the nurses saw fit to assign me. I often worked the night shift because of a 30-cent hourly pay differential.

One man would blow in on Fridays, smiling, and scoop up his paraplegic wife to go home to their three children for the weekend. He was handsome; he laughed and joked. Her injury had been caused by an automobile accident in which he was driving intoxicated, and their youngest child, an unrestrained baby, flew through the windshield and died. The nurses privately spoke of his drunken womanizing during his wife's convalescence. Wellbeing, I learned, is fragile, situated individually, in families and in communities, in place and in time.

I also assisted with autopsies. My first was a beautiful four-year-old boy deceased from influenza. His parents did not realize how compromised his little airway had become until it was too late. How did they go on after this avoidable tragedy? Another case involved an elderly woman with complete procidentia: the desiccated tubular structure protruding from her perineum was her atrophic uterus in the distal end of her prolapsed and everted vagina. (The "distal" end means that it is situated away from the point of origin or attachment.) What circumstances of discomfort and embarrassment led to such a chronic, hidden malady that must certainly have affected her self-image and activities? In each case, the body told secrets and alluded to others.

Emily also worked as an autopsy assistant at a hospital and as a nurses' assistant at a nursing home. Like me, she was exposed to the sights, sounds, touches, and smells of health care. In the nursing home, she learned to care for people physically and emotionally. She helped them move the bodies over which they had lost control. One day she was sent in to sit with a dying person, having had no preparation for this role and no prior experience with death—other than the highly stylized manipulation of stiff, silent morgue denizens. "I figured that if I could do all those things, I probably would be able to handle anything related to medicine." Placing trust in young, unprepared persons to competently perform emotionally and technically demanding roles based on self-identification as interested in medicine cultivates self-confidence, if not bravado, early in the journey to becoming a physician: it is expected of me, I must do it, I can do it, I did it. I can and will do anything required of me.

Medical School: Choosing a Path

During medical school, my first clinical rotation was Medical Psychiatry—discerning how mental and physical health are intertwined. My team was asked to consult with a young woman said to be suffering from depression. She was dying of acute leukemia subsequent to chemotherapeutic agents taken years prior to treat a malignant ovarian tumor. The woman expressed surprise that her providers thought she was depressed. She also expressed profound gratitude that she had lived to see her young daughter grow to be a teenager. I left her room sobbing at the grace with which she faced her imminent end, feeling indebted to the one upon whom I was supposed to bestow therapeutic reassurances. She died that evening. The following morning, I participated in her necropsy. In the hospital's cold, bright morgue, opening and examining the body of a woman so recently warm, alive, and communicative was jarring. Although I had assisted with many autopsies, had dissected human and non-human cadavers, I had never interacted with a live person prior to their systematic disassembly. I would have that opportunity again, examining the physical remains of men, women, babies.

The first birth I participated in as a medical student during my six-week obstetrics and gynecology rotation was on my 25th birthday in the same hospital, assisting the same obstetrician who had attended my own birth, quite possibly in the same delivery room in which I was born. All went as planned: a healthy baby was born to a healthy woman on a surgical table in the dorsal lithotomy position, probably just as I had entered the world. There was a wide range of private practices in that hospital at that time, from an old obstetrician who insisted on doing a complete manual uterine exploration after every delivery (ouch!) to one who quietly assisted deliveries in the dark, in accordance with the Leboyer method. Water birth had not yet become popular. That private hospital served private patients cared for by private physicians. Medical students were tolerated but not exactly welcomed, and then usually only to watch, not to speak or to touch. We had little experience interviewing, let alone examining, actual birthing persons. Still, I decided to specialize in obstetrics and gynecology as a balance of internal medicine and surgery, which would allow me continuity with my patients over their (my) lives.

Emily considered becoming a pediatrician, but realized during her pediatric rotation that working with unhappy children and their parents day in and day out might not suit her. She engaged in a surgical internship after her first year of medical school, in which she learned to repair skin incisions and to write surgical orders. Although Emily excelled at surgery, she did not want to enter general surgery, favoring obstetrics and gynecology as incorporating both internal medicine and surgery, and as perhaps being more accepting of female physicians. She recalls hearing surgical residents refer to their ob/gyn colleagues as "just hacks" as far as their surgical capabilities were concerned. The stereotype of the "cheerful but inept" obstetrician has roots in the earliest days of medical specialization, as related through the fictionalized description of biomedical education described by Sinclair Lewis in *Arrowsmith* (1925), written after the publication of the 1910 Flexner Report, which had exposed major problems with the content, quality, and lack of standardization of biomedical education. Emily thought that "perhaps one could improve on this stereotype and become a meticulous surgeon." So she did, applying her excellent sewing skills in new ways.

Following Divergent Paths: Obstetric Training

Emily trained in obstetrics and gynecology in a busy, well-respected community hospital program with a strong gynecology component: "There was always a lot of surgery going on." If a resident expressed interest, arrived earlier, and stayed later than the others, that individual saw, and was allowed to do, more. Emily recalls that as a first-year resident, a fourth-year resident informed her, "You are going in on this [vaginal] twin delivery and you are going to do a total breech extraction." Her senior resident walked her through the process:

> After delivering the first baby, she said "Stick your hand up there and find a foot. Be *very* sure it is a foot. Break the bag of waters as you gently pull down. The baby will come out with the rushing water." Everything was fine! Baptism by fire, a lot of times. We were encouraged to be prepared for everything.

Emily describes a great breadth of experience, with gradually increasing responsibility for complicated and critical cases. According to her, understanding the natural process of birth and paying attention to detail are essential to facilitating good outcomes and to avoiding complications. "Pay attention to details and you're never going to get caught with your pants down!" Emily admonished. In this context, being "caught with your pants down" refers to missing important clues of impending trouble, taking actions that contribute to problems, or being (or perceived as being) liable for adverse outcomes.

The high volume of routine and intensive cases in which residents on clinical rotations participate fosters expertise in caring for persons with a range of normal and pathological conditions and surgical challenges, yet continuity of care during training is often lacking. During her residency, Emily encountered the same patient twice for normal deliveries: "To be there twice for the same patient was very unusual." Private attending physicians ("attending" physicians have completed their residencies and are practicing their specialties in hospitals or clinics) are "supposed" to catch babies; doctors impressed upon nursing staff the importance of being summoned to arrive not too early but certainly not after the delivery. The precise timing of birth, however, may be difficult to discern. Emily recalls caring for a woman with an epidural at complete cervical dilation, waiting for the attending physician to arrive. Emily, the patient, and the nurse talked and laughed, and with the laughing, the baby was born. "It was very natural, very normal, very calm." The attending doctor, arriving after the fact, was not amused.

I trained in obstetrics and gynecology at a large, overcrowded, underresourced public hospital that served a diverse population of low-income persons. Although the setting and many of the circumstances are similar to those described by Khiara Bridges in *Reproducing Race*, our vantage points and perspectives differ on the basis of many complexly interrelated factors including age cohort, education, location, and skin color (Bridges 2011). As a resident physician, I experienced that hospital as a "total institution"—one that closes an individual off from other activities and situates daily routines and behaviors (Goffman 1961). On my first day as a new doctor in clinic, July 1, 1987, I found myself alone to interview, examine, and treat live persons. The main labor area was comprised of a large room containing seven gurney beds on wheels (plus one that was permanently located in the "fire escape" spot in front of a window on the hospital's fifth floor). Striped fabric curtains could be drawn between the beds for a modicum of privacy. The epidural rate was about 15%; there was demand but insufficient supply. Despite the high-risk status of many patients, the primary cesarean birth rate was less than 10%, and the forceps rate was about the same. We seldom used vacuum delivery because the suction machine was broken during much of my training.

Support persons were allowed to visit laboring persons periodically. "Husbands coming!" the nurses exclaimed, quickly drawing the curtains between beds. Visitors tentatively entered, peeking behind the curtains to identify their loved one. After about ten minutes, they were all marched back out and the curtains were re-opened. Just before a person was about to give birth, her bed was hastily rolled down a long, narrow corridor to a delivery room equipped with a steel surgical table, on which she was strapped in a dorsal lithotomy position (semi-reclining on her back), her perineum was bathed in betadine disinfectant solution, and she was draped with clean green sheets for delivery. After saying a quick "hello" to their mothers, all babies went to a central nursery for at least eight hours of observation before being returned to their waiting moms. This is how it was at that hospital well into the 1990s. Through moonlighting at private suburban hospitals, I learned that there definitely were other approaches.

During my residency, I cared for persons seeking pregnancy and gynecologic care of all descriptions from around the world, whose commonality was poverty. We cared for incarcerated women. Yes, I have assisted birthing women who were mandated to be handcuffed to their beds, accompanied by prison wardens. One female warden would hold the birthing woman's hand and sing to her, blurring the lines of care and control (Sufrin 2017). I have cared for wildly intoxicated laboring persons who clawed and screamed, birthing their growth-restricted babies through thick meconium, and who afterward would cry and apologize. I have delivered dead babies—tiny ones whose bodies have become rubbery yellow, bigger ones whose skin is slipping, recently demised fetuses who look like sleeping angels. I have delivered macerated bodies with disarticulated heads. I have seen a baby's scalp, stuck from shoulder dystocia, turn from pink to purple to blue as it died there on the mother's perineum, the obstetric team unable to either bring it forward or replace it into the uterus for cesarean delivery. I have seen women die of amniotic fluid embolism, infection, and trauma.

The midwestern county hospital in which I worked in the 1980s was the last safety net in that region and still is today. Conditions were difficult. The physical facility was in decay. There were insufficient staff to contend with the workload. As one co-resident put it: "You feel like you are the last rat on a sinking ship. If you do not do something heroic, it will all go down." It was common to find employees sleeping in dark corners at night. All the nurses were women, many of whom had heavy domestic responsibilities as well—their "second shift work" (Hochschild and Machung 2012).

I worked with midwives who were capable and compassionate and with those who were difficult and callous. One repeatedly compared patients of cultural groups different from her own as "more primitive forms of humanity"; I will spare the details. Another midwife nearing retirement had become jaded: "Most people prepare more to bring a kitten home then they do to have a baby." Yet most of the time, most of the midwives strove to provide personalized, compassionate care to the single person under their watch at a time. This left the remainder of the patients, however many there were, to the care of the residents. I was present the night one of my (male) co-residents was escorted out of labor and delivery, handcuffed, by armed police after sexually assaulting a patient by forcing her to fondle his genitals in the delivery room immediately postpartum. We were required to measure blood pressure with a cuff and stethoscope after birth, so her hand was conveniently in the vicinity. Yes, this happened.

After my ob/gyn residency, from 1991 to 1993 I specialized in perinatal medicine down the road at an esteemed "ivory tower" hospital, which at that time provided highly dichotomized services for private "haves" and public "have-nots." Separate and non-equal care was the order of the day. The labor and delivery unit had been founded in the early 20th century by an influential advocate of prophylactic forceps over large episiotomies. His highly interventive legacy reverberated through the nascent profession during his time in the early 1900s, enduring in this institution and beyond. All residents were expected to have several cesarean hysterectomies under their belts. Although the delivery volume was a fraction of that at the county hospital, the incidence of cesarean hysterectomy was higher, largely related to how ruptured uterine scars from previous cesareans were approached. One of the attending physicians would often say "It's easier to teach monkeys to do surgery than young men! Women are much better at surgery." "Yes," I thought. "That makes sense. I have been sewing since I could pick up a needle."

For my Fellowship research project, I examined the respiratory effects of cocaine use on newborns. I reviewed mountains of paper charts. Many of my study subjects were themselves born at the same hospital. I saw how critical elements of their mothers' and sometimes their grandmothers' birth stories were often repeated in their own, vividly illustrating transgenerational biosocial patterns of birth outcomes. During these years, I did not fully understand how the almost battlefield-like conditions that I trained in affected my outlook on obstetrics and public health, but I did witness how local politics, social policies, structural constraints, and cultural practices contribute to individual, family, and community health—or to the lack thereof.

Private Practice: Out in the "Real" World

After completing her residency, Emily entered private obstetric and gynecologic practice in a small community. She felt well prepared for obstetric practice and for gynecologic surgery, but needed more experience with office gynecology to contend with the everyday problems and questions of outpatients. She read and researched anything that was beyond routine. When asked about how her interactions with patients changed upon entering private practice, Emily considered: "Instead of thinking of my patients as diagnoses, I began to see them as persons with a life outside of this office interaction." Emily found it interesting to find out what they did for work, what kind of business their family was in, how their kids were doing. "You talk about medical stuff, but you also talk about other aspects of life, which makes the encounter less sterile."

Emily met resistance to practicing in a patient-centered mode. Although the ob/gyn units at her hospital were outdated, the hospital board members could not understand why lighting and wallpaper were important, nor why they should invest money in a new unit. Emily countered that women generally access health care for their entire families: if the hospital looks and functions well, patronage may increase, along with the hospital's market share. The ob/gyn units were eventually remodeled, coincident with increasing pressure from the corporate healthcare systems moving into the area, which were vying for market shares in the lucrative healthcare marketplace of an area with a growing population.

Gender also played a role in Emily's ability to effect change. Of the three ob/gyns in town, two were female and one was male. The first female ob/gyn to arrive in that town, Emily's partner, was greeted by a male family practitioner with "Welcome to town, but I won't be referring anybody to you." If the female obstetrician/gynecologists requested something, administration "sort of blew us off. My nickname was 'Princess Emily' and my partner's nickname was 'Queen Mary.' We really weren't asking for much. For example, I just wanted a hysteroscope that could inflate the uterine cavity so that I was able to see." As different corporations vied for market share in an increasingly competitive healthcare marketplace, pressures for surgical and obstetric "productivity," and reliance on patient satisfaction surveys increased in ways that Emily felt unduly influenced practice and often impeded good care.

Lack of collegiality between obstetricians and family practitioners was one of Emily's greatest challenges. Older, male family practice physicians had been practicing in the community long before the inclusion of staff obstetricians. They felt completely capable of caring for high-risk obstetric cases without consultation or support, including vaginal births after cesarean (VBACs). One of Emily's final cases in this hospital involved a woman whose uterus ruptured on a January night just after a snowstorm:

> I had no notification that a woman attempting VBAC was in labor. We had asked the family practitioners to *please* let us know when such a woman was admitted. They absolutely refused to do so. I was called in emergently to deliver a patient after the baby's heart tones were down for an hour. The family practitioners were not in the house. The baby's head was low—there was no way I could have accomplished an abdominal delivery as fast as I was able to deliver the baby vaginally. I used vacuum and got the head out. There was a shoulder dystocia, which I reduced by sweeping the baby's arm across the chest. It was four minutes between when I hit the hospital to the time this kid was born. When I reached up [into the uterus], I could tell the scar was separated, so I opened her up and repaired her uterus. The baby was transferred to a tertiary NICU and died after about 12 hours. This eventuality maybe could have been prevented had I known about the situation earlier. The patient just seemed numb to the experience—there was never a lawsuit. She recovered and had another baby, delivered by C-section. This is one of the unfortunate parts of practicing with a bunch of family practitioners who felt they could do high-risk obstetrics.

Obstetric care that is "too little, too late" (Ganatra, Coyaji, and Rao 1998; Miller et al. 2016) also happens in the United States when lack of collaborative practice between birth attendants occurs, robust contingency plans are not formed, and provider hubris eclipses quality care.

Navigating insurance protocols became increasingly burdensome to both Emily and her patients over time. Some persons had prenatal care in one setting but delivered elsewhere for reimbursement reasons. Another challenge Emily contended with was "the whole narcotics scene. When oxycontin came out, they were trying to tell us that none of this was addicting. The other side of that equation was with hospital administration and customer satisfaction." Emily did not allow pharmaceutical representatives to directly market to her office during her practice in the 1990s up until the present time: "It was the expectation that when a patient came in for any type of pain, you needed to give them what they wanted—narcotics. The patients would fill out the customer satisfaction survey and say they didn't get what they wanted, and then administration would become involved." Practice is co-created by patients, providers, and structures of care. Unanticipated consequences of "purposive action" (Merton 1936) as it relates to pain management with opioids continue to devastate lives and communities.

Emily found several aspects of customer satisfaction surveys to be disturbing; she said:

> There are protocols you go through to determine what sort of medical services are reasonable to offer a person. What the patient walks in wanting is not necessarily appropriate. Over time, protocols have been refined to treat specific entities. However, not all practitioners followed these protocols. For example, nonsurgical treatment options should be explored before offering a hysterectomy to a patient, even if the patient is requesting a hysterectomy. If there are complications, the legal system will wonder if all protocols had been followed, if nonsurgical options had been exhausted.

The physician is culpable as the individual who provided care that was inconsistent with established protocols. The untrained person (consumer) who requested the intervention and suffered complications is not generally held responsible. In this case as in others, patient choice may compromise care (Mol 2008).

However great the challenges, day-to-day work with patients and colleagues was rewarding to Emily:

> The patients were very nice; the office and hospital staff and nurses were great. Everyone wanted to learn and to care for patients the best they could. Sometimes people expect less adequate care in rural areas. That aspect kept me in this area for my career. My greatest joy was providing good, up-to-date care for people in a small rural community.

One aspect that Emily views as critical to providing excellent maternity care is maintenance of certification in neonatal advanced life support: "We couldn't expect to have a neonatologist or advanced practice nurse there for emergencies"—thus the obstetrician also functioned as a neonatologist for babies, vigorous or otherwise, at birth.

Emily sees the future of obstetrics as gravitating toward greater use of laborists—"deck docs" who assist with births who are always present in the hospital. A labor and delivery unit must have enough deliveries to justify staffing of laborists around the clock. Continuity with prenatal care is lost, but most obstetricians and hospital-based midwives don't attend the births of all their patients anyway. "The benefits are that the laborist has more consistent experience with high-risk problems than what an individual practitioner would see." Other advantages of the dedicated shift work of laborists (who can include midwives) are that delivering persons are cared for by experienced birth attendants who are in no rush, either from office or personal schedules, vacation or evening plans, and are not compromised by sleep deprivation. Thus, laborists can be patient with long labors.

Emily is alarmed by the recent increases in US maternal mortality and morbidity, which she feels are often due to "people thinking they have to do something versus being patient" (see MacDorman et al. 2016). Emily notes that:

> both the providers and the patients often think it's better to intervene than to just be patient and let the process play out. I would rather the patient who had an epidural and was completely dilated but not feeling perineal pressure just wait and let the contractions bring the baby down and not attempt to push. Other doctors need to know immediately that the patient is complete and want her to begin pushing. This can lead to failed second stage and a C-section.

Emily also believes that physicians as a biomedical specialty need to accept some responsibility for causing problems. "There are components of the story which physicians are responsible for. It's not being vigilant. Some of it's because you're overtired. Some of it may have to do with the training to intervene: 'When in doubt, cut it out.'" Another problem Emily identifies is "the 'I am a God syndrome—I'm going to save you.' I don't know what from, maybe yourself. Your job as obstetrician is to make sure everything goes well and not to cause any problems." Although, Emily adds, "one should always think that they might miss something." Unexpected complications are what obstetricians have learned about, have witnessed in a myriad of unfortunate ways, have contended with through participation in many births, and have nightmares about.

Academic Medicine: Practice in the "Hallowed Halls"

After completing residency in obstetrics and gynecology, and Fellowship training in perinatology, I worked at a large, academically affiliated regional hospital in an urban area under a Chairman who was highly supportive of integrated, midwifery-based maternity and well-woman care. The midwifery staff embodied the best attributes of competent, compassionate healthcare professionals. Experiencing collaborative practice among midwives, family practitioners, and private and academic ob/gyns was the highlight of my career. A variety of practice styles were employed there, from non-interventionist "pull up a chair and sit on your hands for a while" to much more interventionist "nothing wrong with the patient that a little cold steel and sunshine won't cure" (a recommendation for cesarean delivery). Every day I felt that I had an opportunity to possibly, just possibly, change the world in some small way. However, I commuted for nearly an hour to the hospital each way to start early and wrap up late, while my husband's commute was over two hours each way in the opposite direction. With babies of our own at home, this lifestyle had become unsustainable.

Thus, I moved to a large academic medical center that serves a relatively more educated, affluent population with a higher proportion of non-minority persons, including many "worried well" who increasingly utilized technological means of assessing their pregnancies through online research and soliciting medical resources, such as ultrasound. Practice was dominated by a hierarchical biomedical model of pregnancy and childbirth, including a midwifery service that was closely directed by a perinatologist, and in many ways, was indistinguishable from the biomedical practice in that institution. The (male) perinatologists with whom I worked were grappling with changes in the profession, including the increasing role of perinatal ultrasound, the restructuring of care provision to better address patient rather than provider needs, and cogently, the increasing proportion of women providers of women's health care, like me. I was told during a perinatology section meeting that "everything should just go back to the way it was before you were here."

In the ultrasound suite, most pregnant people arrive for routine screening studies in a state of excitement, considering the study a fun opportunity to view the fetal genitalia, hands, feet, and face. Often, the patient's stated agenda is to identify fetal "gender." Patients and families almost never say "sex" but use the gentler term "gender," distancing the purity of the unborn baby from the physical act that (usually) brought them into being. People referred from outside facilities under suspicion of or holding a preliminary diagnosis of abnormality were anxious and tense as they considered the possibility that their imagined future family member might have some form of disability. Abortion is the "barely hidden interlocutor" behind prenatal screening for abnormality, as the vast majority of abnormalities discovered through prenatal diagnosis have no cure (Rapp 2000; see also Moses, this volume). Pregnant people, who never considered having an abortion when it was a theoretical thing that other people did, contend with the usually, but not always, anguishing choice of whether or not to end a desired pregnancy as they project alternative futures for themselves, their families, their progeny.

The Not-So-Private Life of an Obstetrician

It is difficult to over-emphasize the lifestyle impacts of the practice of obstetrics on providers and their families. A working woman's "second shift" does not apply when there is no "shift": there are long workdays compounded by longer nights on call. Even while at home, one must be prepared to drop everything and dash into the hospital. Cases follow you, haunt you, are mulled over and researched from different angles. Being a parent is not shift work, either. Children must be cared for, laundry done, meals prepared, schoolwork reviewed or at least inquired about. Stereotypically gendered roles often dominate, even today. When physicians marry other physicians, domestic labor may be divided along a hierarchy between traditional "female" specialties—pediatrics, obstetrics and gynecology, family practice, and psychiatry, with more men practicing surgery and subspecialty care (Vassar 2015). When female physicians marry non-physicians, traditional female roles for care of children and home also may prevail. (For obstetricians, the majority of whom are now women, work is never done; achieving career/personal life balance is an elusive dream. The divorce rate for doctors overall is less than that of the general population; for female physicians, however, it is higher (Ly, Seabury, and Jena 2015). The number of hours worked weekly is directly associated with the probability of being divorced among female physicians (ibid.).

Emily reflected on how her practice impacted her private life:

> I was always tired. My kids commented on that. You miss things too, working that much. I remember dragging my son as a 5th grader to the hospital to do a delivery before I took him to football practice. He came in all his gear and sat in the call room while I delivered the patient. You would get phone calls and have to address things in a timely fashion. My kids heard things that no normal kid needs to hear about vaginal discharge, breast lumps, breakthrough bleeding, you name it. You're always talking about stuff during mealtime to your family.

As her children became less dependent, Emily volunteered to staff the medical rooms at her children's schools, worked pro bono at a free clinic largely attended by migrant workers in her community, and participated in providing cervical cancer screening in Haiti.

My mentor was a caring and compassionate physician who was seldom home. His wonderful, capable wife bought his clothing, made sure he was fed, and raised the kids. My mother is a second-generation college graduate, a dietitian, who stayed home to raise her seven children. Living up to the standards of both work and home mentors was an impossible task. The patients whom I cared for applied pressure as well, directly and indirectly. Women frequently expressed their strong preference for my presence at their deliveries. I wanted to provide that reassurance and continuity of care, to see the outcomes of our combined efforts. However, the personal cost to me and my family was steep. Some women followed their plea for my attendance at their births by sharing their plan to stay home with their children—"It is so much better for the kids, you know"—reinforcing my cognizance of leaving my children at home with a paid provider to care for my patients and their anticipated children. I was often reminded of an attending physicians' admonishment from my residency days: "You will never be the best doctor that you could have been; you will never be the best parent that you could have been." Yes, that is so.

To me, some of the greatest challenges to providing quality perinatal care were threefold: (1) Hostility from male colleagues due to the rapid incorporation of more women into the field. The concomitant shift from unquestioned physician authority to evidence-based, collaborative practice including, most importantly, the patient, but also insurance companies and healthcare conglomerates, forced self-reflection within the mainly male profession. (2) Reconciling the sheer number of hours required for patient care and administrative responsibilities with a desire for a rewarding life outside of medicine became increasingly difficult. (3) I found the constant specter of mal-occurrences during pregnancy and birth—congenital defects, genetic abnormalities, and repeated discussions of risk, uncertain prognoses and alternatives, including pregnancy termination—extremely taxing in light of the often-limited predictability of disease expression and the imprecision of clinical signs, troubling my views of persons living with disabilities. Taken together, some days it was difficult to put one foot in front of the other. I longed for a more circumspect, contemplative life.

What did I actually do? I stepped out of my script. I bought a commercial stable. I developed a riding school, organized summer camps, hosted pony parties. I worked as a perinatologist part-time, performing pro bono ultrasounds and consultations at a clinic for disadvantaged youth. I raised my kids. I found that in the outside world, there is so much more ambiguity in roles and relationships than in the highly structured environment of the hospital. All sorts of things happen on the outside. I experienced dramatically differential treatment by others based on their assignment of my identity. People who knew me in those new roles addressed me very differently, using different vocabulary, than if they had met me as a physician. It was a study in socialization. Eventually, I made another attempt at a more circumspect life: anthropology—another approach to the study of humankind.

New Beginnings: Enculturation into a New and Hostile Tribe

My decision to study anthropology as a returning student after practicing medicine for many years was met with a variety of responses from representatives of the tribe I was ostensibly to join. "Why would you possibly study anthropology when you're making so much more money as a doctor?" "Why not just get a Masters of Public Health—it's only two years?" "Do you realize that the average student in our program completes their degree in 9 years?" (I did not pursue that one.) "What is this—some kind of 'life-long learning' program for you?" I looked at the photo line-ups of graduate students in potential programs, read their bios, and saw no one like me in their midst. Many institutions offer MD-PhD programs—it is quite fashionable—but training a fully-fledged physician in anthropology seemed enigmatic. The program that I decided on was welcoming of non-traditional students and draws on a highly diverse student population in an urban center. I received no credit for any previous courses or experience. I enjoyed my studies and am grateful for the opportunity to undertake them.

The first American Anthropology Association meeting sessions on reproduction that I attended centered on how the obstetricians of the world wrong and harm women. I was surprised, as this was certainly not representative of my experience. I was clearly out of my territory, surrounded by members of a hostile tribe that seemed determined to totalize and essentialize "the other" using a plethora of multisyllabic words and liberal suffixes. Where was the holistic, multi-perspectival consideration of complex issues that I was learning about? I was unsure if it was safe to reveal myself as a perinatal physician. The session was largely comprised of scholars oriented toward activism against obstetric violence. Obstetric violence exists in this country and elsewhere in the world; it is a violation of respect for persons and their autonomy, of justice, and should not be tolerated. However, obstetric violence is also a symptom of larger societal problems, and may even, sometimes, be perspectival, meaning that the interpretation of events is contingent on experiences and expectations that all parties involved bring to their convergence; outcomes affect how preceding events are interpreted and remembered. When all ends well, people tend to be happy.

Complications, disappointments in birth outcomes or increasingly, disappointment that pre-selected birth options either were not or could not be actuated, tend to be reviewed more harshly. The experiences of many women are confounded by a lack of direct experience with the process of birth and by inflated expectations based on social and mass media projections of idealized or caricaturized imagery, affecting their ability to form realistic expectations. Some pregnant persons have constrained physical, educational, and economic opportunities that limit their awareness of and access to quality care options in their locality. And yet, many pregnant persons feel obligated to research and select their options: to make a plan. However, the best of plans can go awry.

As Brigitte Jordan (1993) has noted, birth practices are marked and shaped by society. "Society" is all of us—the structures that we continuously shape and work within and around, including legal systems, social services networks, insurance, pharmaceutical companies, organized medicine, organized labor, hospital systems, and educational systems. More fundamentally, birth practices reflect social valuations of women, children, bodies, sexuality, maternity, and families (see Davis-Floyd 2022). They reflect impulses related to the valuation of anticipated experience, of choice and risk and responsibility, of individuality, of self, familial and cultural continuation, and of internalized constructs of nature and technology. Obstetricians are but one component. It is easy and seems obvious to attribute the causality of inappropriate maternity care, including unnecessary obstetric interventions, to the one wielding the knife, and yet this individual is the final effector of deeply rooted, widely prevalent, and yet evolving social norms. Positive change must be just as broad.

Navigating the Chasm between Biomedicine and Anthropology

Through this chapter, I have attempted to illustrate that obstetricians are individuals who have chosen to care for birthing persons and who have worked long and hard to earn the privilege of doing so. Most are informed and caring people who take their responsibility to provide quality, person-centered care seriously. Medical training and ongoing clinical experience shape how the world is viewed and can lead to case-hardened loss of sensitivity. Alternatively, sensitivity to human suffering and well-being may be increased through exposure to the spectrum of outcomes that occur in the course of medical practice, including birth. Obstetricians participate in unfortunate and tragic circumstances, including failed home deliveries, shoulder dystocias, uterine ruptures, fetal anomalies, and devastating maternal diseases. Unfortunate experiences like these, one after the other, lead to valuable expertise and heightened awareness of the possibility of such occurrences, hopefully providing opportunities to prevent others. Such experiences render an obstetrician more vigilant for pathology, just as participation in selected cases in which all goes well may lead to complacence that human birth is always a benign process. It is not.

Humans are social beings who respond to incentives, including resource acquisition and prestige, economizing their time allocation in the process. Both obstetricians and birthing persons make agentive decisions that are largely rational. At this point in time, many of these motivations converge to increase the propensity toward intervention in the birth process: when trouble is perceived, action must be taken. In obstetric care, that intervention often equates to cesarean birth: "cure by cold steel and sunshine." This approach is socially rewarded by parents who feel that "everything" has been done, by insurance, healthcare, and pharmaceutical industries that monetarily reward procedures and their medicaments, and by the legal system, which is less likely to find cause against obstetricians for "bad babies" when "everything," including a cesarean, is done. Most obstetricians have dedicated large segments of their lives to learning how bodies, minds, and social structures work, what is normal and what is pathological in pregnant and non-pregnant bodies. They have honed technical skills to facilitate healthy births and to contend with potential challenges to wellbeing. By far, most obstetricians I have encountered see themselves as participating in improving maternal and child outcomes.

Is the viewpoint of the obstetrician or perinatologist skewed toward greater awareness of pathology? Yes. Very much so. There is immense joy in birth; there is also terrible pain. There is beauty, but there is also horror. Things just do not always turn out as hoped. Obstetricians are not a homogeneous group to be studied and "figured out." We have individual biologies and biographies, complex motivations, a range of interpersonal skills and technical capabilities—or lack thereof. The values obstetricians hold incorporate the influences, interactions, and experiences of their lifetimes and those of the communities from which they originate and in which they function. The responsibility of healthcare providers, including obstetricians, to promote good outcomes for mothers and babies cannot be overemphasized, but how that is accomplished is situated within the sociocultural conditions in which they learn, work, and live. Changes in the biomedical and social constructs of pregnancy and childbirth will continue to unevenly emerge and to be implemented, reflecting the evolution of broadly based biosocial attitudes and practices.

Kathleen M. Hanlon-Lundberg earned a medical degree from the Medical College of Wisconsin. She completed her residency in obstetrics and gynecology at a large public hospital, followed by a Fellowship in Maternal and Fetal Medicine at an urban academic medical center. She has practiced perinatal medicine in a variety of settings. She completed doctoral studies in medical anthropology at Wayne State University in Detroit, Michigan, where she teaches Public Health and Anthropology.

References

Bridges, K., 2011. *Reproducing Race: An Ethnography of Pregnancy as a Site of Racialization*. Berkeley: University of California Press.

Davis-Floyd R. 2022. *Birth as an American Rite of Passage*, 3rd edn. Abingdon, Oxon: Routledge.

Flexner A. 1910. *Medical Education in the United States and Canada: A Report to the Carnegie Foundation for the Advancement of Teaching*. Bulletin 4. New York: The Carnegie Foundation for the Advancement of Teaching.

Ganatra BR, Coyaji KJ, Rao VN. 1998. "Too Far, Too Little, Too Late: A Community-Based Case-Control Study of Maternal Mortality in Rural West Maharashtra, India." *Bulletin of the World Health Organization* 76(6): 591–598.

Goffman E. 1961. *Asylums: Essays on the Social Situation of Mental Patients and Other Inmates*. New York: Anchor Books.

Hochschild A, Machung A. 2012. *The Second Shift: Working Families and the Revolution at Home*. New York: Penguin.

Jordan B. 1993. *Birth in Four Cultures: A Cross-Cultural Investigation of Childbirth in Yucatan, Holland, Sweden, and the United States*. Long Grove IL: Waveland Press.

Lewis S. 1925. *Arrowsmith*. New York: Harcourt, Brace & Company.

Ly DP, Seabury SA, Jena AB. 2015. "Divorce among Physicians and Other Healthcare Professionals in the United States: Analysis of Census Survey Data." *British Medical Journal* 350: h706–712.

MacDorman MF, Declercq E, Cabral H, Morton C. 2016. "Is the United States Maternal Mortality Rate Increasing? Disentangling Trends from Measurement Issues." *Obstetric & Gynecology* 128(3): 447.

Merton RK. 1936. The Unanticipated Consequences of Purposive Social Action. *American Sociological Review* 1(6): 894–904.

Miller S, Abalos E, Chamillard M, Ciapponi A, Colaci D, Comandé D, Diaz V, Geller S, Hanson C, Langer A, Manuelli V 2016. "Beyond Too Little, Too Late and Too Much, Too Soon: A Pathway Towards Evidence-Based, Respectful Maternity Care Worldwide. *The Lancet* 388(10056): 2176-2192.

Mol A. 2008. *The Logic of Care: Health and the Problem of Patient Choice*. New York: Routledge.

Rapp R. 2000. *Testing Women, Testing the Fetus: The Social Impact of Amniocentesis in America*. New York: Routledge.

Sufrin C. 2017. *Jailcare: Finding the Safety Net for Women behind Bars*. Berkeley: University of California Press.

Vassar L. 2015. "How Medical Specialties Vary by Gender." *AMA Specialty Profiles*, 18 February. Retrieved 15 September 2022 from https://www.ama-assn.org/residents-students/specialty-profiles/how-medical-specialties-vary-gender.

CHAPTER 5

An Awakening

Jesanna Cooper

Introduction: What's in a Name?

When I was 14, I decided to be a physician. At 24, I decided to be an obstetrician and wrote a personal statement that illustrated my calling to women's health. I saw a career in obstetrics and gynecology (ob/gyn) as my passion and my destiny, written in family history and encoded in my very name. "Jesanna, what an interesting name! Where does it come from?" People I meet invariably ask this question. I always laugh and explain that it was a family compromise. Graduate school, a love of learning, and a passion for teaching brought my parents together, despite their different backgrounds. They named me for two great-aunts, joining their two families and cultures. My name represents tolerance, compassion, and the hatred of social injustice that my parents hoped I would embody. My mother, brought up in the Protestant world of the suburbs and country clubs of the US South, chose to name me after her Aunt Jessie, who was generous, well-mannered, and kind. My father, a working-class Jew from New York, named me for his Aunt Anna, who was loving, hard-working, and brave. Yet, as I laughingly speak of my parents' idealism, I omit the darker portion of my name's story.

When my Aunt Anna was 15, she was brutally raped. Viewing herself as "damaged goods," she never fully recovered from the experience. She refused to marry the man she loved, lived in poverty, and died young. Despite these tragic circumstances, Anna was generous and loving. She gave my father his favorite childhood toy, a blackboard, and helped him write, draw, and do math problems. The story of my aunt haunted my childhood and fills me with an overpowering sense of responsibility. My father told me that I am to lead the life that was stolen from Anna. My life is to be rich and full, not only for my own benefit, but also for hers.

Choosing My Career Path

The task of creating a life that is rich and full presents its own set of problems. In college, I agonized over my career path, deferring my matriculation to medical school so I could further consider my options. There was no question that I wanted to have a positive impact on the lives of others, but what was the best approach? My gifts seemed to lie in the realm of liberal arts. Perhaps I should follow my parents' footsteps and become a teacher? Or I could go to law school and defend the constitutional rights of US citizens. What about social work or public health? But my father's battle against colon cancer, which occurred when I was 14, and my family's interactions with his oncologist, left me with a strong belief that a career in medicine would provide me with the opportunity to be a positive influence both socially and individually. I was convinced that, as an obstetrician/gynecologist, I would be given the opportunity to become a teacher and social advocate as well as a healer. I believed that the values woven into my name would help me to perform these roles.

The story of my aunt raised my awareness of social injustice. I am angered that Anna lived in a society that defined women by gender rather than as individuals. I am angered that she did not know that her worth as a person extended beyond her perceived value as a wife. I am angry that any sense of control over her body and over her life was taken from her. Though our society has progressed, these issues continue to confront women. If I am in a position to fight these problems, I will do so. Sometimes, the fight feels good. It is rewarding to volunteer as a big sister and participate in tutoring programs. Other times, my position has been less satisfying. I have acted as an escort at Planned Parenthood and have defended the right of a sorority sister to work at a gentleman's club without compromising her membership in our organization. In these cases, I put my own distaste aside, focusing on my belief that women should be free to make decisions concerning their bodies and health.

Compassion joins tolerance as necessary qualities for any medical professional working with patients and their families. I once believed that such qualities applied only to non-surgical specialties. I was horrified when my best friend chose to do a residency in general surgery, thinking her kindness would be wasted. I realized my mistake when I myself became a surgical patient. A torn ACL bothered me less than the prospect of surgery. I felt frightened, helpless, and more vulnerable than I had in any previous interactions with the biomedical profession. A compassionate, kind surgeon became important to me. My parents named me after women who were compassionate and generous. They named me hoping I would have a strong sense of social responsibility.

I have tried to live accordingly and was excited to choose a career that emphasized my values.

My Experiences of Medical Training: The Dementor's Kiss

The personal statement that I wrote at age 24 illustrated the passion, idealism, and naïveté that many medical students possess when they begin their education. Biomedical training suppresses those qualities, replacing kindness with toughness, empathy with stamina, and intellectual curiosity with rigidity. During residency, I worked 120 hours a week. I was mocked for incorrect answers, repeatedly told that I didn't "have what it takes" to be an ob/gyn, and once awakened during my precious six hours of sleep to be chastised for missing a breech on exam (which is easier to do than it seems). There were no mental health days or even sick days. We threw up in garbage cans in empty patient rooms and kept going. The cruelest moments were when we had poor outcomes. There was no "safe place" to "process," and they were not opportunities to learn and improve. Rather, we faced accusations and blame. I returned to the floor after a particularly bad shift and was told by the nurse that our patient from the previous night was in the ICU and that it was my fault. I had "killed her." I think back and remember that I was a trainee and that I had appropriately called my attending for help. Sometimes you do everything in your power and yet it ends badly. I wish someone had told me that. It would have helped to hear it.

Completing an ob/gyn training program requires mental, emotional, and physical stamina and strength. I often describe the traumas of my own residency in terms of the Harry Potter books, which served as a solace during those four years. The Dementor's Kiss leaves its victims alive but soulless. I graduated residency a shell of my former self, as though kissed by a dementor. Intimidation, fatigue, and fear had extinguished my critical thinking abilities, joy, and love of service. I exited training in June of 2007, a skilled medical professional with a cheerful bedside manner hiding innumerable terrors and anxieties. I practiced obstetrics and gynecology just as I was taught, driven by fear and seeking safety in conformity. If physicians are not empowered, they cannot empower the patients who entrust them with their care.

Learning about My Lack of Essential Skills

Two years later, in 2009, I became a mother. The birth was underwhelming—premature rupture of membranes (PROM), Pitocin, epidural. Breastfeeding was difficult and largely unsuccessful. The experience snapped me awake. Something was wrong. Why had my education left me with this huge knowledge deficit? If I was struggling with breastfeeding, then so were my patients. I didn't have the tools to help myself or the hundreds of women entrusting their care to me. If I didn't have the skills to medically support lactation, what other skills did I lack? I had failed to identify the power structures and biases shaping my education, training, and practice. I was lost. How could I find my way back?

Finding My Way Back

First, I needed to remember who I was before I became a physician. I was Jesanna: a girl who sees problems and works to solve them. She was an advocate who used her strength to defend the rights of others. I saw systemic injustices, and I fought them. I had no business acting as a well-greased cog in the broken maternity care system of the United States. I needed to use my position as a platform for change. I would partner with midwives and doulas. I would create a culture and a team characterized by understanding, compassion, and respect.

The passion was back, but so was the naïveté. I returned to work with evangelical zeal. I thought that physician and nurse colleagues would look at the data and practices I had "discovered" with the same amazement I had. This information was just outside our own bodies of knowledge! If we listened to women, doulas, and midwives, we could empower ourselves and the families we care for! We could change health outcomes for entire communities! At this point, the only practice change I was trying to initiate was immediate skin-to-skin after birth and lactation support regardless of race and socioeconomic status. What could be more obvious or easy?

The physicians and nurses I worked with in 2012 did not share my interests or viewpoints. The nurse manager, incensed by my saying that a baby briefly touching down on mama's chest before being immediately taken to the warmer was not appropriate skin-to-skin practice, initiated a "whisper" and "write up" campaign designed to undermine my relationships with other physicians and to have my privileges pulled at the facility. The pediatricians, neonatologists, and "baby nurses" complained that I was endangering babies' lives by interfering with resuscitation. My fellow obstetricians simply thought I was crazy. No one would speak with me nor exchange pleasantries. Attempting to change practice style had led to ostracism. The hospital CEO stepped in and shut down the written complaints. However, I was heartbroken, and left that hospital the first chance I got. The nurse manager who had persecuted me left the following year and joined the mother-baby unit at our state's largest academic teaching hospital, where I imagine that her leadership style fit in beautifully.

Looking to escape an environment reminiscent of my residency training, I made a quick and ill-advised career change and joined two physicians starting their own practice at a large hospital in town. I still largely practiced medicalized birth, but my partners' intervention rates were even higher. Attempting to conform to their paternalistic style of care, I lost my calling and my sense of self and sunk further and further into a depression. After only four months, I left.

In 2013, I joined Simon Williamson Clinic in Birmingham, Alabama. The clinic's women's department was in disarray, and we attended births at a hospital whose women's services were hanging on by a thread. It was not an auspicious environment for "hanging one's shingle." However, I had been brought in by a pediatrician who shared my values and was willing to build a different kind of program with me. I would take any kind of business challenges if it meant that I could work with a physician who understood and cared about the breastfeeding outcomes I thought we could achieve.

The US maternity care system pays for "delivery," with only token amounts going to prenatal and postpartum care. There is no reimbursement for obstetrician-performed lactation services or other postpartum issues. To cover the overhead costs of practice, which include some of the highest malpractice insurance rates in health care, an obstetric practice must be volume-based rather than outcome-based. Therefore, most prenatal visits with an obstetrician are bare-bones medical screening "check-ins" that do little to prepare patients for birth and motherhood. Additionally, an obstetrician is paid the same for an hour's work performing a cesarean as for 30 hours work supporting a difficult labor resulting in vaginal delivery. My commitment to excellent outcomes and women's empowerment was not a recipe for a successful business. And, in the United States, health care is a business. Since my career goals were now adversely affecting our family finances, my husband started law school while I gambled on families' willingness to choose quality outcomes over a nice facility and amenities. My husband allowed me the freedom to practice according to my ideals without uprooting my family with financial uncertainty.

We started with lactation services. Aided by a seasoned lactation consultant who was accustomed to supporting women from all walks of life, and by a few nurses who saw the potential in our efforts, by 2015 we had implemented skin-to-skin and rooming-in policies. We established the only breastfeeding support group in our community. For the first time since my college days in the 1990s, I began to take pride in my work.

The doula community took note of our changed policies and practices and began to encourage clients to deliver at our hospital. My commitment to breastfeeding support had led me to question all "routine" labor interventions that might affect lactation success. I now asked "Why?" rather than "Where are we on the curve?" before starting IV fluids or Pitocin, and rarely artificially broke membranes. I did not treat "active management of labor" as the gold standard. My newly adopted, critical approach to obstetric protocols was embraced by women seeking a physiologic birth. I began to see birth in ways that I never had before. I began to see myself and my role in a birthing person's room differently. During labor, I became an ancillary player only. However, my medical degree meant that I must play more than a supporting role when it came to advocating for the space and support for these normal, physiologic births.

I decided that my next step was to bring midwives to my practice and community. I was supporting women who wanted physiologic birth, and midwives are experts in physiologic birth. I was no longer a naïve 24-year-old, but I still underestimated the knee-jerk resistance of the biomedical establishment when it comes to change. I thought that presenting safety data on midwifery outcomes while demonstrating an increase in patient volumes related to our policy changes would convince the hospital administration and the medical executive committee. I was wrong. I was called out for "insubordination" and had my medical license threatened. It took three years of advocating, politicking, and coalition-building to credential our hospital's first midwife.

Success!

As I write this in 2022, our hospital is the only one in Birmingham with midwives on staff. We are in an underserved and socioeconomically depressed community, yet boast the highest exclusive breastfeeding rates, lowest NTSV (nulliparous term singleton vertex—meaning a first-time mother with one baby in the head-down position) cesarean birth rates, and highest VBAC (vaginal birth after cesarean) success rates in our state. In 2020, we were recognized by *Newsweek* as one of the nation's best maternity programs based on JCAHO (Joint Commission on Accreditation of Healthcare Organizations) quality outcome scores. My practice has added more midwives, which enabled us to implement group prenatal care, which decreases preterm and early term birth rates.

Our practice fills me with pride and gives me the sense of professional accomplishment and fulfillment that had been lacking in my career for so many years. I wish it were enough.

Paying the High Prices of Success

But it isn't enough. I am more than an obstetrician and an advocate. I am also a mother, wife, daughter, and friend. These relationships help to make me whole. Helping others to achieve empowering and beautiful birth experiences is all-consuming, but it does not lead to a fulfilling life. Even the positive impact of breastfeeding on community health isn't enough to make a person whole. I am tired. Over the past eight years, I have tried, unsuccessfully, to add ob/gyn partners to share in the call load. Hospitals generally aid practices financially in these efforts, but mine wouldn't. Even if they had been willing, how does one find an ob/gyn willing to work more hours for less money practicing in ways they had not trained for? The obstetrics and family practice physicians at my hospital refuse to share call or to back up my midwife partners—though they do enjoy advertising our hospital's strong outcomes, which are due to the midwifery model of care. The compromises that I have made with nursing and hospital administration to credential midwives to practice in this hospital have led to taxing in-person call requirements that do not make business sense for our practice and contribute to my mental and physical exhaustion. My hospital requires my presence in-house most of the times the midwives are working. The personal toll is significant. I have missed innumerable family events, children's school productions, and athletic games. I can't commit to attending family members' weddings. I work when sick with the flu because I have no coverage. I haven't been to the dentist or gotten a mammogram in years. I struggle with depression. I am overweight, have chronic back pain, and never exercise. I continue working under these conditions because my residency trained me to do so. I'm an obstetrician. I can work impossible hours without collapsing, so I do. I realize that I am functional, but not ok. I am cracking.

Working in a Setting of Fear: Why Must We Pay Such a High Price for Humanizing Our Practices?

What drives obstetricians to live like this and to practice the way we do? My story is different, but I believe that I am driven by the same things that drive most ob/gyns, and that I struggle with the same challenges. It is the human condition. Our patients navigate these same drives and challenges. Like them, obstetricians are strong and want birth environments that allow us to be brave. We want birth settings that allow self-control and respect, both for our patients and for ourselves. But, like our patients, we are limited by maternity care systems that impede our ability to realize our potential. Obstetricians work in a professional setting of fear. We fear being "wrong." We fear lawsuits. We fear professional ostracism. We fear bullying. We fear disappointing our patients. We fear disappointing ourselves. We fear the consequences of not meeting standards set by courts, hospital governance bodies, and insurance companies. We fear not being able to support our families financially and emotionally. Alongside our patients, obstetricians suffer from flawed and dehumanizing medical training and maternity care systems. Why must we pay such a price for trying to humanize those systems?[1] That price has now become too high for me to continue practicing as an ob/gyn, as I have been unable to find a physician partner. In 2021, my multispecialty clinic was bought by a "value-based care" company that decided to close women's services. I am now retired.

Jesanna Cooper was a board-certified ob/gyn practicing at Simon Williamson Clinic in Birmingham, Alabama. She has served on the boards of Birthwell Doula Partners and Safer Birth in Bama as well as the state Perinatal Review Committee. She founded Birmingham's first "Baby Café" breastfeeding support group and was the only ob/gyn in Birmingham working with midwives in the hospital setting, providing midwifery-led group prenatal care and acting as backup for homebirth midwives. She is the former Chair of the Women and Infant's Department at Princeton Baptist Medical Center. Her practice has changed the labor and delivery culture at Princeton Baptist, resulting in Baby-Friendly Certification and national recognition for quality maternity outcomes. She is now retired.

Note

1. Editors' note: The answer to Jesanna's poignant question can be found in Robbie Davis-Floyd's (2023) chapter "Open and Closed Knowledge Systems, the 4 Stages of Cognition, and the Cultural Management of Birth" in Volume II of this series, entitled *Cognition, Risk, and Responsibility in Obstetrics: Anthropological Analyses and Critiques of Obstetricians' Practices*, eds. Robbie Davis-Floyd and Ashish Premkumar. New York: Berghahn Books, 2023. (See also the Series Overview at the beginning of this volume, in which that chapter is described.)

CHAPTER 6

Repercussions of a Paradigm Shift in the Professional and Personal Life of a Brazilian Obstetrician

Rosana Fontes

Inside My Professional Path

This chapter tells the story of my entry into obstetrics, the paradigm shift I made, its repercussions—both positive and negative—and, years later, of my exit from obstetrics and then my return in a different form. I've always regarded pregnancy as a magical and even supernatural event. When I was a kid, as the older cousin, I remember watching my aunts' tummies grow, and I stared at their puffy navels for long moments, wondering what was going on inside. As I am finishing this chapter in late 2022, we are still passing through the COVID-19 pandemic that has lasted more than two years. This contact with life and death provokes me to reflect on the extremes we are living in.

My graduation from the most prestigious medical school in Latin America was the result of family teamwork. In fact, collaboration has always been at the center of my life. I decided to be a doctor in middle school, motivated by a sincere desire to help people. It seemed impossible for my parents to pay for private education, but we worked together to make it possible for my sister, also a doctor, and me. I graduated as an MD in 2003 and decided on a residency in gynecology and obstetrics, motivated to discover what was going on inside those big tummies from my childhood.

I studied at the University of São Paulo School of Medicine, then moved to a countryside city, São José dos Campos, when I got tired of chaotic São Paulo City at age 30. I was already stressed and working too much for an average person (and as much as any other physician). By then, I had surrendered to having professional success, and had left behind my initial ideal of "helping people." It took other ob/gyns (obstetricians/gynecologists) a long time to accept my new practice in my new-to-me city; they used to tell me that I "came to take away their patients."

I remember when nurse-midwives were initially hired in my area—the Paraiba Valley in the state of São Paulo, Brazil, just eight years ago. At that time, I was taking shifts in São Francisco de Assis Hospital in Jacareí—the only hospital in the area with a mission that encompassed humanistic values. In São Paulo, I had been used to working with nurse-midwives. Here, the obstetricians objected, saying that midwives would take their place and did not have the technical capacity to perform the same work. In fact, it was the opposite: there was so much work on the maternity ward that we obstetricians could not handle. After nurse-midwives did finally arrive, they took on a great deal of that work, and doctors remained resting in the break rooms while these midwives worked one-on-one with all laboring women. Midwives' inclusion in maternal and childcare was why, in our hospital, normal birth rates dramatically increased and labor interventions decreased, mainly episiotomies.

When the obstetric humanistic paradigm (described in the Series Overview at the beginning of this volume) found me, I had become disillusioned with the kind of obstetrics I practiced, seriously planning to change careers. I had done two postgraduate degrees in business administration to learn how to run my clinic better, and I had come to like the area. Within obstetrics, my practice was not what my heart had planned when I first decided to study medicine. Even though I love normal birth, I was far from performing what I considered the ideal medical practice. My exhaustion after long hours of attending births used to overwhelm both the patients and me. We both gave up. We had neither physical nor emotional support to endure this whole process, and we surrendered to cesarean surgery in the end. No one had taught me in college how to support women. And childbirth is a disease anyway, right? In a country where cesarean births account for more than 56% of all deliveries, no one had explained to these women—nor to me—that it is natural to give birth. The interventions are numerous and not cataloged to know their frequency. Every labor seemed to be a new battle to win. And victory hardly ever happened; my normal birth rate in private practice was 14% at most—the same rate found in the private healthcare sector in Brazil. The normal birth rate in public maternity care services is higher, around 56%. This better rate is probably because, in medical shifts, obstetricians (obs) take turns every fixed hour and share the process with nurse-midwives, allowing more time for labor to unfold.

In 2013, I cared for a woman pregnant with twins, and this woman joined the birth humanization movement in my region. She had a lot of contact with doulas. She came to me to respond to her longing to have a VBAC (vaginal birth after cesarean), even with twins. She managed to give birth naturally and easily to her twin boys, even though I still performed on her the episiotomy that I regret most in my professional life. Since then, women and doulas wanted me to be their ob, and we began a series of extraordinarily kind and trilateral growing relationships.

In 2014, I attended the first SIAPARTO São Paulo, Brazil, annual international normal childbirth conference,[1] organized by well-known holistic homebirth midwife Ana Cristina Duarte. This is one of the few conferences here in Brazil where an obstetrician can come into direct contact with evidence-based information about birth assistance and the people who are practicing it. This first conference changed my views of childbirth, women's power, corporate power, and the work of doulas and midwives. I intensely embraced this new universe I hadn't encountered in medical school, and it satisfied all my needs for the ability to make a professional change.

Inside Birth Humanization

At first, births challenged me a lot. There were prolonged expulsive periods; long nights on hospital watch with women in labor; challenging labor inductions; normal births in high-risk pregnant women; women eager for attention and for their care to be built on scientific evidence. My obstetric theory learned in medical school had to change. Besides, I wasn't alone anymore. I had the support of midwives and doulas—faithful companions in delivery rooms—coffee, and the waiting sofa. I took part in humanistic doctors' groups around the country through electronic media, learning how to attend births humanistically and discussing cases. These contacts with other humanistic obs helped me immensely to open my mind and learn to wait for labor to take its own time. I learned how to use the forceps and vacuum extractor better and more gently to avoid cesarean births. I understood the anatomy and physiology of childbirth more deeply, discovering new and illuminating positional techniques, such as Spinning Babies® (Tully 2001)—a program in which practitioners learn how to encourage the fetus to rotate into and stay in the head-down position, leading to an easier, lower-intervention birth.

However, making all these changes was an excruciating process for me. I felt cheated in my obstetrics training during medical school. How could they hide this whole world from me and everyone else? It was common to hear extremely demoralizing comments about doctors I didn't know who attended normal births in the humanistic model. These comments discredited them and made me not want to approach such obs to see them for myself. Like a Stage 1 (see Series Overview) fundamentalist religious sect, technocratic obstetrics generates fear in its practitioners of searching for answers on their own. The punishment for those who follow another path is severe ostracism. And the "bad patients" who reject the system and ask for "too much" are punished with excessive procedures or cesarean births without an accurate medical indication.

I felt like asking for forgiveness from all the women I forced into unnecessary procedures, even though I acted unconsciously, according to my technocratic training. I forgave myself when I decided to leave the labor room in situations where another ob was working violently. I could no longer bear to see Kristeller maneuvers (pushing hard on the laboring woman's abdomen to try to force the baby out), radical episiotomies, harsh words, cervical dilations performed by finger force, and pulling on the umbilical cord to force the expulsion of the placenta—all dangerous and completely unnecessary practices. As for placenta expulsion, for example, a Cochrane review showed uncertainty around whether there is a difference between active or expectant management, and that women should be given information before birth to help them make informed choices (Begley et al. 2019). Also, I did not know how to help these women and stop all this violence and hostility. All I most wanted to continue in obstetrics was to assist pleasant, normal births. Being escorted into this role by doulas and midwives was filling me with joy. Why didn't they teach us how to work as a team in medical school? Ultimately, midwives were the ones who made the work less solitary for me.

Because of my paradigm shift, my medical procedure changes put me in professional isolation from my obstetrician "colleagues," which took me a long time to accept. Several colleagues approached me through various social networks, asking me to take care in dealing with "this type of patient"—the one who wants normal birth "at any cost." Some hospitals called me to question simple procedures that I had stopped doing, saying that I could not stop performing such procedures because they were "necessary." One day, an anesthesiologist approached me in the hospital parking lot to try to force me to administer Pitocin to augment labor to all patients who had epidurals or other types of labor analgesia. She was trying to take possession of obstetric conduct; it was not an anesthesiologist's decision. Ultimately, I and the midwives and doulas who worked with me ended up working in just one hospital—the only one that was able to give us the freedom to act as we believed.

I was terrified that some pregnant woman I was caring for would seek a doctor on duty for some pain management or an urgent exam. The other obs told them frightening lies about how I was "the doctor who kills babies and puts mothers at risk of death." I had never had any complications in my professional history that justified this label. The more normal births we attended, the more intensively they watched us. Because of this, and because we wanted to practice the best scientific evidence-based medicine, we become more demanding and experienced in "seeing, hearing and perceiving" fetal distress signs, acting before they manifested as actual problems. It is essential to consider that identifying those babies at the highest risk of adverse outcomes requires more techniques than we have now. For example, some studies are questioning electronic fetal monitoring (EFM) to predict fetal hypoxia accurately because its misinterpretation may lead to an unnecessary cesarean birth (see Balayla et al. 2020).

One day, a doctor's group in my region banned me after I complained about an applauded video of an older man assaulting a feminist woman. Then, I had an insight: I did not fit into my Stage 1 professional silo anymore. I no longer shared the idea that the members of our technocratic silo were superior to other professionals and other people. I no longer shared the notion that we need to achieve financial success at any cost. I wished to be an obstetrician who practices based on scientific evidence, no longer performing unnecessary and iatrogenic standard procedures that increase the risk of birth complications (see Liese et al. 2021).

Another critical episode that I remember in my career was a formal dinner sponsored by a pharmaceutical company. I used to attend these events often. This last time, I listened to jokes about doulas in silence while everyone else laughed. They made these jokes intentionally to (metaphorically) slap me in the face. I did not finish my dinner and made up an excuse so I could leave. After that, I stopped relating to most other ob/gyns in my town. These less-than-subtle battles between Stage 1 obstetricians and myself kept happening; many obs denigrated me in front of my patients, other colleagues, and my team of midwives and doulas.

After eight years of humanistic practice, I still worked as the sole obstetrician in my private practice. I could not find other doctors with humanistic behaviors that matched the ones I defended. Finally, I accepted my professional loneliness in my region. I allied myself with other non-medical professionals in the birth environment; other hospital staff called me the "mother of doulas" because I defended them inside hospitals. And I acted on midwives' obstetric suggestions more than on other ob/gyns' opinions.

Observing various birth humanization movements spreading in my region, and seeing pregnant women and doulas acting alone, I realized that nobody was hearing them and that, as a doctor, I could encourage more cohesive groups, creating a more robust and unified network. I changed my work structure, leaving jobs that no longer made sense in this new journey. I structured my private care to respect my new precepts, attending women who wanted normal births instead of scheduled cesareans; we performed these surgeries only when essential. From there, in 2013, I created the Mátria Clinic, along with my partners Milena Fondello, a doula, and Dayane Salomão, a breastfeeding consultant. Until 2020, for as long as we managed it, this clinic represented a reference point in humanized birth care in the Paraiba Valley, bringing together humanistic professionals with similar ideals: obstetrician/gynecologists, pediatricians, nurse-midwives, doulas, breastfeeding consultants, psychologists, nutritionists, psychiatrists, and physiotherapists, among others.

At the beginning of my professional transformation, I predicted many internal and external taboos that I would break and how much I needed to change my learned concepts about birth. Thus this change seemed difficult and painful to me. However, with multidisciplinary support, I quickly established my choices, and the path became much lighter. All the measures implemented in my private practice at that time were low-cost, focusing on the orientations of pregnant women and family members, and causing a dramatic drop in our cesarean rates within a short period. I hired a midwife who had graduated from Brazil's only direct-entry (non-nursing) school—the University of São Paulo Midwifery School, which has existed since 2005. This midwife started to perform initial home care for pregnant women in labor, evaluating them and keeping them in their family environments until they entered the active labor phase, defined as beginning at 6 cm (cervical dilation). This was a huge practice change for me, as latent labor can safely take hours or days. This partnership optimized my time, as I still attended many consultations and performed gynecological procedures in my office. My in-hospital hours decreased, and my patients' satisfaction with labor and childbirth increased.

In our country, everyone sees the figure of a doctor as unique and sovereign in obstetric care. Thus we faced many obstacles to the acceptance of the presence of midwives. Today, that acceptance is much greater, so that many women undergo prenatal care exclusively with midwives. There were then four in our team, which we called Acaiá Urban Midwives. After explaining the risks and benefits, we respected women's choices for cesareans, but I stopped scheduling elective cesarean births (CBs). Instead, we advised the women who wanted them to wait for the beginning of labor to perform the surgery to ensure that the baby was ready to be born. We increased the time allotted for prenatal consultations, conducting discussions about birth options; risks of elective cesarean births and benefits of normal birth for both mother and baby; preparation for birth and breastfeeding; and the guidance of our multidisciplinary team. In August 2016, we implemented a group prenatal care model, changing it to an online model due to the COVID-19 pandemic, which in Brazil began in March 2020. At that time, this group model was still relatively new in Brazil but already well consolidated in other countries, mainly in the United States (Rising 1998; Rising and Jolivet 2009).

This group prenatal care model, called Centering Pregnancy (see Rising and Jolivet 2009), captivated me so much that it became the subject of my Master's thesis in 2018. I was already quite busy; I realized how crazy it would be to go back to school! But anyway, I felt like returning to the academic environment because it was another path to change the obstetric technocratic paradigm. I looked for a university that could offer me scheduling flexibility to continue my practice. At this time, I was attending 12 births per month, on average, at the Mátria Clinic. I met Miria Benincasa, who helped me identify the Health Psychology Graduate Program at the São Paulo Methodist University—UMESP. This program deals with the psychological prevention of diseases, creating a multidisciplinary bridge between psychologists and physicians.

Benincasa's research was on developing psychological prenatal care and full prenatal programs, nonviolent and respectful childbirth practices, and intervention models to support postpartum women. I found myself instantly belonging to these themes. I believe that generating reliable scientific knowledge is necessary to justify obstetric healthcare system transformation in my country. Global humanistic prenatal care objectives are to see and treat women as bio-psycho-social beings, thereby generating benefits for babies and their families. We have a greater chance of fully achieving these proposed objectives when working with a communicative and aligned multidisciplinary team.

During my Master's degree research, I observed the very real benefits of this group prenatal care model. There are usually five to eight pregnant women per group. These women have their individual needs met within a mixed model, with personal consultations (where they can express themselves freely) interspersed with group conversations (where we discuss topics of interest to the pregnant women in the group). I conducted a study on the results of this kind of group prenatal care that included 160 pregnant women; 91 of them were nulliparous (56.9%). This study showed a low frequency of prematurity (5.6%); a high frequency of normal births (72.5%); a high frequency of intact perineum or first-degree perineal lesions in childbirth (74.1%); a short labor duration (mean 8.45 hours; the shorter labor duration was two hours and the longer was 36 hours; standard deviation of 4.02); and a low frequency of neonatal complications (1.9% NICU admissions). We had five NICU admissions resulting from high-risk pregnancies: one was a 31-week-pregnancy cesarean because of maternal HELLP syndrome (a condition related to pre-eclampsia); one was a twin pregnancy with severe maternal hypertension and fetal growth restriction that ended with a 30-week-pregnancy cesarean birth; one was a twin pregnancy delivered in a 38-week-pregnancy cesarean; and one of the newborns had fetal growth restriction and transitory respiratory failure. All five newborns were released from the hospital in good condition. Pregnant women in the group had a high frequency of hiring doulas to accompany them during labor (75.6%). Both participants and practitioners reported satisfaction with this model. We also observed a low frequency of requested cesareans, excellent bonding between mothers, their newborns, and family members, and a high frequency of high-quality scientific information transmitted to group members. These data still need publishing (but see Fontes 2018).

It is essential to highlight that birth complications did not increase as the normal birth rate increased, unlike what most technocratic practitioners predicted. The attention we paid to the mother-baby unit during labor and birth followed guidelines recommended by the World Health Organization (WHO 2018) and the Brazilian Ministry of Health (MS 2014). Our team members accompanied births always with two professionals (usually an obstetrician and a midwife), using only intermittent fetal monitoring during labor and birth. We required EFM only when fetal monitoring alterations needed confirmation. These team members had attended courses in childbirth care, obstetric emergencies, and neonatal resuscitation. We stuck to the three principles of humanized care in childbirth: (1) using a multidisciplinary team; (2) respecting and honoring women's informed choices; and (3) using updated scientific evidence (MS 2014).

Even within a country where the rate of cesarean births in the private system is so high, increasing the rate of normal births is easy to achieve through low-cost measures. For me as an obstetrician, the great advantage of interdisciplinarity was the relief in my workload. To get these results, I had to leave existing prejudices behind. Education for entering this kind of Stage 4 humanistic culture (see Series Overview, this volume) is essential; we could not hire a technocratically trained practitioner and just expect them to adapt overnight.

A possible disadvantage of our model was that we had to limit the number of clients we attended to give the needed time and attention to those we did attend. Between 2013 and 2020, when I sold the Mátria Clinic, our team attended 700 births. Our rate of normal deliveries in 2013 was 14%. In June 2014, our cesarean rate was still high, at 47.8%. But in 2015, when we had implemented all changes, we delivered a normal birth rate of 68%; in 2017, we ended that year with 73% normal births and 27% cesarean births—in a country with an overall cesarean rate of 56%. We are still working on publishing our statistics.

In 2015, I started attending home births with the Acaiá team because it was something that became very intriguing to me, and because we were still having to deal with hospital restrictions. Over the last eight years of our practice, 19.4% of the births we attended were planned home births; the (planned and unplanned) home birth rate in Brazil as a whole is only around 1% (Cursino and Gomes 2020). For me, accepting and respecting childbirth at home was another challenging process. I got my medical education in a technocratic system that insists "there are no births without risk." But as I attended home births, I found that I was a watcher most of the time, learning over and over that most births don't need medical interventions. The most crucial factor for all births was our emotional support team, which consisted of doulas and midwives. Others kept surveillance and acted as hospital backup on standby. I went to the family's home and cleaned, cooked, and functioned as technical support. It is impossible to describe my feelings in being in these women's family environments. They opened their doors to me—to someone outside their family in whom they put so much trust. As for me, I felt like a stranger there, outside of my known clinic routine. The truth is that these experiences were delicious! But then, unhappily, I had to suspend attending home births, serving only as a backup for the midwives. I feared having my right to practice obstetrics suspended because the Regional Council of Medicine in São Paulo (CREMESP 2010) had prohibited doctors from attending home births (see the chapter by Robbie Davis-Floyd and Eugenia Georges [2023] in Volume III of this series [Davis-Floyd and Premkumar 2023b]). There was increasing pressure against us, so much that I couldn't take this risk anymore.

Difficulties with my colleagues and hospitals continued, regardless of the good technical reputation I may have had among them. Once, a hospital practitioner verbally banned me from accompanying a birth that required hospital transfer. We had to change to another hospital that did let me in. The first hospital didn't ban me formally because they knew they couldn't: there was no ethical or professional reason. They just told me that they were upset about the type of care I performed. I took their words as just an "invitation" for me not to come back anymore. However, I know many other humanistic ob/gyns who do get formally banished elsewhere in Brazil (for example, see Jones, this volume).

Inside Brazil's Obstetric Realities

The causes of Brazil's high cesarean birth rate are numerous, covering economic, social, political, technical, and cultural reasons. Economically, health insurance companies made the cesarean the easiest and fastest way for institutions and physicians to make money. They don't properly pay for the countless hours spent attending normal births. Depending on certain contracts, a Brazilian ob/gyn can receive only around 110.00 USD for a vaginal birth. Socioculturally, given Brazil's more than 50 years of high cesarean rates, people in general no longer see normal childbirth as natural. Mothers of currently pregnant women consider the cesarean as a "prize" because they see the vaginal births "suffered through" by these new grandmothers as not "normal": the CB seems the only solution for their daughters to escape what they see as the violence and pain of childbirth.

Technically, most Brazilian obs have forgotten how to attend normal, physiologic births—if they ever learned. Such attendance requires their presence, as well as training in perceiving abnormalities. And they don't allow the company of other obs or midwives who can do what they no longer do. We have often seen obstetricians who disapprove of doulas and midwives in the labor room sleeping for hours on end in their cars while their patients labor without any fetal monitoring. Then they attribute bad outcomes arising from this carelessness to the process of normal childbirth itself, which, according to them, "kills babies," or to the "misplaced" desire of women seeking to fulfill their right to have a normal vaginal birth.

Brazilian obs tend to consider their techniques—primarily the performance of cesareans—superior to any natural biological process. According to Barbara Katz Rothman (2000), ideologies are political, residing on a power base. When an entire social system of values, attitudes, beliefs, and morals supports the dominant order, Antonio Gramsci's concept of "hegemony" is often applied (see, e.g, Gramsci 1957; Pearson 2014). When people internalize this technocratic consciousness, it becomes part of common sense.

The common sense in Brazilian obstetrics today is that "women can't stand the pain," "childbirth is difficult," and "the doctor needs to be the savior of birth." Within these concepts, interventions occur—as Suellen Miller and colleagues (2016) put it, either "too much too soon" (TMTS) (to "fix" the supposedly dysfunctional process of birth) or "too little too late" (TLTL) (in Brazil, often as a specific punishment for a "recalcitrant" childbearer who does not willingly cooperate with obs' demands). The path of childbirth humanization is based on obvious, truly commonsense scientific evidence. Interventions should be performed in "the right amount at the right time in the right way"—RARTRW (Cheyney and Davis-Floyd 2020). Nevertheless, even the mountain of scientific evidence *against* TMTS interventions and *for* the facilitation of normal physiologic birth cannot break the hegemony of the technocratic paradigm.

As I reported earlier, I suffered many repercussions from my colleagues until I finally got away from them to feel happy with my new, entirely humanistic, obstetric practice. I was getting great results and seeing satisfaction in the women I attended. But I still needed to find theories that could explain why we had so much difficulty undoing this technocratic paradigm.

Then, I decided to study the Anthropology of Birth. In 2016, I discovered one of Robbie Davis-Floyd's publications (Davis-Floyd 2001). In that article, she delineates three contemporary birth care models: technocratic, humanistic, and holistic. The technocratic model looks at the body as a machine that allows possession and needs repair; obs' hegemonic power allows them to control women's bodies and birth processes. For them, it is difficult to understand the process of childbirth as natural and not as dysfunctional, as humanistic practitioners do. After all, obstetricians are used to dealing with problems, so, in the 1–2 Punch described in the Series Overview (Punch 1: mutilate a natural process via technology; Punch 2: prosethetize—fix—the problems thereby created with more technology), obstetricians create problems via technological interventions and do not allow childbirth to simply flow. They are not a necessary part of the process and should refrain from acting without need.

I learned from Robbie's work (Davis-Floyd 2003) that rituals are essential for human culture. As Robbie describes in her chapter on the "4 Stages of Cognition" in Volume II of this series (Davis-Floyd and Premkumar 2023a, which is summarized in the Series Overview in this volume), rituals can help people move beyond rigidity and think more openly and fluidly. They can also make people shut down cognitively and ground themselves in rigid beliefs and practices, as the rituals of hospital birth quite effectively do, for both patients and practitioners (Davis-Floyd 2022; see also Davis-Floyd 2018a; Davis-Floyd and Laughlin 2022). Birth is an essential rite of passage to motherhood that has long been accomplished via the rituals of hospital birth—the standard obstetric procedures that serve, as all rituals do, to enact the core values of the culture from which they stem (Davis-Floyd 2018a, 2022), thereby socializing both birthing women and their practitioners into a technocratic worldview. Robbie (Davis-Floyd 1987, 2018b) has also analyzed obstetric training as a rite of passage, during which the technocratic model is implicitly taught and explicitly modeled via rituals to heavily socialize incipient physicians into that ideology and its hegemonic control of the obstetric profession.

Reading Robbie's work helped me to understand my transition from the technocratic to the humanistic paradigm. I could see my own work from a very different perspective. When I joined ReHuNa—the Brazilian Network for the Humanization of Birth—I received an offer to intern with Robbie in the United States. My new paths could not take me anywhere else than to Robbie's house in Texas. And there I went, and she welcomed me. She shared with me her home, her family, her friends. In her loving home in Austin and in her ancestral house in northern Louisiana, I could find some peace for my spirit, arriving from Brazil so tormented after my divorce and too much work. We shared many good times. I loved learning from Robbie about what she has studied her whole life—birth and midwifery cultures and all the anthropological, medical, social, and political issues around them. I loved reading her book *Ways of Knowing about Birth: Mothers, Midwives, Medicine, and Birth Activism* (Davis-Floyd and Colleagues 2018), which is a great compilation of much of her work and ideas. I especially loved her concept of "informed relativism"—the ability to incorporate various ways of knowing about birth and to pick and choose among them for what works best in a given situation—and her careful distinction between "superficial" and "deep" humanism (see Series Overview, this volume). This distinction enabled me to understand why some obstetric practices appeared to be humanistic on the surface, and how my deeply humanistic practice differed from those. I also took the opportunity to visit places that held group prenatal care programs within the CenteringPregnancy® model.[2]

Additionally, I found a great deal of relief in the written works of the well-known former Brazilian holistic ob Ricardo Jones (2009, 2012), as he had also made a paradigm shift and had experienced the same professional torments as I had (see Jones, this volume). Yet despite reading the works of both Robbie and Ric, which comforted me greatly in my paradigm shift, I still could not understand this blind obedience that obstetricians and other doctors give to the technocratic paradigm, notwithstanding the large amount of evidence favoring the humanistic paradigm.

In the process of getting my Master's degree in Health Psychology, I met the "nature of power and evil" by Hannah Arendt, and "social totality" by Theodor Adorno (see Batista 2014). These theories seemed well-suited to explain the internal and external taboos that I had to stand up to in my years of obstetric practice. According to these philosophers, the atrocities committed in the name of totalitarianism throughout the 20th century destroyed our moral judgment criteria. By teaching with violence and repression, we intensify both barbarism and tyranny. We null subjectivity, and the individual must adapt to the existing model to keep existing. In this system, criticizing technique and science is obsolete; science must solve all problems. The apparent comfort and wellbeing that the system offers make people live an illusion of freedom and autonomy.

There are no logical reasons to justify the violent control of human birth and women's bodies as technocratic practitioners often do (for many examples, see the chapters in Part 1 of Volume III of this series called *Obstetric Violence and Systemic Disparities: Can Obstetrics Be Humanized and Decolonized?* [Davis-Floyd and Premkumar 2023b]). Nevertheless, this model justifies the practice of cruel acts through science and authoritarianism. As the technocratic model cannot fully explain the mechanisms of physiologic birth, its practitioners feel the need to manipulate them. By supporting implicit violence and discrimination among practitioners and women, this Stage 1 model excludes those who do not practice this blind obedience. Women's autonomy in judgment and ability to make choices freely is compromised. "The system" promises you a free life and social status (as it does to the physician). Still, in actuality, it takes away your liberty to think freely outside of "science" and outside of the Stage 1, fundamentalist and often fanatical technocratic box. (Again, please see the Series Overview for explanations of the "4 Stages of Cognition" and "Substage.")

In medical school, the students learn supposedly "scientific" knowledge, and they stop thinking, judging, and understanding the effects of the scientific; in this fundamentalist, Stage 1 thinking, they transform living people into objects. The physicians become nothing more than bureaucrats who submit to this production process logic, committing atrocious acts justified by the system they obey. That's why biomedical education attracts me so much. I believe that education is the way to change the obstetric technocratic paradigm. According to Adorno, we must think of an education that prevents adhering to barbarism and practicing cruel acts. According to Arendt, we should be concerned about teaching care and responsibility, unconditionally defending the plurality that defines us as beings. (See the chapter in Volume III of this series on "Decolonizing Medical Education in the UK" [Lokugamage, Ahillan, and Pathberiya 2023]). Both philosophers emphasize the importance of reflective thinking, which is supplanted today by scientific language. Being aware of these processes and of how much they determine our ways of thinking and being are necessary conditions for resisting socialization into rigid models.

Inside My Personal Life

I have directed myself onto other paths over the past two years, intending to leave obstetric care. However, I did not wish to go without transmitting my knowledge to different generations (previous, current, and coming). I want to help other practitioners make these painful paradigm shifts. I love teaching. However, I have not had access to the medical schools of my region; they block me from getting in—they may think of the harm "new" thoughts such as mine can cause, of the cracks in the technocratic paradigm that such thoughts can create. Thus, I have only been able to run free classes for students' leagues when they come to me.

Recently, while I was teaching one of these classes, a coordinating professor didn't accept the idea of doing an instrumental (forceps or vacuum) vaginal birth without episiotomy. It was not enough for him to show that 75% of the normal births I had attended were via intact perineums, or had only first-degree perineal lacerations, which are less extensive than an episiotomy. It would be worth improving instrumental birth techniques without the perineal injury of an episiotomy. He could not conceive of this kind of conduct and formally attacked me with no scientific basis in front of my students—yet another attempt to demoralize me within an educational institution.

It took me a few days to emotionally re-establish myself from this event. I felt momentarily weakened in my struggle to change biomedical education. In this moment of my life, after I have given up on so many personal choices to be an instrument of change, I feel that I have lost precious time. This time costs me much more today than before. At the age of 42, with no children, I am beginning to wonder if these fights still make sense to me.

For eight years, the Mátria Clinic was my life goal, consuming me in all areas, professional and personal. I was distant from my marriage, and my husband had an affair, so we separated in 2016. I truly understand that we were both guilty in this process. Like a humanistic obstetric practice, a relationship needs care and time to bloom. I have postponed too many personal choices because of my deep commitment to obstetrics; I was rarely at home. I have lost too many important family events to birth care. In 2019, I went on vacation with my sister, and I received from her an outburst about me never being present in her life, or in the lives of my nieces and of my parents.

I was also devastated by many other guilts. In her above-mentioned chapter in this series (Davis-Floyd 2023), Robbie states that Stage 4 cognitive opening isn't easy to maintain, especially in conditions of (dis)stress and overload. Although the midwives I worked with took a lot of stress off me, I was the only Stage 4, humanistic ob in my region. I couldn't refuse to help a pregnant woman wanting a birth. So, the volume of births I personally attended was absurdly high! I was under so much stress and overload in my work that I couldn't be humane anymore.

When this overload comes, how can we be compassionate with others if there is no humanity for ourselves? In Robbie's terms, I had "lost it," had descended into "Substage." I was highly irritated, losing patience with family, friends, staff, and patients. Any out-of-plan situation took me out of self-control, which cost me a lot to maintain when I could. When work injustices showed up—the ones I had long been used to dealing with—I now acted without thinking, without compassion, and without holding back. After making so many political concessions so that I could work in peace, I was no longer willing to make any more. I didn't want to attend to the phone anymore; it wouldn't leave me alone or let me sleep! I learned that what is humanizing for laboring women is *not* always humanizing for their obstetricians; it's not a two-way street—as Jesanna Cooper explains in more detail in the preceding chapter.

Natalia Ronque is one of the midwives who worked with me in the Acaiá team; below I use her words to portray the limits of our work reality:

> Availability is cruel! I committed myself to offer evidence-based assistance, placing women as protagonists of their processes. Being pregnant can be powerful, but it also brings insecurity, fear, and doubt, especially for the first time. Hiring a team that offers humanistic assistance does not guarantee a normal birth without interventions. We are stuck to strict hospital protocols, which don't always allow us to do what we want.
>
> When I decided to work with births, I knew I wouldn't be home on commemorative dates. I missed my best friend's wedding, a midwife; she knew I was where I needed to be. I knew it would be donated time that often goes beyond what I'm willing to offer.

Sometimes my body reaches its limit . . . and the desire is to run without looking back. The COVID-19 pandemic devastated us; it took away smiles, hugs, lip-reading, coffees we used to drink together while waiting for the babies to be born. It took away the ability to speak into one another's ears softly—it could make us scream instead, so we stopped expressing important things, things that would help our bodies reach their limits more slowly.

WhatsApp both makes life easier and promotes confusion in patients' understandings of our professional availability. I get a message at 2 a.m. asking to confirm a consultation that will take place in a month, another on Friday at 11 p.m. to know if she can dye her hair. I just ask to be seen as a human being, as a person with my individualities. I also eat, sleep, go to the market, take care of a home. I have a father, mother, and husband—they are my biggest support network, and without them, I probably would have given up in my first year as a midwife. I ask everyone to see me as a person who makes mistakes, has feelings, cries, and wants to reach those expectations that involve birthing a baby. This anxiety creates emotional stress, especially in this kind of assistance.

In this work, I *chose* to be available! It's an amazing, unique work of powerful and incredible energy . . . To be an open-hearted midwife, we must externalize the difficulties and delights of this crazy life: no time, too many interrupted nights, going out in the cold of dawn, eating poorly, ignoring your own health to take care of others! I constantly try to put myself in a women's place [to try to feel as she feels. And I want to ask her] "And what about you? Have you put yourself into your caregivers' place?"

I (Rosana) feel the same, and I want to ask women the same question. I too have paid a high price for being available to my patients, for caring for them as I have long done. At some point, it all becomes just too much. And I wonder when Jesanna will reach that place, as I have. [Editors' note: In fact, Jesana did reach that place; as she explains in the preceding chapter, she is now retired from her obstetric practice.]

Even within the birth humanization movement itself in Brazil, there are disagreements. As in politics, we also see a polarization: you are on one side or the other; there is no middle ground. I understand that shifting paradigms does not necessarily make you an out-loud activist who marches in the streets. I realized that I had to obey certain basic norms of the technocratic system. I would lose my power of action by overexposing myself, by moving too far into holism—and if that happened, the women I attended would lose an essential piece of their direct assistance. I tried to be tactfully political in my attitudes to counterbalance proposals in favor of both sides (women and hospitals). I avoided getting involved in conflicts. Because I refused to go to a public hearing on obstetric violence—this topic hits the technocratic system's face with a boxing glove!—I suffered another ostracism, now by the people in the same humanization movement to which I had long belonged. My proposals and lectures were no longer accepted for humanistic congresses. I started not to agree with midwives who did not update themselves and who made tragic mistakes; for this, I was considered a traitor. Now, I belonged neither to one model nor to the other. I felt homeless, and it made my emotional state worse.

In 2020, after much criticism and resentment about my decision on the part of my staff, I walked away from my job for almost six months. I chose to take a break from my profession: after 20 years of practice, obstetrics had been responsible for the best and worst of my life. Because of my overwhelming commitment to obstetrics, I had lost my personal and reproductive lives. I couldn't conceive of being a half-mother, so I was a full doctor. I needed time away for reconciliation, to prevent believing that my profession was to blame for my life dissatisfaction.

My partners and I sold the Mátria Clinic, and we gave up this project permanently; we decided it was too much, and our personal lives were calling to us. It is a pity that after the sale, the Mátria Clinic couldn't keep the care entirely humanistic because the buyers needed to make a profit. They could no longer have the luxury of selecting the practitioners they let in, as we used to do, so even Stage 1 obstetricians work there now.

Finding a Balance

Today, after experiencing so many extremes, I live in search of balance: "Not so much to sea, not so much to earth" (Portuguese proverb). Financially, obstetrics has brought me much stability; that was one of the upsides of my profession. Those other priceless parts were the wonderful births I assisted, the reborn women, and the best-welcomed babies coming into this world. Thanks to my financial planning, I can now enjoy not needing the job and working only for pleasure. My colleagues have made a lot of financial speculations, saying that I must have charged high fees for normal births, driving away women who thought about seeking me to assist them. The truth is that for most of my obstetric career, I've always met the values agreed on health insurance contracts without getting more than that. It was the midwives who worked with me who received this extra charge from patients.

I believe that birth care humanization should not privilege those who can afford a differentiated team; that is why I have always provided access to my assistance to the general population. Serving only in the private healthcare system bothered me because of its distance from economically vulnerable people. These women suffer the most significant violence in childbirth, and they have less access to everything: information, rights, compassion, and care. They can only have access to the public healthcare system, which is as patriarchal and technocratic as the private system but allows fewer options for perinatal care—you just get whoever is assigned to you and must accept whatever care they give, which is often TLTL rather than TMTS. Reaching this audience is my goal today. For the past two years, I've been studying about the "third sector" economy. A non-governmental organization seemed to be the solution to realize a dream and do social good through well-directed resources.

In 2020, the midwives and I started an independent social project to insert intrauterine devices (IUDs) in economically vulnerable women in the city where we live to help them in their family planning efforts. Another project's objective is to train other practitioners, such as midwives, to insert these devices. In Brazil, the professional nursing council endorses them, but they do not have physicians' support. By August 2021, we had inserted 200 IUDs. We obtain our income through crowdfunding.

My obstetrics downside was an excessive dedication in such a short, critical period, specifically my reproductive life. Time passed me by so fast that it doesn't even seem to have existed outside offices, hospitals, and the Mátria Clinic. Only now do I desire a pregnancy, considered a high-risk one due to my age. After four years with a new partner, between turns and twists, we ended up having an unplanned pregnancy, which became a much desired one, and then a miscarriage. After recently and quickly going through my first pregnancy experience, I was able to experience what I had only witnessed in my professional life. After suffering the miscarriage, I cannot describe my new pain experience in words. It has allowed me to live another moment that we cannot understand as caregivers unless we live in it.

The three months of pregnancy that I lived were enough to cancel my doctoral plans abroad and for me to reconcile once and for all with obstetrics by returning to ob/gyn attendance in a sensible way—three to five births per month, only with women referred to me by the midwives. My partner and I decided to live together to form a family while there's still time. I still have work conflicts. Many of them are about fears of losing myself again to births. It is simultaneously a highly seductive and sick world.

When I made my paradigm shift, it felt like I was walking a lonely path as a traditionally trained obstetrician becoming a humanistic practitioner. I felt alone because I was leaving behind people who mattered to me. When I got out of the Substage phase I had entered due to overwork and over-stress, and opened up again to feel empathy for what my patients pass through, I felt that I was going back to the past, when, full of naïve idealism, I first chose to be a doctor. As I have changed, I realize that I have stopped battling with others and myself to be "right." I am learning to plan better to achieve all the goals I desire, without leaving any aside in my professional and personal lives.

Today, within this paradigm of humanistic care, my body extends its limits to feel the millennial strength of all women. I share this magical ability to transport a new body from the immaterial to the material universe, even when I am in the labor room without being pregnant. I feel oxytocin in me too. I feel part of something far more extensive than me, something that is ineffably infinite. Now in attending others, I somehow feel that I am reclaiming my own procreative powers.

My partner and I try to have an egalitarian relationship. I want to know his contrary opinions to share our realities and build our lives together. That's not easy at all. The need to always be right is in our blood! We discuss a lot about sexism and misogyny. Women have been oppressed, voiceless, and without rights for so very long. But men have also suffered a great deal from oppression, hiding their pains and weaknesses to be strong in a world that does not tolerate "losers." They are also victims of violence because the patriarchy oppresses men and women alike.

In antiquity, childbirth had always been a woman's event only. Acting with violence, men took birth for themselves through hospitalization, interventions, and surgery. I believe in a different context, where women resume their power with men at their sides, and RARTRW evidenced-based care is provided instead of TMTS or TLTL practices.

According to Robbie's delineation (see Series Overview, this volume), one of the basic tenets of the humanistic paradigm is achieving "balance between the needs of the institution and those of the individual." The sort of balance I seek can now be summed up in one word: *family*. Helping to form a family for others means that I also care for building one of my own. In learning to balance, I can express all the rights I stand for: maternity and paternity; birthing and breastfeeding; activism and pacifism; equality and respect; education; and character formation. I no longer see women, men, and babies as separate; instead,

I am often privileged to see a family being born in my much smaller obstetric practice. Now, I am focused on seeing my own family being born.

Rosana Fontes is a practicing obstetrician/gynecologist who shifted to humanistic practice and is the founding partner of Mátria Clinic in Brazil, where she worked with midwives attending woman-centered births, with excellent outcomes. She conducted her residency in Gynecology and Obstetrics at the Clinical Hospital of the Medicine College of the University of São Paulo (HCFMUSP—2008) and received a Master's degree in Health Psychology at the Methodist University of São Paulo; she also has a Specialization in Medical Acupuncture from Van Nghi Institute (2004). She holds an MBA in Health Services and another MBA in Business Management, and a certification from APMG International in Social Project Management (PMD Pro Level 1-2019). To study medical and reproductive anthropology, she carried out a two-month, live-in internship with Professor Robbie Davis-Floyd.

Notes

1. See "Simpósio Internacional de Assistência ao Parto." Retrieved 15 September 2022 from www.siaparto.com.br.
2. "Improving Health, Transforming Care and Disrupting Inequitable Systems through the Centering Group Model." *Centering Healthcare Institute*. Retrieved 15 September 2022 from https://www.centeringhealthcare.org.

References

Balayla J, Lasry A, Gil Y, et al. 2020. "Theorem and Protopathic Bias: Methodological Concerns When Addressing the Impact of Fetal Heart Rate Patterns on the Cesarean Section Rate." *AJP Rep.* 10(3): e342–e345.

Batista J. 2014. *Thinking and Judging: An Education Against Barbary and Evil Banality*. Curitiba, Brazil: Appris.

Begley CM, Gyte GML, Devane D, et al. 2019. "Active versus Expectant Management for Women in the Third Stage of Labour." *Cochrane Database of Systematic Reviews* 2: CD007412.

Cheyney M, Davis-Floyd R. 2020. "Birth and the Big Bad Wolf: A Biocultural, Co-Evolutionary Perspective, Part 2." *International Journal of Childbirth* 10(2): 66–78.

CREMESP—CFM. 2004. "Resolution n° 111/04." 23 November. https://sistemas.cfm.org.br/normas/arquivos/resolucoes/SP/2004/111_2004.pdf.

Cursino TP, Gomes MB. 2020. "Planned Home Birth in Brazil: A Systematic Review." *Cienc Saúde Coletiva* 25(4): 1433–1444.

Davis-Floyd R. 1987. "Obstetric Training as a Rite of Passage." *Medical Anthropology Quarterly* 1(3): 288–318.

———. 2001. "The Technocratic, Humanistic, and Holistic Paradigms of Birth." *International Journal of Gynecology & Obstetrics* 75, Supplement No.1: S5–S23.

———. 2003. *Birth as an American Rite of Passage*, 2nd edn. Berkeley: University of California Press.

———. 2018a. "The Rituals of Hospital Birth." In *Ways of Knowing about Birth: Mothers, Midwives, Medicine, and Birth Activism*, Davis-Floyd R and Colleagues, 45–70. Long Grove IL: Waveland Press.

———. 2018b. "Medical Training as Technocratic Initiation." In *Ways of Knowing about Birth: Mothers, Midwives, Medicine, and Birth Activism*, Davis-Floyd R and Colleagues, 107–140. Long Grove IL: Waveland Press.

———. 2022. *Birth as an American Rite of Passage*, 3rd edn. Abingdon, Oxon: Routledge.

———. 2023. "Open and Closed Knowledge Systems, the 4 Stages of Cognition, and the Obstetric Management of Birth." In *Cognition, Risk, and Responsibility in Obstetrics: Anthropological Analyses and Critiques of Obstetricians' Practices*, ed. Davis-Floyd R, Premkumar A, Chapter 1. New York: Berghahn Books.

Davis-Floyd and Colleagues. 2018. *Ways of Knowing about Birth: Mothers, Midwives, Medicine, and Birth Activism*. Long Grove IL: Waveland Press.

Davis-Floyd R, Georges E. 2023. "The Paradigm Shifts of Humanistic and Holistic Obstetricians: The 'Good Guys and Girls' of Brazil." In *Obstetric Violence and Systemic Disparities: Can Obstetrics Be Humanized and Decolonized?* ed. Davis-Floyd R, Premkumar A. Chapter 9. New York: Berghahn Books.

Davis-Floyd R, Laughlin CD. 2022. *Ritual: What It Is, How It Works, and Why*. New York: Berghahn Books.

Davis-Floyd and Premkumar eds. 2023a. *Cognition, Risk, and Responsibility in Obstetrics: Anthropological Analyses and Critiques of Obstetricians' Practices*. New York: Berghahn Books.

———. 2023b. *Obstetric Violence and Systemic Disparities: Can Obstetrics Be Humanized and Decolonized?* New York: Berghahn Books.

Fontes RS. 2018. "Implantation of a Group Prenatal Care Model in Assistance to Pregnant Women in the Private Sector." [In Portuguese.] Master's thesis. São Bernardo do Campo: Universidade Metodista de São Paulo. http://tede.metodista.br/jspui/bitstream/tede/1819/2/Rosana%20Seleri%20Fontes.pdf.

Gramsci A. 1957. *The Modern Prince and Other Writings*. New York: International Publishers.

Jones R. 2009. "Teamwork: An Obstetrician, a Midwife, and a Doula in Brazil." In *Birth Models That Work*, eds. Davis-Floyd R, Barclay L, Daviss BA, Tritten J, 271–304. Berkeley: University of California Press.

———. 2012. *Entre as Orelhas—Histórias de Parto* [Between the Ears: Birth Stories]. Porto Alegre, Brazil: Editora Ideias a Granel.

Liese K, Davis-Floyd R, Stewart K, Cheyney M. 2021. "Obstetric Iatrogenesis in the United States: The Spectrum of Unintentional Harm, Disrespect, Violence, and Abuse." *Anthropology & Medicine* 28(2): 1–16.

Lokugamage A, Ahillan T, Tharanika SDC. 2023. "Decolonizing Medical Education in the UK." In *Obstetric Violence and Systemic Disparities: Can Obstetrics Be Humanized and Decolonized?* ed. Davis-Floyd R, Premkumar A, Chapter 6. New York: Berghahn Books.

Miller S, Abalos E, Chamillard M, et al. 2016. "Beyond Too Little, Too Late and Too Much, Too Soon: A Pathway towards Evidence-Based, Respectful Maternity Care Worldwide." *Lancet* 388(10056): 2176–2192.

MS (Ministério de Saúde do Brasil) (Health Ministry of Brazil). 2014. *Humanization in Prenatal Care and Birth*. Brasília, Brazil: Autor.

Pearson N. *Antonio Gramsci: The Concept of "Hegemony."* New York: Achilleus Ralli.

Rising SS. 1998. "Centering Pregnancy: An Interdisciplinary Model of Empowerment." *Journal of Nurse-Midwifery* 43(1): 46–54.

Rising SS, Jolivet R. 2009. "Circles of Community: The Centering Pregnancy Group Prenatal Care Model." In *Birth Models that Work*, eds. Davis-Floyd R, Barclay L, Daviss BA, Tritten J, 365–384. Berkeley: University of California Press.

Rothman BK. 2000. *Recreating Motherhood*, 2nd edn. New Brunswick NJ: Rutgers University Press.

Tully G. 2001. "Spinning Babies." Retrieved 15 September 2022 from www.spinningbabies.com.

World Health Organization (WHO). 2018. *WHO Recommendations: Intrapartum Care for a Positive Childbirth Experience*. Geneva, Switzerland: WHO.

CHAPTER 7

The Bullying and Persecution of a Humanistic/Holistic Obstetrician in Brazil
The Benefits and Costs of My Paradigm Shift

Ricardo Herbert Jones

The Origins

I was never an easy child. My father always treated me like "the rebel"—the indignant one, and the one who was very difficult to impose orders on. The second son of a middle-class family in southern Brazil, I carried with me my father's dream that his children could attend university—something that poverty had prevented him from doing in his youth. The dream of studying medicine had been present in my life since the age of 15. When I turned 18, I took the entrance exam (*vestibular*—the national competition for admission to the university) for medicine at the public university in my city and was approved.[1] That was when my trajectory began within a field of knowledge as rich and passionate as it was contradictory and, at times, cruel.

During my medical school years, I was always a very odd student, different from the rest of the class. I was the one who always asked the questions, bothered the teachers, and tried to find out the ultimate meaning of the treatments. Restless and inquisitive, I was not well regarded by colleagues and professors. And at the age of 22, and in my third year of medical school, my first child, Lucas, was born, and his arrival indelibly marked my entire perception of human birth and, ultimately, of biomedicine itself. The birth of my son was marked and shaped by the violent births that occurred in Brazil at the beginning of the 1980s—and often still do. Everything that I, a few years later, started to question and denounce was present in Lucas's birth. Isolation (they allowed me to be present at the birth only because I was a medical student), invasive maneuvers, the supine position, episiotomy, multiple small aggressions to my wife's autonomy, in addition to the pediatrician's insensitivity, were events that will remain forever in my memory. Above all, they are constitutive elements of my transformative process—my break from the technocratic model of childbirth care in which I was taught. The scenes of my son's birth showed me that there was something profoundly wrong with the way we handled birth in modern societies, but it was only after my graduation that these thoughts changed from ideas to attitudes and practices.

At 22 years old, I was both a student and a father. Very early on by today's standards, I needed to care for and support my family. Due to this responsibility, I began to work in several places long before my colleagues and I, during our official training, started to see "real" medicine as it was practiced daily. I worked in general hospitals, pediatric and cardiology emergency services, nephrology services, and in a small maternity hospital near my city. It was in this small obstetric hospital that I was touched by the ravishing magic of births, and where I could see that childbirth is controlled by powers beyond science and under the aegis of patriarchy. This experience gave me the opportunity to enter obstetric residency having already attended around 200 births, while most of my colleagues had participated in only about three or four.

Residency

The years of residency are the last part of a long transformative process. As noted by Robbie Davis-Floyd in her brilliant article "Obstetric Training as a Rite of Passage" (1987), it is important that the obstetric resident who reaches the end of his education reproduces, now as an obstetrician, the contents and, in particular, the values that guarantee meaning to and reinforce the social importance of the obstetric profession. These values, which are determined by technocratic ideology, stem from beliefs in the essential defectiveness of women, their inability to deal with their specific physiologic events—pregnancy, birth, breastfeeding—and the importance of biomedical professionals who will, above all, fix their defective body-machines. (See the Series Overview at the beginning of this volume for descriptions of the technocratic, humanistic, and holistic paradigms of birth and health care.)

When I joined the residency program in obstetrics, my daughter Isabel had just been born. In fact, she was born during my last shift as a student, just two weeks before my graduation ceremony. Thus I started my residency with two close and personal experiences with birth and parenting, while many of my peers were just starting to date "seriously." This put me in a very different situation than those of my colleagues, especially regarding maturity and personal experiences. It was in this turmoil of transformations that a particular birth I attended early on in my residency produced a revolution in me, due to what I experienced as a thunderous epiphany. On this occasion, a woman from the countryside who had just walked into the hospital gave birth to her baby under her own power, and did so by snubbing, smugly, and haughtily ignoring the mistaken, arrogant, unwanted, unscientific, and unauthorized actions that I tried to impose on her. With her back pressed against the wall, this woman gave birth on the floor in a squatting position in the emergency room, despite my efforts to get her to move to the table and lie down, mortally offending my youthful arrogance. The impact of this "disobedience" was catastrophic to the image of an obstetrician that I had been building for several years. The scene of an empowered, determined woman who refused to obey the absurd and arrogant commands of a young obstetrician never left me. The upheaval it produced in me turned out to be the seed for my personal transformation and for my passion for the humanization of childbirth, but also the source of my personal tragedies.

First Steps

I left my residency still with the reputation of being the "odd" obstetrician, the one who did not accept the norms and rules. My fellow doctors had condemned me to a kind of ostracism. While still in residency, I heard mockery of me in the corridors simply for attending births in a squatting position and authorizing the presence of the father in the delivery room. My fellow residents called these "Indigenous" childbirths, and along with this derogatory observation came the prejudices of "primitive," "ignorant," "uneducated," and "savage." "Indian childbirth" was seen as a relic of the past, a model that no longer had space nor place in a modern and technological world.

In the early 2000s, cesarean rates in Brazil were already dangerously approaching 40% and it was clear that, without a counterpoint, that rate would continue to grow indefinitely. That is exactly what happened in the last 20 years, but already I had been concerned with offering alternatives to this trend. Thus, at the beginning of my career as an obstetrician in the 1990s, I created a model of childbirth care that was based on the midwifery model of care. My model contained six fundamental points that I would use in my private practice and in the public hospital shifts that I attended at the time. These were:

1. Favorable environment
2. Upright positions for birth
3. Physical and emotional support
4. Restriction and strict selection of drugs during labor and delivery
5. Restriction on the use of "routine" interventions—episiotomies, forceps, Kristeller (pushing down hard on the abdomen to try to get the baby out faster—a commonly performed maneuver across Latin America), fasting, enemas, pubic shaving, etc.
6. Use of doulas—from 1998 onward

I incorporated this sixth item when my work with doulas began. Although all my other interventions had decreased dramatically, my cesarean rate stubbornly remained at 25%. Then a patient of mine, Cristina, who, as she had wished, had a normal physiologic hospital birth with me in attendance, came to my office to tell me that she was a doula and wanted to work with me. Once she explained to me what doulas did and how they did it, I realized that this kind of hands-on care would be essential to lowering my cesarean rate and providing my patients with more satisfying and fulfilling birth experiences. Then, from watching Cristina and me work together at births, my wife Zeza, already a pediatric nurse, decided to study midwifery and became a nurse-midwife (*enfermeira obstetra*). I describe our 34-year-long practice in my book chapter "Teamwork: An Obstetrician, a Midwife, and a Doula in Brazil" (Jones 2009).

Returning to my list above, it was much more of a "list of principles" than a protocol. In fact, I already believed at the time that the humanization of birth could not be considered a "method" or a list of procedures to be avoided or encouraged, but above all was a particular attitude toward the birthing process. I also believed that "humanization" meant how professionals positioned themselves in the face of the magnitude of these events. Therefore, much more than specific rules, I was concerned with establishing a respectful perspective on this process from its inception, guided by the belief that the vast majority of women have the full capacity to handle it themselves. Above all, I believed that our performance as guardians of maternal and fetal well-being should be restricted to cases where the process strays from the safe path of physiology. At the time, I was fully delighted with the possibility of offering an appropriate synthesis of the Technology versus Nature dilemmas, and so I wrote:

> The Humanization of Birth brings the synthesis between recent achievements in science, which offer us security, with the evolutionary and adaptive forces of the millennia that preceded us. This rereading of human birth is necessary to accommodate the affective, psychological, and spiritual needs of women and their children with the achievements that knowledge has brought us through the growing acquisition of technology. (Jones 2012:7)

Little did I realize how much and how often this posture and my practice would produce profoundly negative reactions from other obstetricians. There was a silent discomfort each time a woman under my care gave birth without intervention at the hospital where I attended births. I was often called to the accounts department of the hospital to explain why I did not use episiotomies, needles, threads and sutures, or saline solution in an absolutely physiologic birth. My attitude as an obstetrician even affronted the wheel of capitalism, as the births I attended did not produce the excessive and unnecessary expenses that births attended by other obs did. From the beginning of my private practice, I was aware of the gossip that ran through the hospital corridors. This gossip was perpetrated not only among obs, but also among nurses and other hospital staff who did not accept that a doctor would question the work that they had been doing for so many years and believed to be the most correct.

After some time, and due in part to the fact that the hospital's pediatricians and neonatologists did not accept my approaches—especially keeping the cord intact until it stopped pulsing and allowing patients to remain connected to their newborn babies in skin-to-skin contact—the aggressive tactics slowly changed. In this hospital, where non-compliance was highly visible, the head of pediatrics informally told his peers that all babies born from "humanized births" (in the squatting position, with the presence of the husband, using delayed cord cutting, with no directed pushing efforts, etc.) were to be kept longer in the observation room, away from their mothers. Due to that informal policy change, which was intended to punish me for my disobedience, my patients questioned me, asking whether something bad had happened in the birth that justified this longer separation. No, nothing had happened to harm the baby, but the strategy was to undermine the trust patients placed in me by creating imaginary problems in non-problematic births.

By this time, I should have been more aware that my attitudes and questions about—and my rejections of—current obstetric practices were offensive to the officialdom of obstetrics. Questioning the abuses committed by these practices means attacking the very ideological structure that supports it. It did not occur to me that in so doing, I was creating this huge wave of contempt and resentment of which I, being mostly confined to the privacy of my office, was not fully aware.

Over the years, the ways in which this disapproval manifested went from subtle to explicit. From colleagues who turned their faces so as not to greet me, to an anesthesiologist's refusal to help in an emergency case, the fact is that they preferred not to deal with the kind of patients who arrived at my office: pregnant women who made it clear that they wanted to have the leading role throughout the whole process of birth. The doctors in my city not only detested the "new order" that I brought, but also despised the "new patients" who emerged, who no longer accepted a passive position regarding the conduct determined by the doctors. Some doctors claimed that the attitude of these pregnant women was based on a "brainwashing" produced by a "leftist" doctor whose only objective was to pit patients against professionals, creating "disagreement where peace had always reigned." However, as Sheila Kitzinger (2005:132) has said, "You don't make a revolution with pats on the back," and in childbirth this could be no different. As was easy to perceive, the future I envisioned for childbirth resembled the futures desired by all other social movements that aim at profound change in the hegemonic paradigm. That can never happen without conflict.

I should explain here that, for some years, I was the only humanistic ob practicing in this hospital, which had a 90% cesarean rate; the other 10% were vaginal and violently attended births, or precipitous births that allowed no time for interventions, and some humanized births with me and the two other colleagues who decided to humanize their practices after knowing me and my work. For many Brazilian doctors, "normal birth" means "vaginal birth + epidural," because many obstetric professors created the idea that "humanization means no pain," and use the term to create this conceptual confusion: "humanization = hyper-medicalization."

In any case, I continued my work and, as previously noted, created a transdisciplinary birth care team in the late 1990s, consisting of a doula, a midwife, and an obstetrician. Despite the animosity of hospital staff—both obs and nurses—we included the full team in all the births we attended. This practice fully counteracted the values of the biomedical corporation and infuriated the people on the medical board.

Also at this time, I joined ReHuNa—the Network for the Humanization of Childbirth—a diversified collective of birth care providers and receivers who were interested in reforming the obstetric care system. At the time I joined in 1999, little was said about the goals and strategies needed for transformation, and much more was discussed about our nonconformity with how the public and private systems managed maternity care. We had annual meetings where these discussions gradually took shape, starting with inappropriate, non-evidence-based practices—episiotomy, Kristeller (hard fundal pushing to expel the baby faster), lithotomy position, excessive cesareans, and more—and leading to our elimination or minimization of these practices and to the presence of husbands/partners and the introduction of doulas into the birth room. It was at these meetings that I first heard the term "obstetric violence" and gained the understanding that these practices were sheltered under a great umbrella related to the chauvinist views of biomedicine under the domain of patriarchy.

In November of 2000, ReHuNa held an extraordinary event that indelibly marked the entire movement to humanize birth in Brazil—the I International Conference for the Humanization of Childbirth in the city of Fortaleza, Ceará, northeastern Brazil. We expected around 600 attendees, yet almost 2,000 people attended, taking us all by surprise. Thus that conference marked the official beginning of the movement to humanize birth in Brazil, and created a ripple effect, with many other South American countries then holding their own humanization conferences to promote these ideas in their own countries. This first conference entailed the opening of floodgates of ideas that had long been dammed up about the need for changes in childbirth care, and that is why its success was so astounding. The attendees were diverse—epidemiologists, pediatricians, neonatologists, obstetricians, professional and traditional midwives, doulas, and nurses. Of the speakers, six were invited from abroad: Marsden Wagner and Jose Vilar of WHO; Lesley Page from the UK, then President of the Royal College of Midwives; water birth pioneer Michel Odent; famed holistic midwife Ina May Gaskin; and the American anthropologist Robbie Davis-Floyd, whose works had made a strong impact on the small group of Brazilian obstetricians who had carried out a paradigm shift from the technocratic to the humanistic model of childbirth care. Robbie's talk on the technocratic, humanistic, and holistic paradigms has shaped our discourse and our ways of thinking and practicing ever since. In her closing talk, Lesley Page stated that Robbie's presentation was the most important of the entire conference, for she had helped us to understand what "humanizing birth" truly means. Right after Robbie finished speaking, a group of humanized obstetricians, including me, lined up carrying armloads of her books for her to sign: *Birth as an American Rite of Passage* (1992), which had shown us precisely what was wrong with technocratic birth and *why* we needed to change; *From Doctor to Healer: The Transformative Journey* (Davis-Floyd and St. John 1998), which showed us *how* we could change; and *Childbirth and Authoritative Knowledge* (Davis-Floyd and Sargent 1997), which gave us fresh perspectives on the fact that just because a given knowledge system is authoritative doesn't mean that it is correct. We told her that we were "the good guys and girls"—the ones who didn't do unnecessary cesareans—that we called ourselves "the Floydettes," and that we competed with each other to see who could quote her the most! We thanked her for the important work that cemented our knowledge about the deeper meanings of childbirth. Robbie's books and articles made it clear to us that anthropology could make a huge difference in practitioners' ideologies and practices. Her work was remarkable for opening our eyes and our hearts.

Moreover, that was also, for Robbie and me, a meeting of shared pains. Three months prior to this conference, Robbie's daughter Peyton, age 20, had died in a car accident on the same day that a patient of mine had suffered an acute amniotic fluid embolism (see below). Our twin tragedies and our open wounds brought us close and fortified a friendship and exchange of ideas that has lasted for decades. My encounter with Robbie at the beginning of this century marked a turning point in my life and opened paths I could never have imagined taking.

Through ReHuNa, and often at Robbie's invitation, I started to attend, as an international guest speaker, the CIMS (Coalition for Improving Maternity Services) annual meetings and the conferences held by DONA International, Lamaze International, and Midwifery Today, in the United States and Mexico. This international experience and Robbie's help gave me opportunities to contribute publications to journals such as *Midwifery Today* (Jones 2016a); to Robbie's coedited, groundbreaking collection—the first book to call attention to highly functional and fully humanized birth practices, called simply *Birth Models That Work* (Davis-Floyd et al. 2009; Jones 2009); and to Sylvie Donna's *Promoting Normal Birth* (2011) (Jones 2011). I also contributed publications to books published in Brazil, such as *Breastfeeding: Scientific Bases* ([2010] 2016), edited by my colleague Marcus Renato de Carvalho (Jones 2016b). I wrote two books—collections of ideas and birth stories written in the first person—first *Memoirs of the Man Made of Glass: Reminiscences of a Humanistic Obstetrician* (Jones 2004) and later *Between the Ears: Birth Stories* (Jones 2012). The title of the first book stemmed from my experience of attending that woman whom I described above who gave birth in the emergency room in a squatting position: when I had entered the room and commanded her to get off the floor and onto the table, she had looked right through me as if I were made of glass, making me realize that for her, my presence was both irrelevant and completely unnecessary.

This kind of public exposure that I was slowly receiving as I gave lectures, seminars; radio, TV, and newspaper interviews; and was featured, along with Robbie and other experts, in documentaries such as *Orgasmic Birth* and O *Renascimento do Parto* (*Birth Reborn*)—only increased the biomedical corporation's discomfort with a professional who questioned the deepest values of the technocratic practice of childbirth assistance. Certainly some revenge, eventually, would come.

An Acute Amniotic Embolism

In the year 2000, when I was starting my career as a speaker and beginning to write about birth from a humanizing perspective, a tragedy occurred. I was providing prenatal care for Vania, an important feminist leader of our region. We had a total harmony of ideas about childbirth, to the point that in her "baby shower," she innovated by asking me to give a talk on the humanization of childbirth for her friends and associates. She was around 35 years old, pregnant with her first child, and planning to have a natural birth in the hospital with me.

Her pregnancy went smoothly. I was called to the hospital when the contractions were already quite strong, with 5 cm of dilation. Vania was accompanied by her husband, a friend, and the doula who worked with us at that time. The labor had lasted exactly six hours when the baby's heart rate dropped abruptly when dilation was already complete. (I did not know it at the time, but later it became clear that she had an amniotic fluid embolism—a rare but life-threatening condition, known as the most insidious of obstetric diseases—that no doctor can predict nor prevent.[2]) I immediately began maneuvers to improve fetal oxygenation. I changed her position several times to see if that was related to cord compression. I began fluid infusion. I didn't give the mother oxygen because there's no proof that it can produce any benefit (see Thurlow and Kinsella 2002; Raghuraman et al. 2021). But after attempting for ten minutes, the heartbeat did not return to normal. An anesthesiologist was called (since there were none on duty in the hospital) and I performed the cesarean 38 minutes after the indication—a value within international expectations of "D-I" (decision-incision).

At the entrance to the operating room, Vania had a seizure. The baby was born in very bad condition; it was possible to recover his heartbeat, but that wasn't enough, and he died after more than 30 days in the hospital NICU. The mother, no longer under my care, was taken to the ICU, where she responded well to the treatment. But after around a month, at a point where she was just a few days away from discharge, she succumbed to an infection caused by chickenpox, which she acquired from a friend who came to visit her. Because her immune system was very weak from the corticosteroids administered and other factors, no visitors should have been allowed. She overcame her underlying illness and died from a breach in the biological safety of the ICU.

Given that most women die from amniotic embolisms, it was a miracle that she survived and was recovering well, and a tragedy that she died from an entirely preventable cause. Her death turned into a scandal because a local political figure had "died in childbirth"—or so the story went. And who was the obstetrician? The infamous one who advocates for normal births and for the humanization of birth. For my opponents, this seemed to be the perfect opportunity to destroy the "heretic," the "traitor" to the biomedical order. It was evident that such an event had been long awaited by the obstetric establishment in my city. During the investigation carried out at the hospital, a nutritionist heard the following comment from the head of pediatrics: "This is our opportunity to destroy this guy!"

It did not matter that the world literature explained the unpredictability of an acute embolism caused by amniotic fluid. There was little interest in the unanimous studies asserting the impossibility of predicting or preventing this type of occurrence. And here was my big mistake: imagining that my medical colleagues, however much they hated me, would be faithful to the truth. Unfortunately, this is not what happened, and the case was used to violently attack the premises of normal birth and turn public opinion against the professionals who practiced it. My accusers did not spare lies, distorted versions, or legal technicalities to place blame on a doctor who had faced the most terrible nightmare of obstetrics—an amniotic embolism—that, even now, many years later, still has no solution.

I ended up convicted in courts of criminal and civil justice. I worked for three years in a daycare center providing medical care for children—a deeply rewarding experience—and paid a large sum of money as a fine. The local Board of Medicine initially sentenced me to a 30-day suspension and public censure, but when I went to the court of appeal at the Federal Council of Medicine—at the national level—I was surprised by a much older panel of judges who realized that it is a very rare condition against which there is no prevention nor prediction. I received a minuscule punishment for minor failures in filling out the documents, with a private letter sent to my house. Unfortunately, this sentence, which affirmed my innocence, had the result of infuriating local obstetric authorities. My almost insignificant punishment at the federal level, and without the severity that they had expected, ended up disallowing the sentence I received at the local level. This would end up reinforcing the idea to "discipline and punish" (Foucault 1975) me. It took ten years for a new chance to arise.

My Ongoing Obstetric Persecutions and My Advances in the Humanistic/Holistic Model

The years following Vania's death were filled with intense persecutions at all levels. One of the many ways in which my supposed "colleagues" took their stands against me was through the construction of fictitious labels and characters such as the doctor "against cesarean sections," the "fanatic for normal birth," the "militant against technology," the guy who "puts his patients at risk" driven by a "fixed idea" on vaginal births. The proposal was to classify all professionals who opposed the barbarity of excessive and dangerous cesareans as part of a "sect"—a "mystical cult" that defended anachronistic hypotheses about normal births.

The attacks against me were also combined with the defense of the dangerous or useless medical procedures applied in childbirth care, even when the international community had long established their inadequacy. Thus, my refusal to routinely perform "standard obstetric procedures" was part of this constructed image of a doctor who questioned the most basic foundations of the field of obstetrics, attacking the heart, the deeper structure, that sustains this biomedical specialty. In Robbie's terms (see Series Overview, this volume, and Davis-Floyd 2023), I was a Stage 4 humanistic obstetrician practicing within a Stage 1, silo-oriented, fundamentalist, and often fanatical obstetric system. And as Robbie cogently points out, Stage 4 global humanists are anathemas to Stage 1 fundamentalists, who believe that "our way is the only right way," and fanatics, who believe that "our way is so right that everyone who does not accept it should be assimilated or eliminated." Thus, as I could not be assimilated, I was constantly a target for being eliminated. Yet despite the attacks I continuously received, my attitude was not one of containment, but of radicalization. Many would have expected me to back down on my ideas and begin to move closer to a more interventionist and more lenient model with the procedures I had criticized and refused to perform for so many years, but what happened was exactly the opposite.

Home Birth: The Ultimate Offense

In the early 2000s, a few months after the deaths of Vania and her baby, I attended to a patient whom I will call Adriana, who was giving birth to her second baby. Adriana's prenatal care was uneventful, and labor began smoothly and spontaneously. In the hospital, my team and I could see that her relationship with her husband seemed to be built through genuine partnership, respect, and connection. The labor went smoothly and quickly, and the baby was born through a physiologic birth without any intervention. Immediately after delivery, the midwife put the newborn directly into Adriana's arms while her husband sheltered them both in a warm embrace, where the baby remained for quite a while without any interruption.

Eventually, the pediatrician who was present (as required by law) stated that the baby should be sent to the nursery. Adriana, her husband, and I then spent a long time talking, especially about the ease of this delivery compared to her previous one, but also about the importance of emotional states in determining the quality of the birth process. I called these issues "soft factors"—the calmness, the connection, the tranquility, the confidence, and the atmosphere—which I call the *psychosphere* of birth (Jones 2009)—an ambience in which the atmosphere/energy in the room must be kept clear and clean, with no negative energy that could impede the birth. (According to Robbie's definition of the holistic paradigm [see Series Overview, this volume], this focus on energy puts me in the realm of holistic practice.) I compare these soft factors to the "hard factors" related to the physical aspects that obstetricians normally value, such as blood pressure, the baby's size, position, and heartrate, the progression of labor on a predetermined curve, and so on. At one point, Adriana turned to me and said, "Do you know what's the only thing I think I didn't need in this birth?" She then smiled and pointed upwards, saying: "This hospital. I cannot see anything it could have helped me with. I think I would have given birth much more easily if it weren't for being here, surrounded by strangers who are even responsible for the fact that the baby is not here with me now."

Her words made me extremely thoughtful. In the early 2000s, there were no doctors attending home births in the entire country. The very mention of an out-of-hospital birth caused an immediate reaction of rejection, as if the birthplace were a "civilizing" colonial conquest (see

Lokugamage, Ahillan, and Pathberiya [2023] in Volume III of this series) and trying to return to the roots of human history was nothing more than an absurd setback that would immediately put mothers and babies at risk, without access to the multiple "advantages" that the techno-medicalization of birth offered them.

However, my project of "smoothing birth" through the simple and practical protocol that I had created easily resolved this dilemma: couldn't I understand the hospital as one of the technologies applied to childbirth with the greatest iatrogenic effect? Isn't the displacement of the pregnant woman to an "inhospitable," unfamiliar environment one of the greatest activators of the adrenaline cycle of fear-tension-pain so well described by Grantly Dick-Read (1933, 1942)? Wouldn't the de-hospitalization of childbirth be the last barrier, the ultimate taboo, and the ultimate challenge for the humanization of childbirth?

From that moment on, I began to question the issue of childbirth outside the hospital more intensely. At the beginning of this century, the discussion lists on humanized childbirth on the internet were already fully functioning, and we had very intense debates about this issue. Little by little, reports came to us of women who gave birth at home in foreign countries, especially in the Dutch system, and after my entry into the international circuit of humanization of birth, I started to listen to similar narratives from American women and their midwives. At the same time, I continued to listen to the old arguments that tried to obliterate any debate about the place of birth. The reason for this, they said, was that "time could not be turned back" and that science had already progressed far enough to definitively demonstrate the superiority of hospital births conducted by obstetricians as compared to care provided by midwives in birth centers and at home.

Even today, this debate only makes sense if we are aware that science does not behave like a boat that moves on a placid and immobile lake using evidence and proof as oars. Quite the contrary: the boat is at sea, tossed around by the winds of cultural energies, balancing on gigantic ocean currents, the flows of which are determined by capitalism and patriarchy (and according to some, also by imperialism [see Rothman 2021])—the main forces that move the waters of behaviors, but also of data, research, and studies. Thus, it is legitimate to understand that the safety of home birth is not an exclusively medical debate, even though medicine and obstetrics can produce science that seems to show the non-safety of home birth—such as the notorious study by JR Wax and colleagues, which falsely showed a three times greater neonatal mortality for home births. This study has been widely refuted (see Anderson, Daviss, and Johnson 2021; Lokugamage and Feeley 2023), but many obstetricians still use this study to justify their fear of and resistance to home birth.

With this perspective, it was very clear to me that the questions about home birth were only apparently linked to science and the protection of mothers and babies. They were, in fact, clearly conditioned by a worldview, a way of understanding birth from an essentially defective female anatomy perspective, as if for a woman to give birth she would have to yield to a rite of submission to the patriarchal order. Questioning the birthplace was basically sacrilege, an act that challenged the deepest foundations of the very existence of biomedical obstetrics.

Despite the constant threats from the biomedical corporation, I decided to dedicate myself to home birth, based on the growing demands from women who came to us precisely because they wanted to escape the hospital and its interference in the otherwise free-flowing course of labor and delivery. For 16 years, from 2000–2016, we attended home births, which ultimately came to constitute the majority of our practice. One of our team of doulas would go to the family's home when the woman was in early labor and stay with her to support her until it was time to call myself as the obstetrician and my wife Zeza, our team nurse-midwife. If a hospital transfer became necessary—which it rarely did—we would all go together, and if needed, I would do the cesarean, providing complete continuity of care.

Our outcomes were outstanding. I have not calculated them for all our years of practice, but I have for the years 2001–2013. During that time, we attended 312 births—around two per month—sometimes more, sometimes less. We would have liked to attend more, but during those years, there was (and still is) a campaign to discredit home births and "natural" births after Vania's death in 2000, and my bullyings and persecutions were ongoing, so we had to be extremely circumspect in the number of clients we took on. Of these 312 births, around 95% took place in upright positions, including hands-and-knees—a position that opens the pelvic outlet to its maximum capacity. Our episiotomy rate was 3%; 45% were planned hospital births and 55% were planned home births. Of the home births, 13% required hospital transfer. Of those transfers, 45% of women went on to have a vaginal birth, while 55% needed cesareans, leading to an overall cesarean rate for our practice of 16.5%, in a country with a cesarean rate of 56%. My persecution by the obstetric establishment in my city continued, but, sustained by our excellent outcomes and the high satisfaction rates of our patients and ourselves, our practice flourished, and our outcomes remained outstanding. With the exceptions of the death of Vania's baby as described above, and the neonatal death I will describe just below, our perinatal mortality rate was 0.

The End of My Practice: How They Finally Got Me

In 2010, a woman came to our office saying that she had searched for us specifically because she wanted to give birth at home. She told me that she had another obstetrician for many years, but that she would not have the birth under his care because he did not accept out-of-hospital births. Her pregnancy was normal, and she went into labor spontaneously. However, as it was her first pregnancy, we went too early to her house, at nightfall. As the labor did not evolve and she was able to sleep, we all decided—obstetrician, midwife, and doula—to sleep in the living room to wait for her entry into the active phase of labor, which only occurred toward the end of the following morning. At around 5 p.m. the bag of waters broke, and at 7:42 p.m. the baby was born, calmly and receiving an Apgar of 7 and 9. The family, gathered in the living room, was thrilled to hear, in the distance, the baby's cry. The new grandmother hugged me, saying "Thank you for existing." From there were photos, more hugs, and socializing.

However, after a few minutes, we noticed that the baby had tachypnea (increased breathing movements), which occurs in almost all babies because of the need to reabsorb the fluid that normally accumulates in the lungs. This moisture needs to be absorbed little by little, and this makes breathing efforts increase—all this is within the framework of normality. However, as time passed, the tachypnea continued and the newborn's respiration did not stabilize, although the baby remained hydrated, flushed, and with preserved muscle tone. His breathing movements were above expectation (tachypnea), but his breathing pattern was below expectations.

I decided to comply with international protocols and wait for two hours for full normalization. In the meantime, I tried to call colleagues and exchange ideas, but as it was a local holiday, I was unable to contact any of them. When the two hours had passed, I told the family that we were going to the hospital because the baby had not developed a calming respiratory rate, and that in the last few minutes he had a slight fluttering of the nostrils, which was abnormal. With some reluctance, the new mother accepted. I called an ambulance, but the service seemed to be congested, so I decided that it would be much faster to go in my car. We arrived at the hospital at midnight. I spoke directly to the pediatrician on duty, telling her about the tachypnea condition and the newborn's general condition—ruddy, hydrated, with preserved tonus and with more than 90% saturation. She told me the child would be under observation. The mother went to a hospital room to sleep, and my team and I went home.

The next day when I went to the hospital to check on the baby, I was aggressively received by the child's pediatrician. During the night, the situation had become very seriously complicated. When I looked at the baby's medical record, I realized that after he had been admitted to the NICU, it had been three and a half hours before he had finally been given an antibiotic for the streptococcus infection he had been diagnosed with—but not the one indicated. Only four hours after arriving at the hospital did this newborn finally receive the appropriate medication for the infection. Nevertheless, this head pediatrician was as angry with me as if I were to blame for the errors that occurred during that night.

The child died that same night, 24 hours after birth. Immediately the chief pediatrician—who already had a lot of friction with me—filed an accusation to the medical board, saying that all the problems were due to a home birth. That is when my new dramas began. For six long years, during which I kept on practicing, I spent money I did not have on lawyers, court fees, plane flights, and supportive reports from other obstetricians. I lost my hair and my tranquility. I lost my health and my hope. I also lost the court battles. I was tried by the same local judges who, ten years earlier, had sentenced me and who had seen their sentence eased at the national level. Now they had the opportunity to finish me off. After all, this time the "final offense" had occurred—a home birth.

It did not matter that the hospital's neonatologists had made huge mistakes nor that the baby had arrived at the hospital in good condition. A home birth, without the control of doctors and their technologies, and having the supreme offense of the baby being born into the hands of a nurse-midwife, could not go unpunished. During the entire process, it was clear to me that the verdict had already been decided from the beginning, and that the legal procedures were just ritual enactments to display the proper formality of what was actually an Inquisitorial act. I was condemned to lose the right to serve as a doctor, and the same sentence was confirmed when I appealed at the national level. My license was revoked in 2016, preventing me forever from working as a doctor in any capacity. I was beyond devastated.

Epilogue: My Ongoing Story and the Persecutions of Other Humanistic Obstetricians in Brazil

Since then, after recovering some psychological stability, I have been involved in writing, teaching, offering courses in various places, and going back to school. My family and I decided to move to a small farm where others, including friends and my son and daughter and grandchildren, have formed an intentional community involving a "minimalist" approach. I decided to return to university to study anthropology so that I can keep on learning and growing and can better learn to understand human behavior and beliefs. However, I feel that I will never disconnect from childbirth—I will never stop being a humanistic obstetrician, even though I am unable to attend births. Every single night, I dream of my patients, the babies I have seen being born, the joy on their parents' faces, the wonderful feeling of seeing life emerging in a birth.

After my elimination as a doctor, a series of nationwide attacks on other professionals began. What was not given much importance before has become something very serious. Humanistic obstetricians have been sued for ridiculous reasons, such as allowing parents to cut the cord of their newborn children without wearing gloves. Others were attacked for not performing episiotomies, as I had been. Countless such attacks began in the country, configuring a true "witch hunt." Not by chance, in this exact period, Brazil had a juridical-media coup with the forced removal of a president from the left—Dilma Rousseff. From that moment on, other coups in sequence were made with the association between a biased judiciary and a media massacre that culminated in the arrest and prevention of the leftist candidate, Lula da Silva, from running for the presidency, leading to the ascension to power of the far-right candidate Jair Bolsonaro. In this entire process, which took around four years, many fundamentalist doctors—a very far-right segment of the society—sided with the coup plotters and with Bolsonaro, either through direct and open support or by supporting the government's denial of the coronavirus pandemic.

In this situation, all practitioners who supported women and their claims to reproductive and sexual human rights (humanized childbirth, abortion, presence of doulas, etc.) placed themselves on the left of the political spectrum, and thus in the position of enemies of those who control what Barbara Katz Rothman (2021) has called "the Biomedical Empire." The result could only be an increase in attacks on such humanistic practitioners, with the absolute impunity that allows members of this "Empire" to make the most unreasonable accusations, politically motivated and without any kind of accountability. The field became open for the most reactionary and conservative forces in biomedicine to hold the power in their hands. All obstetricians were prohibited from attending home births, so none do. Today (2022), we are living in the midst of an epidemic of attacks on humanized professionals (see Davis-Floyd 2023)—not only in Brazil but also in many other countries—and there is no possibility of reversal in the short term.

During all these years, I have acted as if moved by what I think of as "an imperative of conscience." I have always known that I would be attacked and misunderstood by my peers—just not how much nor how profoundly. Sometime after my graduation from medical school, while walking with Moysés Paciornik's book *Learn to Give Birth Like the Indians* (1979)—a book about Indigenous techniques to assist squatting birth—through the corridors of the hospital where I was doing my residency, a colleague noticed the book I was carrying and, after taking it from my hands, he quickly leafed through it and, frowning, shot off the words, "From where you are, it's impossible to go further down." At that pivotal moment, I could envision that my whole life as an obstetrician would be marked by attacks and persecutions. Yet at the same time, I had the clear feeling that more obs than Paciornik and a few others like him needed to be among the first to take this path and to expose the unworthy ways in which technocratic childbirth was conducted. It fell to me to be one who pointed to the noble lord walking without his robes and shout, "The Emperor is naked!"

Despite everything I have been through, I consider myself a huge optimist. Many of the ideas that supported my practice for over 30 years are now considered "mainstream" in many countries, not yet including Brazil. The father's or partner's presence in the delivery room, the abolition of episiotomies, vertical positions for childbirth, the abandonment of violent and/or humiliating practices such as enemas, pubic shaving, frequent cervical exams, supine births, Kristeller, and infantilizing discourses with pregnant women—all these and more were flags I had been carrying for three decades and only now are being slowly adopted by young obstetricians in my country. It is in them—the young professionals, many of whom are members of ReHuNa—where I notice much more openness to reassessing their practices, questioning obstetric myths and taboos, and accepting the breath of humanistic renewal in childbirth. And in Brazil, a new legion of professional midwives (both nurse- and direct-entry midwives) is in the process of "invading" large urban hospitals, producing with their sweetness, softness, skills, and professionalism the necessary counterpoints to technocratic institutional births, which retain their violent approaches in my country.

I have (mostly) withdrawn from the birthing scene, leaving more than 2,000 articles written on my blog Orelhas de Vidro (in Portuguese),[3] most of them about medicine, childbirth, exams, routines, rituals, short stories, chronicles, fiction, obstetric violence, and many other topics. I am still going to face criminal trial for the last case, which has been delayed due to the COVID-19 pandemic, and I have no idea what will happen to me after that.

I simply say that I did what my conscience determined was right, and I did it because, by respecting women and their babies, I wanted to offer them the best of both worlds—the biomedical and the social. Throughout my obstetric career, I was fully aware that, while defending the human rights related to childbirth, I would be touching the exposed wound of patriarchy and its control over female sexuality. As many experts agree, childbirth is part of women's sexual lives: oxytocin flows through their bodies while they are making love, birthing, and breastfeeding. Thus the idea of protecting women from bodily invasions seemed to me to be worth fighting for. All the suffering that my family and I went through, especially my wife and partner Zeza, was worth it, given the milestones that my journey in obstetrics facilitated in the lives of so many families. To them, the brave women who radically resisted an oppressive system to give birth in peace, I dedicate this work.

Ricardo Herbert Jones attended home and hospital births for 34 years in his private practice as an obstetrician/gynecologist in Porto Alegre, Rio Grande do Sul, Brazil, with his midwife and doula team, and is also a homeopathic practitioner. He is author of two books—*Memórias do Homem de Vidro: Reminiscências de um Obstetra Humanista* (2004) and *Entre as Orelhas: Histórias de Parto* (2012)—and of numerous articles and blogs. He is also an international speaker, doula trainer, and perinatal education teacher in Brazil, Portugal, and other countries.

Notes

1. The processes of biomedical education differ greatly in Brazil from those in high resource countries, in which students attend four years of college, followed by entrance into medical school, and then residency. In Brazil, high school graduates who wish to become doctors enter straight into medical school, which takes six years and into which some non-medical courses are incorporated. Thus in Brazil, medical school graduates—now MDs—are generally much younger than those in the US and other high resource countries that can afford for students to attend four years of college before entering an actual medical school.
2. An amniotic fluid embolism occurs when amniotic fluid or fetal material, such as fetal cells, enters the mother's bloodstream. A likely cause is a breakdown in the placental barrier. When this breakdown happens, the immune system responds by releasing products that cause an inflammatory reaction, which activates abnormal clotting in the mother's lungs and blood vessels. This can result in a serious and usually fatal blood-clotting disorder.
3. Jones RH. "Orelhas de Vidro." Retrieved 16 September 2022 from www.orelhasdevidro.com.

References

Anderson DA, Daviss BA, Johnson KC. 2021. "What If Another 10% of Deliveries in the United States Ocurred at Home or in a Birth Center? Safety, Ecomics, and Politics." In *Birthing Models on the Human Rights Frontier: Speaking Truth to Power*, ed. Daviss BA, Davis-Floyd R, 205–228. Abingdon, Oxon: Routledge.

Carvalho M. R. (2010) 2016. *Amamentação, Bases Cientificas* (Breastfeeding: Scientific Bases), 4th edn. Rio de Janerio, Brasil: Guanabara Koogan.

Davis-Floyd R. 1987. "Obstetric Training as a Rite of Passage." *Medical Anthropology Quarterly* 1(3): 288–318.

———. 1992. *Birth as an American Rite of Passage*. Berkeley: University of California Press.

———. 2023. "Open and Closed Knowledge Systems, the 4 Stages of Cognition, and the Obstetric Management of Birth." In *Cognition, Risk, and Responsibility in Obstetrics: Anthropological Analyses and Critiques of Obstetricians' Practices*, eds. Davis-Floyd R, Premkumar A, Chapter 1. New York: Berghahn Books.

Davis-Floyd R, Barclay L, Daviss BA, Tritten J, eds. 2009. *Birth Models that Work*. Berkeley: University of California Press.

Davis-Floyd R, Sargent C, eds. 1997. *Childbirth and Authoritative Knowledge: Cross-Cultural Perspectives*. Berkeley: University of California Press.

Davis-Floyd R, St. John G. 1998. *From Doctor to Healer: The Transformative Journey*. New Brunswick NJ: Rutgers University Press.

Dick-Read G. 1933. *Natural Childbirth*. London: Heinemann.

———.1942. *Childbirth without Fear: The Principles and Practices of Natural Childbirth*. London: William Heinemann.

Donna S. 2011. *Promoting Normal Birth: Research, Reflections and Guidelines*. Chester-le-Street: Fresh Heart Publishing.

Foucault M. 1975. *Surveiller et Punir: Naissance de la Prison*. Paris: Gallimard.

Jones R. 2004. *Memórias do Homem de Vidro: Reminiscências de um Obstetra Humanista* (Memories of the Man Made of Glass: Reminiscences of a Humanistic Obstetrician). Porto Alegre, Brazil: Ideias a Granel.

———. 2009. "Teamwork: An Obstetrician, a Midwife, and a Doula in Brazil." In *Birth Models That Work*, eds. Davis-Floyd R, Barclay L, Daviss BA, Tritten J, 271–304. Berkeley: University of California Press.

———. 2011. "Reasons for Intervention . . . but No Justification." In *Promoting Normal Birth: Research, Reflections and Guidelines*, ed. Donna S, 113–120. Chester-le-Street: Fresh Heart Publishing.

———. 2012. *Entre as Orelhas: Histórias de Parto* [Between the Ears: Birth Stories]. Porto Alegre, Brazil: Editora Ideias à Granel.

———. 2016a. "Birthcraft in Brazil: An Update on the Brazilian Humanization of Birth Movement." *Midwifery Today International Midwife* 118: 40–45.

———. 2016b. "O Continuum da Amamentação" (The Continuum of Breastfeeding). In *Amamentação, Bases Cientificas* (Breastfeeding: Scientific bases), 4th edn., ed. Carvalho MR. Rio de Janeiro, Brasil: Guanabara Koogan.

Kitzinger S. 2005. *The Politics of Birth*. London: Books for Midwives.

Lokugagamaje AU, Ahillan T, Pathberiya SDC. 2023. "Decolonizing Medical Education in the UK." In *Obstetric Violence and Systemic Disparities: Can Obstetrics Be*

Humanized and Decolonized? ed. Davis-Floyd R, Premkumar A, Chapter 6. New York: Berghahn Books.

Lokugagamaje AU, Feeley C. 2023. "Cognition, Risk, and Responsibility: Home Birth and Why Obstetricians Fear It." In *Cognition, Risk, and Responsibility in Obstetrics: Anthropological Analyses and Critiques of Obstetricians' Practices*, ed. Davis-Floyd R, Premkumar A, Chapter 11. New York: Berghahn Books.

Raghuraman N, Temming LA, Doering MM, et al. 2021. "Maternal Oxygen Supplementation Compared with Room Air for Intrauterine Resuscitation: A Systematic Review and Meta-Analysis." *JAMA Pediatrics* 175(4): 368–376.

Rothman BK. 2021. *The Biomedical Empire: Lessons Learned from the COVID-19 Pandemic*. Stanford CA: Stanford University Press.

Paciornik M. 1979. *Aprenda a Nascer com os Índios: Parto de Cócoras (Learn to Give Birth like the Indians: Squatting Birth)*. Brazil: Brasiliense.

Thurlow JA, Kinsella SM. 2002. "Intrauterine Resuscitation: Active Management of Fetal Distress." *International Journal of Obstetric Anesthesia* 11(2): 105–116.

Wax JR, FL Lucas, M Lamont, et al. 2010. "Maternal and Newborn Outcomes in Planned Homebirth vs. Planned Hospital Births: A Meta-Analysis." *American Journal of Obstetrics and Gynecololgy* 203: 243e1–8.

CHAPTER 8

Hungarian Birth Models Seen through the Prism of Prison
The Journey of Ágnes Geréb

Ágnes Geréb and Katalin Fábián

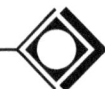

"Geréb!"

Who is calling me? And why? "Geréb" is my family name. Nobody except my very best, long-time friend calls me by this name, and she calls me Geréb only ironically because the pretense of "official" distance invoked by the family name makes our closeness all the sweeter. But my family name rang out in the Budapest municipal prison on a frigid October day in 2010. Accused of professional negligence, I was shackled and imprisoned without bail on October 5, 2010. My trials have spanned many years, and by the Prosecutor's request, cases were combined to make me appear incompetent and criminally negligent. While awaiting trial and supposedly still under the presumption of innocence, I was imprisoned for 77 days followed by house arrest for an additional three years and two months, lasting until February 2014.

The sentencing phase started in October 2015, and the judge rendered her decision on November 25, 2015, with a suspended sentence of one year of prison, three years of prohibition from practicing as an obstetrician, and destruction of the medical equipment (such as two cardiotocography scanners) that the authorities confiscated from my office in October 2010. Both the prosecutor and my legal team appealed. The prosecution demanded a longer prison sentence and prohibition from ever working as a doctor in any capacity, and my team asked for the reduction or elimination of the punishment meted out. But on September 26, 2016, the Appeals Court not only upheld the guilty verdict in the five combined cases, but also extended the suspended prison sentence from one to one-and-a half years, while also increasing the ban to work either as a doctor or midwife from three years to five years. In February 2012, my legal team and I appealed to the President of Hungary for clemency in the cases of the shoulder dystocia and the twin birth (both described later in this chapter). President Áder first stated that he would decide after the final verdicts appeared in the other cases in criminal courts, and then on April 13, 2017, he rejected my appeal. These decisions made me feel sad because of the blatant injustice involved in being singled out and treated differently from how similar current hospital birth deaths (shoulder dystocias and others) are processed without any criminal aspect. I am also saddened by the changes in the homebirth world in Hungary, where the services, because of high costs, are now not available to everyone, and in many ways, I see "the soul of home birth" as having gone missing.

My legal team requested the reopening of two remaining active court cases (the shoulder dystocia and the twin birth) in a special court. The punishment in these two cases was two years in prison, ten years prohibition to work as a doctor or midwife, and paying (along with Ági Király, another midwife) the cost of 1,748,300 HUF (about 7,000 USD) for the legal proceedings. On April 20, 2017, the Court of First Appeals (Fővárosi Ítélőtábla—the court of appeals just below the Supreme Court—the Kúria) accepted the reopening of the lawsuit in the case of the twin birth, but not the shoulder dystocia. A Hungarian medical expert had come forward to defend my professional actions at the twin birth that revised the earlier expert testimony, and thus the case had been reopened in court following the approval of the Healthcare Scientific Council (Egészségügyi Tudományos Tanács). On that same date, the court in charge of the reopened investigation of the twin birth suspended my two-year prison sentence for a five-year probationary period, reduced the professional prohibitions from ten to eight years, but further increased the cost of legal proceedings that I alone had to pay. In addition, my applications for a passport were rejected twice. I appealed this decision four times without success. Since July 2017, the spokesperson for the Prosecutor's Office (Fővárosi Fellebbviteli Főügyészség) repeatedly and publicly called for reinstating the previous prison sentence (Medvegy 2017).

The six years that I spent in prison, house arrest, and under continuing severe restrictions on my movements and the prohibition to exercise my profession have all been part of "preliminary detention." During my 1,128 days of house arrest, the police checked on me unannounced, four times every 24 hours. With three days in house arrest counting for one day in prison, I would have already served more time than my sentence. However, the various forms of imprisonment do not count as punishment because these were preliminary, so-called "protective" measures (óvintézkedés).

The Accusations and Their Results

After graduating from medical school, I started working as an obstetrician/gynecologist on September 1, 1977, in the Szülészeti és Nőgyógyászati Klinika (Obstetrics and Gynecology Department) of the University of Szeged Hospital. During my 15 years of employment at the University Hospital, I often accompanied more than 10 births during one shift, accounting for around 7,000 births. (Although the 7,000 births are a conservative estimate during my employment at Szeged, I record this number because the documentation for the number of births during my hospital work is inaccessible.) On April 10, 1992, I took maternity leave, and officially left my employment at the Szeged University Hospital in 1994. I began to attend home births in 1989 as an obstetrician. In addition to my medical doctor training, I became a certified midwife (in a three-year-long training) at the University of Debrecen in 2005. In 2010, I obtained a Bachelor of Science degree in Midwifery (a four-year-long training) from the Budapest-based Faculty of Health Sciences of Semmelweis University. Over the course of my career, I have assisted in the births of more than 10,000 children, of which 3,500 were home births with me acting as an independent midwife at the mothers' sides.

In 2007, two years after I had become a certified midwife, my license to practice obstetrics and gynecology was revoked for three years—the result of an event that happened in 2000. This case was that of baby Zita, who suddenly stopped breathing in the arms of her mother, with me in attendance while waiting for the emergence of the placenta. Zita was born without any complications and apparently healthy. She cried a little and started to suckle, and her mother covered her with a blanket, holding her close. Zita was out of my sight in her mother's arms for a couple of minutes, and nobody noticed that she had stopped breathing. She was successfully resuscitated, but only lived to the age of 14 months (Geréb 2000) and died of what was considered to be Sudden Infant Death Syndrome (SIDS). In this case, I was acquitted at the Court of First Appeals, but the prosecution appealed and won. The sentencing judge, Ágnes Czene, later handed down unusually severe punishments in my subsequent cases.

By 2012, I was facing a set of five cases. The Public Prosecutor had pressed charges against me in three birth cases and in two other "criminal offenses." The first court hearing was on December 6, 2012, at the 3rd District Court. The first criminal charge was "quackery," which means that a person performs activities for money falling under the scope of biomedical practice without authorization to do so. This charge built on that 2007 binding court order barring me from practicing as an obstetrician/gynecologist for three years, from October 26, 2007, until 2010. This prohibition is significant, as it prohibited me from prescription privileges, referrals, and prenatal and post-natal service provision, all of which only doctors can offer. The criminal quackery charge stemmed from proof that I had taken part in 200 planned home births.

After my arrest in 2010, the police searched the *Napvilág* Birth House and found a file folder documenting 200 cases of birthing mothers. We never kept our patients' files at the Birth House for security reasons, but this folder was left there by accident. Therefore, the police had these 200 cases as evidence. When accompanying home births, however, I exclusively performed activities falling under the scope of a midwife's competence—activities I had been certified to perform through my training at the University of Debrecen. Families only paid the Alternatal Foundation for Undisturbed Birth (Alternatal Alapítvány a Háborítatlan Születésért, Szülésért), not me directly, between 0 and 50,000 HUF (about 240 USD) plus tax, for the one-week prenatal course. This price included as many consultations as necessary during the pregnancy and in the postpartum period. The 200 mothers listed by the authorities made written statements that they were aware that the accompaniment of the birth did not include the services of an obstetrician/gynecologist, and that I neither requested nor received payment for accompanying the births. When I was working in the hospital, my practice of not accepting patients' payments (*hálapénz*, "gratitude money") directly conflicted with what had become an endemic part of the Hungarian healthcare system until 2021. In that year, the government declared it illegal for doctors to accept such untaxed income from patients. Consequently, midwives in hospitals have started to replace the doctors to provide more individualized attention to the birthing mother and the newborn (Wiedemann 2021). The 2021 law likely will increase the number of pregnant women choosing an independent midwife and home birth, because they remain at liberty to choose their healthcare provider, in contrast with the now-prohibited financial incentives paid to doctors.

The second charge was incitement to falsification of documents based on a February 2009 complication-free birth at *Napvilág* Birth House. In the case of an out-of-institution birth, the midwife must report the birth to the municipality of the place of residence. For the birth to be registered, the parents must state the place of birth. In this case, the family gave the address of their own place of residence instead of the address of the Birth House when they registered the birth; thus, false data was registered. Subsequently, the family gave the true information to the municipality, stating that they felt uncomfortable about not giving accurate information when they initially registered the birth. The couple claimed that I had convinced them to give false information in the first place, yet I had not. On the contrary, at the time of the birth, the couple had very simple practical reasons to give false data: namely, that the one-time lump sum maternity benefit (*anyasági támogatás*) can only be obtained with a birth certificate, and such a certificate was much easier to get from the local government where they lived.

The third case was a birth fatality at the Szent István Hospital on September 3, 2009, involving a 38-year-old first-time mother. I was the only person charged in this case for allegedly having committed a professional error by agreeing to accompany the birth of a first-time mother falling into the high-risk age group, and for allegedly waiting too long before bringing the mother to the hospital. The mother intended to have a planned home birth after a problem-free pregnancy. Labor began and proceeded without complications until I noticed meconium in the amniotic fluid. I immediately went with the family to the Szent István Hospital in Budapest, and I remained with the mother as a doula throughout the birth. The family arrived at the hospital at 8:40 p.m.; the attending medical personnel decided that the child should be born vaginally. After stimulation of contractions with synthetic oxytocin and applying pressure to the abdomen, the child was born at 10:35 p.m. with the help of vacuum suction. At birth, the child's condition was poor, and resuscitation was immediately necessary. Unfortunately, all attempts were unsuccessful, and the child died the next day, on September 4, 2009, due to oxygen deficiency. I had acted in compliance with the international standards of midwifery by immediately bringing the mother to a hospital at the first warning sign. A mother giving birth for the first time at age 38 should not be considered high-risk.

In the fourth case, I was accused of having failed in my duty to provide continuous supervision of the newborn, not providing the child with appropriate care while waiting for the ambulance to arrive, and failing to treat the infection in time and to refer the mother to hospital care. On May 17, 2010, a mother expecting her fourth child went into labor at her home in her 38th week of pregnancy. She had given birth to her first three children at home without complications and planned to give birth to her fourth child in a similar manner. Labor began earlier than expected and proceeded very rapidly, as the mother informed me by telephone. I went to see her immediately and arrived when the child was born. Shortly after the birth, I noticed problems with the child's breathing. I called for a newborn ambulance, attended to the newborn, and began ventilation. The child was taken to the Pediatric Clinic of the Semmelweis University in Budapest, where she was diagnosed with a newborn streptococcal infection. After receiving appropriate medical care, the child (Eliza) was discharged from the hospital. She is 11 years old (as of 2021) and completely healthy.

In two previous cases, I had already been sentenced to two years in prison and ten years of prohibition from working as either a midwife or an obstetrician. One of these cases involved a baby who died in 2007 due to shoulder dystocia, a condition linked to high mortality even in hospitals (Hope et al. 1998). In the other case in which I was sentenced, one of a pair of twins died at seven months of age in 2004. The first of the twins was born without any complications. The second became ill in utero; he turned correctly with his head toward the birth canal, but suddenly his heartbeat deteriorated. We attempted to hasten birth by administering oxytocin, and the baby was born with the next contraction. We started resuscitation and called the ambulance immediately upon birth. The prosecution could not prove that I was professionally negligent but maintained the charge that I should not have accepted a twin birth under my care.

In four of the five cases, the birthing mothers supported me in court. The couple involved with the charge of forgery feared for their own safety if they were to stand with me. The family whose baby had the shoulder dystocia continued to charge me in a civil action for damages related to professional negligence surrounding the death of their child. At the time of writing (October 2022), my appeal was rejected, and I am obliged to pay the compensation of 21 million Hungarian Forints (approximately 50,000 USD) for the loss of their daughter.

The Hungarian and International Birth Movements

Profound indignation over my imprisonment and subsequent house arrest spurred the development of numerous formal and informal organizations comprised of thousands of mothers who gave birth or wanted to give birth with my assistance, fathers, family members, other independent midwives, doulas, and human rights and feminist activists. Thousands campaigned for my release from prison and my exoneration. My continued imprisonment and trials propelled the gradually emerging Hungarian homebirth movement to lobby even harder for regulations to create a framework for independent midwifery. We have been partially successful in pressuring the government to re-establish independent midwifery as a legitimate profession, and home birth is not illegal in Hungary.

Our movement began in the early 1990s when various informal networks started to connect the ideas of regime change and democratization at the macro-level with more freedom and evolving non-hierarchical norms in personal behaviors. Around this time, there was an increasing recognition of the oppression experienced during everyday practices connected to important life events such as birth. My arrest and subsequent imprisonment became catalysts for one of the most notable transnational activist campaigns waged in contemporary Hungary, which burst onto the world stage during the winter of 2010 and continues to this day. From our ostensibly single-issue cause of wanting to humanize the alienating and oppressive birthing practices widely used in Hungarian hospitals, we extended our focus to human rights and women's issues and, most importantly, to freedom and democracy. Taken in the context of current serious threats to democracy in Hungary, it seems that the charges against me were harbingers of the new era of authoritarian limitations on individual freedom and democratic rights. The European Commission increasingly expressed concerns over anti-democratic trends in Hungary (Tavares 2013), while Prime Minister Viktor Orbán endorsed an "illiberal democracy" in the country (Simon 2014).

In the spring of 2014, the Court of First Appeals ruled that my house arrest should be relaxed for health reasons, allowing me to leave the house for an hour a day, like the daily one-hour walk permitted in prisons. Until then, I was not even allowed to go out to the yard (see Figures 8.1 and 8.2).

As of February 20, 2014, a ruling by this same court permitted me to move freely within the Budapest city limits. However, this same decision entirely stripped me from practicing my only remaining income-generating activity: to advise or consult with pregnant women and their partners as they prepare for the arrival of their child. This last small but critical method of income was essential in supporting me and the two youngest of my four children. My legal team could not appeal this ruling because it was not a sentence against me, but rather a "protective" order toward others, and one cannot challenge the decisions of the Court of Appeals. It took until the Court of First Appeal's ruling on April 20, 2017, to invalidate this "protective" order issued in 2014.

The transnational aspect of our movement's activities appears much more optimistic than my still very difficult legal situation in Hungary. Yet throughout my house arrest, I continued to garner recognition and even accolades from abroad; for example, in 2013, I received a prize from the Danish foundation En God Start i Livet (A Good Start to Life). Thanks to the extensive transnational outreach of homebirth activists, major international organizations such as the United Nation's Convention on the Elimination of All Forms of Discrimination against Women (CEDAW) Committee and the European Union's Petitions Committee, headquartered in Brussels, expressed concern over my treatment (Ig-

Hungarian Birth Models Seen through the Prism of Prison ♦ 151

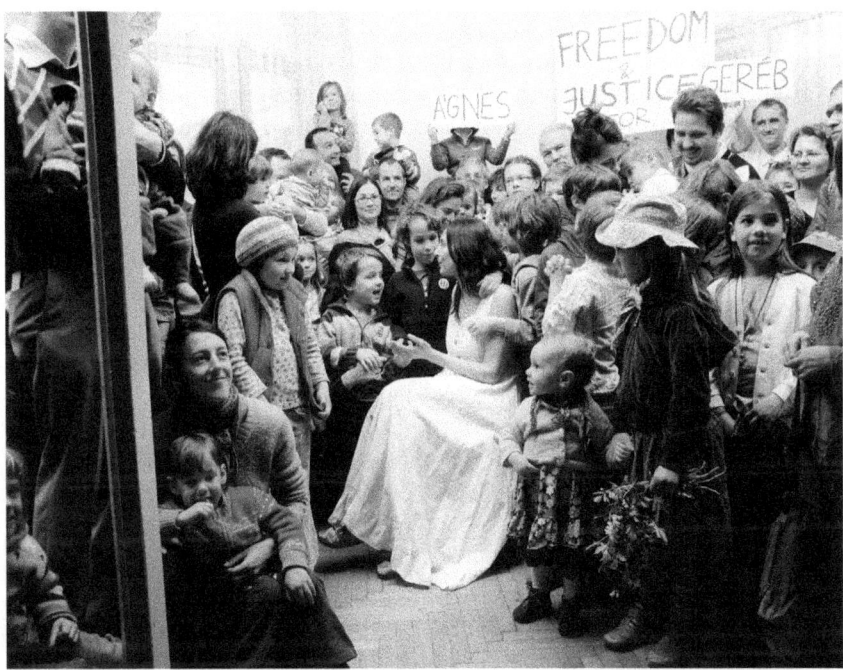

Figure 8.1. Ágnes's chair inside, surrounded by supporters inside her home during her house arrest, April 2013. © Éva Ágnes Molnár

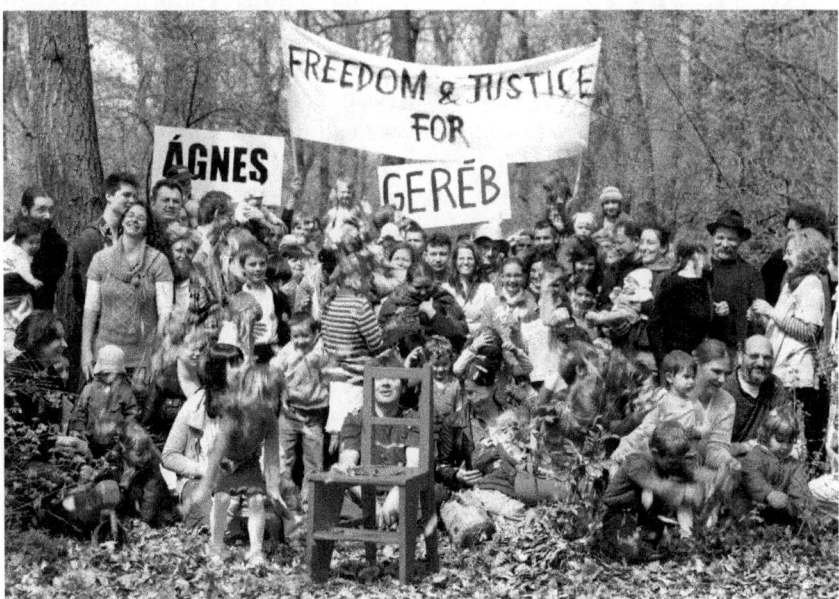

Figure 8.2. Ágnes' symbolic empty chair outside, surrounded by her supporters during her house arrest, April 2013. © Éva Ágnes Molnár

azságot Geréb Ágnesnek Mozgalom and Születésház Egyesület 2013). However, the Hungarian home birth movement is not about me and should not be seen as such, although I am heartened and encouraged that my persecutions have motivated others to pursue and achieve unexpected gains for all women.

A Major Victory in the European Court of Human Rights

The most far-reaching legal outcome of our movement is dated to 2010. An expectant mother, Anna Ternovszky, assisted by the Hungarian Civil Liberties Union (Társaság a Szabadságjogokért), filed an action against the government of Hungary with the European Court of Human Rights, alleging that her right to privacy had been violated, as she was unable to legally give birth at home with me in attendance due to the prohibition under Hungarian law for biomedical personnel to attend out-of-hospital births in Hungary. Anna won her landmark case: the court ruled that Hungary must recognize a mother's right to choose where and how she wishes to give birth as a human right (Ternovszky 2012). This case has since become an important part of what is now called the "Mothers' Revolution," as it has major implications for women, the interpretation of human rights, and expectations toward governments in the provision of health care. Even during pandemic times in 2021, Hungarian women marched to demand more humane treatment and elimination of violence against and mistreatments of newborns and mothers in hospitals both before and during giving birth (Csengel 2021). Activism to create opportunities for a safe and what we call *háborítatlan* (undisturbed) birth in post-communist Hungary is a natural extension of a worldwide movement that started many decades ago (see Goer 2004; Daviss 2005). I maintain that the birthing mother's own inner perception of safety is central to the success of giving birth. If she feels safe in the obstetrics department of a hospital and elects a cesarean birth, then this is an undisturbed birth for her. I now turn to a discussion of the "prison-hospital nexus" as I experienced it.

The Prison-Hospital Nexus: Applying Foucault's Analysis to Contemporary Hungary

"Geréb!"

It took several days for me to understand even a few of the rules in prison. When the prison guard called my family name, it meant that an attorney was there to see me or that I had to sign for a certified letter. On the other hand, the exaggerated first syllable of the word "Séééééta!" ("walk") signaled that I should be fully dressed in a coat and with a hat on, standing in silence, ready to step out of the door of my prison cell. It meant that I was allowed to leave my cell and walk in the courtyard of the prison for 60 minutes in this dreary October. Yet another shout meant that I could take a shower. I did not know any of this. How could I? Nobody bothered to tell me. You might miss the chance to go out of the cell this time, but when will the next time come? You do not know. You cannot predict. You eventually learn, however, that there are other signs that prepare you in advance. For example, there is the "pre-opening" when the guards open most of the locks on the main door to let the Head Prison Guard proceed to open the last lock so that the boss can move on without wasting time. Or, we can be waiting lined up for hours all dressed in winter clothes because there was a call—but the doors do not open. There are rules, but there is no instruction on these rules, and you are left behind if you do not follow the rules: no shower, no walk, nothing but the bare prison cell, in front of which many of my supporters gathered (see Figure 8.3).

This situation is eerily familiar and stunningly reminiscent of the hospitals where I trained as a doctor and worked for nearly two decades.

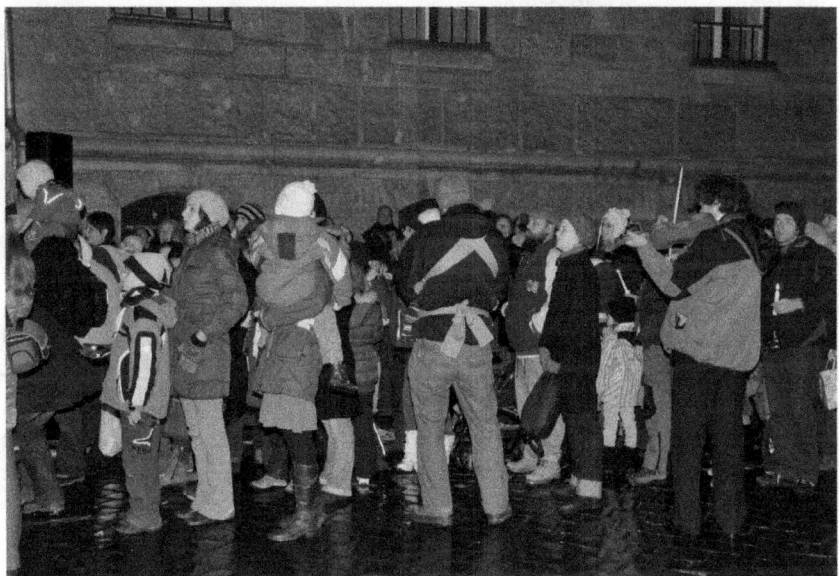

Figure 8.3. Protest in front of Ágnes's prison cell with hundreds of participants, December 20, 2010. © István Csintalan

Right before the Chair of Obstetrics and Gynecology starts his daily rounds with his entourage of subordinates and young doctors in training, an orderly rushes into the ward, alerting all the new mothers to clean up, take off their panties immediately, and tidy their surroundings, to be ready for the all-important whirlwind visit. There is no particular reason for the patients to clean up and be on their best behavior because only their charts are consulted: a quick look, then on to the next case. With younger medics in attendance creating a self-referential and insulated entourage, the patients' preparation does not substantively matter as far as their treatment is concerned. The patients do not understand the doctors' language; they live in very different worlds.

Prison was quite similar to the hospital. The rigidity of hierarchy separates the prisoners from the guards, although both are cut off from the outside world. This segregation reflects the insulation of staff from patients in hospitals. The power and information hierarchy are palpable, neatly separating the two classes. There is a clear pecking order within each of these institutions. The Chair of the Ob-Gyn Department occupies the highest level in the hierarchy of knowledge, then come the other specialists, then the young residents. The doctors' and prison guards' tight-knit communities are very much alike. Both prison guards and doctors cover for their colleagues, not only to maintain professional standards, but also for individual economic gain—similar to what Marsden Wagner (2008) described as "tribal obstetrics."

For example, I remember my immediate supervisor instructing me as a young doctor that not only was an episiotomy required at all births, but that the incision should not be sewn up too neatly. (Damaging episiotomies are routine in Hungary and many other countries, most especially in low-to-middle income countries, but they are much less frequently performed in Canada, the United States, and Western Europe; see Davis-Floyd 2022). Failure to suture meticulously creates further damage. I was told that a neatly sutured incision would require no further attention from a doctor in later years, which results in a loss of income for doctors. As long as a pregnant woman is seen as a source of income, doctors collude to ensure that more techniques and surgical instruments are used, which unethically drives up costs to the patients. A trained midwife can help avoid episiotomy altogether, saving the woman from a lot of suffering in the future (Wagner 2000). The independent midwife is thus perceived as economic competition and a serious challenge to the rigid and even abusive obstetric practices in hospitals.

The need to ensure continued revenue explains in part why doctors and prison guards have a tradition of protecting each other against any outside intervention. Their funding depends on them maintaining trust in the necessity of their work. Society trusts that they are working for the common good. This trust forms an invisible and exceptionally strong layer of inscrutability around both doctors and prison guards. They oversee life and death; they can tell you what is wrong with you, treat you in whatever way they feel is appropriate, and tell you when you can go home. All others—such as nurses, patients, and their families in a medical facility, or prisoners and the visitors in a prison—lack this sanctified knowledge, elevated responsibility, and importance. I realized this in prison as I saw the guards acting as if they knew everything. No one could question what they did or how they did it. Prisoners must follow orders, just like patients.

There are many layers of communication between biomedical professionals and patients, and only one of these is the spoken word. Doctors communicate with patients on multiple levels: delivering meaning, writing shorthand symbols, and performing silent yet real actions that produce the strongest emotional responses in patients, ranging from fear, humiliation, and dependence to security, joy, and pride. I see a similar use of verbal and non-verbal communication in this prison, this "total institution" (Goffman 1961), and I am part of it. These layers of communication and the corresponding social hierarchy feel strangely and comfortingly familiar, yet totally alien. I rejected this type of hierarchy and mode of communication after 17 years of practice at the Department of Obstetrics and Gynecology of the University of Szeged. Writing about France, Michel Foucault (1978) presented the emergence of the modern prison as a form of discipline enhanced by a new technological power that regulates the body and limits the questioning of power. He described this logic as applied to places such as schools, the military, and even hospitals, and my experiences in a Hungarian prison and in hospitals further highlight these parallels. In addition, my case highlights an unfair legal prejudice also found outside of Hungary: midwife-led adverse birth incidents become the subject of routine criminal investigation, whereas doctor-led hospital-linked adverse incidents are occasionally investigated by doctors' professional peers and rarely referred to the police for criminal investigation. No doctor in Hungary has faced such charges, much less been sentenced to prison or faced house arrest as I have.

A Very Personal Story of the Hungarian Homebirth Movement

I began to attend home births in 1989, and of the approximately 3,500 home births I have attended (about four to five per week on average[1]), no mother has suffered from birth complications. There was one birth fatality (the 2007 shoulder dystocia case), three cases of hypoxia (in 2000, the 2003 twin birth, and the case in 2010 that led to my arrest), and approximately 10% ended in hospital births (a typical figure for homebirth practices, including some cases requiring emergency hospital transfer). (The international average of planned home births that require hospitalization ranges between 10–20% [Johnson and Daviss 2005; de Jonge et al. 2009; Janssen 2009; Cheyney et al 2014]). Compared to general infant mortality rates in Hungary (5.04/1000 in 2009), one would expect about 18 infant deaths among these 3,500 births.

Above, I described the two cases of hypoxia. The third case led to my imprisonment. The mother of this boy was expecting her third child and planned to have a home birth when she contacted me after having taken the prenatal course that I organized. I advised against this plan because of the mother's health issue (a high thrombocyte count). When the mother arrived at the *Napvilág* Birth House for a fetal heartbeat check-up, she suddenly went into labor. When I arrived, she was already in the final (pushing) stage of labor. The child had a high birthweight and was not breathing at birth. Two midwives began normal resuscitation and called the paramedics specialized to take care of newborns, who took charge of resuscitation upon their arrival.[2] The child suffered permanent hypoxic damage. While the newborn was being resuscitated, the police arrived. Once the child had been taken to a hospital, the police arrested me and the two midwives who had taken part in the resuscitation. I was imprisoned without bail while awaiting trial, while the other two midwives were released after interrogation.

The newborn who died because of shoulder dystocia on the day of her birth on September 15, 2007, was the only neonatal death that occurred during more than two decades of my assisting home births in Hungary. Every mother I attended at home is healthy and well. Two mothers suffered from postpartum depression, and both were treated at home and able to continue breastfeeding—contrary to the usual Hungarian approach of hospitalizing the mother, treating her with medication, and separating her from her baby. In the home births that my colleagues and I attended, the connection between mother and baby was usually very healthy and strong, and we saw cases of postpartum depression extremely rarely. I believe that this rarity is also because we honored the natural birth process by waiting for physiology to take its course. We did not intervene unnecessarily, shame the mother, or rush her to "PUSH!"; we did not threaten that if she "breathes wrong she will kill the baby." Instead, our holistic birth practice offered unconditional support that reduces the fear of birth. Gentle birth can fundamentally empower women—a testament to the value of the homebirth movement in Hungary and to the strength its activist members found when connecting to similar movements all around the world.

I did not call what we were doing a "homebirth movement," but I now understand why others do. My incarceration in 2010, my house arrest, continued limitations on my movement and profession ever since, and the many years of parallel legal prosecution I have endured, make it even more obvious that the obstetric practices that I and others advocate for have indeed presented challenging alternatives to the existing biomedical, economic, social, cultural, and political orders, just as other social movements do. My series of punishments are part of an important message from the powers-that-be: "Do not attempt to challenge the status quo." But I did, although I only fully realize that in retrospect.

Our practice offered unconditional support and freedom of choice to individuals and communities. This triggered immense resentment and rejection among those who try to assert control over the people to whom they are supposed to be providing a service. What I understand now, having experienced the (mostly official) aggression toward me and other independent midwives, is that: "We, women, give birth knowing that everybody who is born will die, whatever we do. We, independent midwives who attend births, admit, and represent this fact and confront people with it. And this is a frightening fact until we are able to yield to and accept it" (Geréb 2013). I have argued that the freedom of a country can be measured by the freedom of birth it offers—and in this respect, we have a long way to go, and not just in Hungary. Since 1992, I have collaborated with other healthcare professionals and midwives to develop a set of values for holistic practice. From there, we established a few central points that became some of our most deeply treasured statements; for example, *Szabadon szülni, szabadnak születni* ("To be born free is to live free"); *A születés minősége az élet minősége* ("The quality of birth is the quality of life"); and *AprÓnként változtatjuk meg a világot*, which literally means we change the world step-by-step, but alludes to the tiny baby born as the step—we change the world baby-by-baby.[3]

It is difficult to explain but important to note that the education and biomedical training that I received in the Communist Era did not make it easy for me to establish such principles. I was trained as a biomedical doctor specializing in obstetrics and gynecology, one of a handful of women who chose this specialty in the 1970s in Hungary. It took a long time for me to develop my own approach, but I quickly realized that many others shared my thoughts on undisturbed birth and the importance of a balanced, non-hierarchical doctor-mother relationship. I learned to allow mothers to choose their birthing position and I advocated for this practice in the hospital. I slowly started to see that there were alternatives to the prevailing hospital practices in Hungary—alternatives that provided a less painful and less alienating birth experience. What fundamentally confirmed my way of practice was a set of three interconnected events.

First, a Hungarian doctor who had emigrated to the United States but came back to Hungary when expecting her ninth child asked me to attend her birth. She had given birth to eight children in the United States with her midwife in attendance and did not want to go to a hospital in Hungary. As there were no other options at that time, she was referred to me. After I attended the successful birth, she suggested that I visit her midwife, Bea Haber, in California, and they invited me in 1988 for a yearlong study tour.

Second, while we were waiting for the US visas, I voluntarily resigned from my position at the Department of Obstetrics and Gynecology at the University of Szeged. I had three small children at that time; thus, my family and I had to travel together, and this condition caused extensive delays in getting the visas. All the while, many expectant mothers who had been under my care still wanted to give birth with me in attendance. Because I no longer had hospital privileges, I could only attend these births if they took place in these expectant mothers' homes. These early homebirth experiences in 1988 and 1989 formed the foundation of my practice.

The third stage in the development of my medical philosophy took place during my four months of studying midwifery in the United States (only four months were left from the one-year leave by the time we got the visas). My experiences there did not create but rather confirmed the conclusions I had drawn from assisting home births in Hungary. I believe that we independent midwives speak a common language. The best thing about meeting independent midwives in the United States and at international conferences is speaking this common language—learning about various techniques is the icing on the cake. We support the birthing mother's natural processes and help her and her baby on their journeys. In our practice, we found that if this natural process is disturbed, the mother cannot go through the birthing process as easily and her child may experience distress. In Hungarian hospitals, birthing women are denied emotional support, food, and drink, and are subjected to shaving of the pubic area, enemas, frequent obtrusive vaginal examinations, fetal monitoring that immobilizes the woman, uncomfortable birthing positions, stirrups, threats both overt and subtle, and often extensive physical pressure on the abdomen to squeeze the baby out. These routine practices create disruptions and make the process a nightmare instead of a welcome passage through a changed consciousness toward the birth of one's child.

Nurses, teachers, psychologists, economists, midwives, mothers, and fathers have formed a collective of thousands of like-minded homebirth supporters in Hungary. There are also a few biomedical practitioners with a more humane approach to birth than the factory-like pseudo-scientific approach perpetuated in hospitals. In the early 1990s, I became one of the few obstetricians in Hungary (and possibly in Central Europe) who wholeheartedly supported what in Western Europe and North America became known in the 1970s as "alternative birth practice" (Goer 2004). I was becoming aware of this international movement because information about social movements and new scientific challenges to existing medical birth practices and birth-related psychology, history, and anthropology had just started to become available (DeVries et al. 2001). Because the required second language in our schools was Russian, our generation did not learn English and thus did not have access to such information.

In the late 1980s, there were already a few Hungarian nurse-practitioners who had worked in Western Europe; they most often had great difficulty finding a suitable place in the oppressive hierarchy so pervasive in hospitals. These harbingers of what would much later become a modern midwifery movement initially worked in isolation from one another. Despite a long history—as Deáky and Krász (2005) have demonstrated—and the well-established training and certification of independent midwifery, this profession had totally disappeared in Hungary and in much of the rest of then-Communist Europe by the 1950s. It is stunning to note how, during one generation, the repercussions of World War II and the Communist drive to control the population in every aspect succeeded in eradicating trust in home birth. In my practice, I often encountered grandparents and parents of women wanting to give birth at home who themselves were born at home with the help and support of a midwife. Because of the extensive propaganda that hospitals are the only safe place for a mother to give birth, even these close relatives who were themselves the obvious results of successful home births were often adamantly against their daughter or granddaughter giving birth outside of a hospital—even when an experienced obstetrician was able to attend.

A year after I started to work as a doctor at the Szeged University Hospital in 1977, I began to allow husbands in the delivery room. This practice was much welcomed by the mothers and their families, but it caused uproar among my colleagues—both doctors and obstetric nurses—and I faced sanctions at the university hospital for six months in 1980–1981. They were delighted when I became pregnant and took maternity leave in 1992. (Ironically, years later, the Director of this hospital declared proudly that his institute was the first to allow fathers into the labor room.) Because my supervisors threatened me with dismissal early in my medical career for my unorthodox views, I decided to expand my training. I gained a Master's of Science in psychology in 1982–86 and, as previously noted, qualified first as a certified (*okleveles*) midwife, and then in 2010, after a four-year training period, as an obstetric midwife (*diplomás szülésznő*).

The emerging demand to change birth practices seemed to echo the many freedom-oriented social and political changes in Hungary in the late 1980s and early 1990s. We as mothers, along with our families and interested biomedical professionals, were used to living in what became known as a "grey society," analogous to a "grey economy" in which workers are paid "under the table," leading to the development of an organic network of homebirth supporters. As BBC's Hungarian correspondent Nick Thorpe used to say, the situation was "a-legal, but not illegal." Developing under these constraints, the homebirth movement had reached thousands of supporters by the turn of the millennium.

In 1992, after many confrontations—both major and minor—with colleagues and the Szeged Hospital administration, I decided to organize an International Conference on Childbirth (Nemzetközi konferencia a születésről) in Szeged. At this conference, Kitty Ernst, Sheila Kitzinger, Michel Odent, and others discussed alternative birth practices. It was probably the first forum on this topic in Hungary; indeed, in the whole post-Communist region (Nemzetközi konferencia a születésről 1992). At this conference, I met many others who shared my beliefs. Kitty Ernst, a well-known nurse-midwife and internationally recognized expert and lecturer who helped to start accredited nurse-midwifery educational programs in the United States, held a workshop entitled "How to Establish a Birth House." This is where I met Kati Domján, a teacher of English and mother of six, who, at the end of Kitty's seminar, passed me a note: "Would you like to establish one too?" The answer was obvious, but with my attitude toward money, it was not an easy undertaking. Obstetrics is one of the highest-earning biomedical professions in Hungary. Although it pays a relatively low official salary, nearly all patients pay a significant amount of gratuity directly to the doctor. Much to the chagrin of my colleagues, I never accepted gratuities because I consider them to be bribes. Based on these values, establishing a new, "deeply humanistic" practice of birth meant more work and less income. (See the Series Overview at the beginning of this volume for a description by my friend and colleague Robbie Davis-Floyd of the differences between "superficial" and "deep" humanism.)

My colleague and friend Kati and I (along with our husbands) established the Alternatal Foundation (Alternatal Alapítvány), the first

Hungarian NGO dedicated to "woman- and child-centric" birth practices. Alternatal became a training center, hosting many internationally known midwives and biomedical experts as trainers. In 1993, Parliament allocated the sizable sum of 32.6 million Hungarian Forints in support of Alternatal, worth approximately 350,000 USD in 1993 prices, and about 720,000 USD in 2022. Thanks to a Soros Foundation loan, we were able to start the Birth House before the Parliament transferred the money. However, the Hungarian Board of Obstetricians and Gynecologists refused to issue an official review of the plan, thereby permanently blocking the transfer of funds. We had to sell the Birth House and repay the loan. For the next ten years, Kati's family gave a home to the birth house, called the "Daylight Birth House" (Napvilág Születésház). In 2007, with personal loans—and considerable physical help—from families whose children were born with me or with the other independent midwives, we bought an apartment and turned it into a birth house.

This fiasco of blocking the transfer of legislatively approved funds was just the first in a series of escalating conflicts with the biomedical establishment and eventually with the legal and political authorities. Instead of direct confrontation with that establishment and those authorities, Alternatal and associated NGOs, such as Mérce Egyesület, started publishing guides for the women who found their way to childbirth workshops because, beyond hearsay, there was very little information about the services in hospital obstetric departments (Mérce 1999, 2001). Alternatal's screening of normal pregnancies, courses for expectant parents, and efforts to establish a support structure by training a small group of independent midwives, plus extensive publishing activities, led a few thousand families to choose home birth. These individuals, along with their families and friends, were the ones who came out to protest my imprisonment in October 2010—the culminating event after years of escalating harassment by the police, the biomedical establishment, and the administrative authorities.

Pink Walls: Less than Half-Hearted Official Responses

The independent midwives and I often tried to speak with my former bosses at the Szeged University Hospital, with the administrators of hospitals in Budapest, and with the national government, about reforming the exclusively hospital-based, highly medicalized birth practices in Hungary. We had no policy success either prior to my imprisonment or in its aftermath, despite the worldwide attention that my incarceration had generated. What has taken place in response to both domestic and international pressure is what I call "painting the walls pink"—an example of "superficial humanism," resulting in little change, if any.

Since the passage of a seemingly major legal change in 2011 in Hungary regulating midwifery, only four midwifery practices (each of which consists of two midwives) have been able to overcome the obstacles created by the law. While the pressure from domestic constituents and international experts and organizations compelled the conservative-nationalist government to legalize home birth in March 2011 (*Magyar Közlöny* 2011), the price of legalization was strict regulation with prohibitively high insurance premiums and the requirement that participating doctors and midwives have a decade of specialized hospital experience. On December 11, 2011, the Hungarian government reduced the requirement from ten years of hospital experience to two years or supervised attendance at 50 home births. The price of midwifery service has become so high that only very well-to-do clients can afford it. Instead of becoming part of basic care, midwifery has become the privilege of a select few. Also, the midwifery service must be incorporated and running continuously, thereby causing a lot of stress to the provider, given that there are few clients. Midwives are excluded from attending births, leaving only pregnancy and postpartum care to which they can (legally) attend. Last, midwives' work is impossibly curtailed: midwives can only work with clients whom the gynecologist had pre-approved as low risk in their first trimester. The supposedly new, EU-conforming independent midwives have remained totally subordinate to the biomedical establishment. One of the consequences of the strict regulations has been that the independent midwives are so concerned about the precarity of maintaining their licenses that they adjust their homebirth practices to fit the hospital-presuming framework of the law. Even the best midwifery practitioners in Hungary have become excessively risk-averse and avoid collaboration with each other.

In response to increased interest in home birth and Hungarian media attention, a few hospitals started to offer alternatives to the highly regimented and alienating standard birth practices. These actions amount to less than half-hearted attempts to consider the birthing mother's and the newborn's needs. The "alternative" obstetric departments have started to allow birthing mothers to eat, drink, and walk around with their epidurals. Birth stools also appeared, but birthing women are advised not to use them for fear of "excess bleeding." Birthing pools made an appearance too, but the laboring women have to leave the water for all the examinations and the birth. Similarly, vaginal birth after cesarean (VBAC) has made an appearance in Hungarian hospitals, but only the best-prepared client may be able to avoid a second cesarean. A December 2015 VBAC case unfolded, in which a pregnant woman adamantly refused having her waters broken and undergoing an emergency cesarean, making the hospital staff so angry with her that they left her alone in the room, where she could peacefully and vaginally give birth to her child.

About 30 years ago when I attended a birth, someone asked me to "cut the umbilical cord only when and where it has to be cut." I did not understand the request, so the person explained that she wanted me "not to cut into the aura of the newborn." Well, I did not share such New Age-y beliefs, but I decided to wait and observe what was happening. I had never seen anything like it before. About 45 minutes after the birth, approximately 3–4 inches from the newborn's body, I saw a clear border on the umbilical cord, separating a thick, blue, warm, pulsating side from a lifeless, white, collapsed side that used to link to the mother. I was surprised that I had never noticed this separation before, although I had increasingly tried to distance myself from the time schedules dictated by clinical obstetric practice. Since then, I have always placed the clamp on the dead part of the umbilical cord, and to my knowledge neither I, nor any of the independent midwives, have incurred an infected umbilical cord, possibly because of this practice.

The Hungarian media carry only parts of the information that matters to the health of the mother and the newborn, and such news items create new demands. These new public demands tend to get a half-hearted response from the bureaucratic realm of Hungarian maternity care providers, leading to more problems than solutions. With Hungarian parents increasingly learning from the media to ask maternity care providers not to cut the umbilical cord while it is still pulsating, obstetric nurses now show the cord to the mother and check with the father that the umbilical cord has stopped pulsating. Then the nurse tends to cut the cord an inch from the baby's body, right into the part that is still fully open and connected to the newborn, thus risking infections even when the highest-quality instruments are used. Instead of half-hearted, superficial, and potentially risky gestures to satisfy demand, further medical studies and analysis of the practice of cutting the umbilical cord when and where it has already collapsed would be a useful step to consider so that we could provide better care to newborns (see ACOG 2020).

The Rejection of My Appeal and Its Consequences

On January 9, 2018, my appeal for the cases' de novo review was rejected, and the court reinstated the previous sentence, confirming the two-year prison sentence (as my 77-day-long prison and three-year-long house arrest were all preliminary, "protective" measures) and the ten-year-long professional prohibition to practice midwifery or obstetrics. While acrimonious debate followed across much of Hungarian media, local and international support mobilized with the message crying out, "She does not deserve a prison sentence!" On January 20, 2018, more than 2,000 supporters each brought a flower symbolic of gratitude, which were then placed on the Liberty Bridge over the Danube in Budapest, covering it in spring colors (see Figure 8.4). Activists in Budapest filmed the events and posted personal testimonies and pictures of the "flowers of gratitude" from all over the world.[4] More than 40,000 individuals signed a Change.org petition, and thousands of others sent a direct appeal in support of a Presidential clemency on my behalf, while notable international scholars and organizations (such as the International Confederation of Midwives and the International Federation of Gynecology and Obstetrics) issued public statements to help me gain my freedom after nearly a decade of prison, house arrest, and severe limitations on my movement and livelihood.[5] On the video documenting the collective action in January 2018, Joan Baez's "Carry It On" accompanies the thousands of bright flowers falling from the Liberty Bridge to the Danube. I hope we indeed carry on. I remain hopeful and grateful for the support.

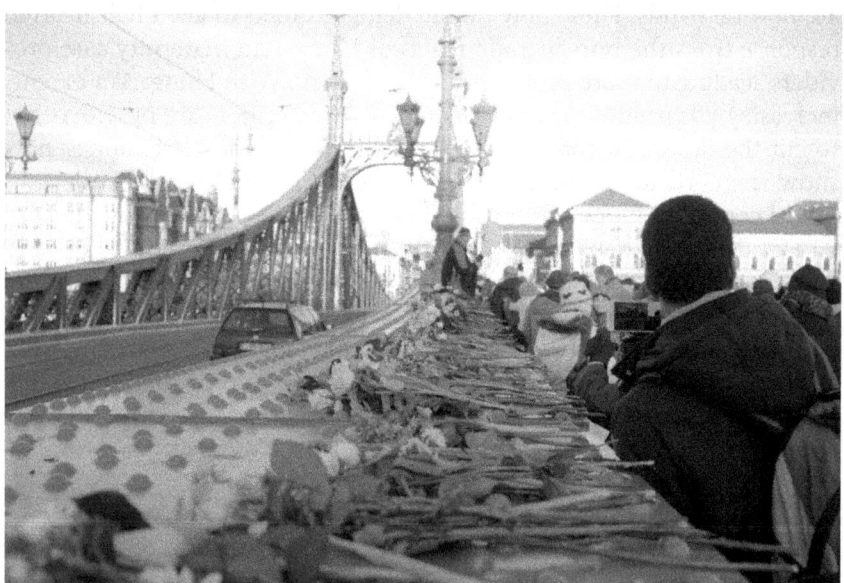

Figure 8.4. "Flowers of Gratitude," January 2018, Freedom Bridge, Budapest. © Jakab Erdély

Conclusions: Where Can We Go from Here?

"The freedom of a country can be measured by the freedom of birth" is a statement that I have often used to describe the importance of independent midwifery. Although it was difficult in many countries to re-establish the legitimacy of modern midwifery, to many observers both inside and outside Hungary, the many charges against me echo the Communist-Era show trials of the 1950s and are reminiscent of Inquisition-Era witch hunts (Varró 2009). My supporters and I believe that my trials created fears that have no factual basis; they are indicative of resentments toward midwifery and a rejection of women's freedom of choice. Both midwifery and freedom challenge hegemonic control. My trials sent out a powerful symbolic message to Hungarian society, expressing a strong "NO" to women claiming ownership over their own bodies and to an emerging small yet powerful trend of substantiating individual rights and democratic freedoms.[6]

Women wishing to give birth outside of hospitals are a fraction of a percent of pregnant women in Hungary. Such a small group, even with all their supporters, could not possibly pose a significant challenge to the biomedical establishment nor shake the foundations of their substantive economic interests. However, the political and biomedical authorities in Hungary perceive even the tiniest challenge as potentially lethal to them. In Robbie Davis-Floyd's terms (see Series Overview, this volume), this type of thinking represents a "Stage 1" authoritarian mindset that is fundamentally fearful and uncertain.

What could be the rationale of the political and biomedical authorities to engage in such oppressive practices? It is quite possible that the authorities' aim has never changed: to strengthen and re-establish control by creating fear even among those who are not directly affected. In Central and Eastern Europe, my case may be the most extreme at the moment, but it is surely not the only one against independent midwives. Independent midwives such as Lithuania's Jurgita Swedas and Czech midwives Ivana Königsmarkova and Zuzana Stromerova have also faced charges (Cameron 2011).

Despite, and perhaps because of, my continued and extensively publicized prosecution, our movement has achieved a great deal: people in Hungary now know about the problems of hospital birth, and many have heard about the gentler alternatives that we continue to advocate. And the right of a woman to choose the place and way she gives birth was established in 2011, thanks to Anna Ternovszky's case before the European Court of Human Rights.

At the same time, there is a great deal of work ahead of us. My imprisonment has created a deep sense of fear that has affected many people besides me and my immediate friends and family. The fear of being caught if they give birth at home has replaced the healthy and important questions that pregnant women used to raise at my prenatal workshops. The state with its disciplining apparatus has made its way even into the dreams of these pregnant women. It would be a life-affirming change if both pregnant women and I were rid of this waking nightmare and could truly live free.

On June 28, 2018, the President of Hungary, Dr. János Áder, granted me clemency so that I didn't have to serve another two years in prison. He did not, however, lift the ban on practicing for ten years. The "Free Ágnes Geréb" Facebook site had this to say about the announcement:

> Dr. Geréb has made the freedom of childbirth the centre of her life's work. Part of this work was her contribution to legislation that empowers the autonomy of women in childbirth. One result of her four decades of work is that the presence of fathers at childbirth, once forbidden, is now commonplace. Dr. Geréb has made a significant and lasting impact on Hungarian society by introducing undisturbed birth and fighting for the rights of women and their babies.[7]

After 40 years of dedicated work, my monthly retirement income does not reach 400 USD. I continue to advocate for undisturbed birth, to volunteer and work as a presenter, consultant, advisor, and expert on various reports and podcasts. I am a regular contributor to online trainings and have collaborated with other independent midwives to organize the first Hungarian Homebirth Conference. Within the network of homebirth supporters, I have been reviewing bills and regulations that our movement proposes to the Hungarian biomedical authorities and the government. I yearn to once again fully assist women who choose home birth. As my ten-year prohibition on attending births ended in 2022, I pursued every avenue to fulfill that yearning and satisfied every regulation to become reinstated in the profession. But I needed to sign up for the obligatory insurance coverage for midwives. Generali is the only insurance company in Hungary that has the permit to enter into such a contract and they refused to enter into one with me, thereby stopping me from attending births for the rest of my life. To slightly balance my sense of total defeat, in October 2022, I had the great honor of receiving the David Chamberlain Award of The Prenatal Sciences Partnership for having the bravery to advocate for the rights of unborn children at birth (see https://www.prenatalsciencespartnership.org/about-1). Although I now know that I will never again be able to attend births, I will always think of myself as a midwife, and will remain grateful for all the births that I have attended and for the women and their families who placed their faith in me to attend their births safely and respectfully.

Acknowledgments

We would like to thank Marie-Josée Sheeks for a very careful and caring review of this text. Relying on her scholarship and their many years of conversations, Katalin wrote this chapter in first person singular to best represent Ágnes' experiences, while Ágnes carefully reviewed and factually corrected the text.

Ágnes (Ági) Geréb graduated from the University of Szeged as a Doctor of Medicine in 1977. She finished her obstetrics residency in 1982. Between 1977–1994, Dr. Geréb worked as an obstetric resident and then as an obstetrician at the Albert Szent-Györgyi Clinical Center in the Obstetrics and Gynecology Department of the University of Szeged. In 1986, she obtained a Bachelor of Science in Psychology at the Eötvös Loránd University, Budapest. In 1989, she started an independent midwifery practice. In 1990, she participated in a six-month training in professional home birth practice in Livermore, UK. In 1994, she became a staff member of Daylight Birth Center. In 1997, Geréb was elected an Ashoka Fellow. In 2005, Geréb became a certified midwife (University of Debrecen). In 2010, she obtained a BSc in Midwifery from the Semmelweis University, Faculty of Health Sciences (Budapest). She founded the first and second birth centers in Hungary. She also founded the Hungarian Alternatal Foundation (1992) and co-founded the European Network of Childbirth Associations (1993) and the Association of Independent Midwives (2008). In 2022, Agnes was recognized for her bravery by the Prenatal Sciences Partnership with the David Chamberlain Award, offered to those who advocate and support the rights, health and wellbeing of the (un)born children, healing primal traumas, or working in the direction of gentle primal experiences.

Katalin Fábián is Professor of Government and Law at Lafayette College, Easton, PA. Her book *Contemporary Women's Movements in Hungary: Globalization, Democracy, and Gender Equality* (2009) analyzes the emergence and political significance of women's activism in Hungary. She edited *Globalization: Perspectives from Central and Eastern Europe* (2007) and *Domestic Violence in Post-Communist States: Local Activism, National Policies, and Global Forces* (2010). She coedited, with Ioana Vlad, *Democratization through Social Activism: Gender and Environmental Issues in Post-Communist Societies (2015). With Elżbieta Korolczuk, she coedited *Rebellious Parents: Parents' Movements in Central-Eastern Europe and Russia* (2017). Her most recent publication is *The Routledge Handbook of Gender in Central-Eastern Europe and Eurasia* (2021), coedited with Janet Elise Johnson and Mara Lazda, which earned the 2022 Heldt prize for Best Book in Slavic, East European, and Eurasian Women's and Gender Studies.

Notes

1. Editor's note: This number of home births that Agi attended—4–5 per week—is far higher than those of most other homebirth midwives working in high-income countries; they usually attend 2–5 births per month. Given what most other such homebirth midwives would experience as massive overload and stress, we find it amazing that Agi achieved the good results that she did.
2. The events on October 5, 2010 developed with intense succession. At birth, the baby did not begin breathing spontaneously. With the resuscitation administered by the two midwives, he became pink but was toneless. Immediately at birth, we called the Peter Cerny Alapítvány paramedics specialized in treating newborns. It turned out that they were busy and sent another type of ambulance trained to work with children. But before this latter ambulance arrived, I looked out the window and saw an ambulance. I assumed that it was the one that was trying to find its way to the Birth House, but as I only learned much later, it was just an ordinary ambulance with a driver and a trainee medic that happened to be there. I immediately sent out the father to show them the way. They came in and took charge of the baby, continuing the resuscitation. We were shocked to see that they lacked the skills necessary to work with a newborn, and the baby became blue. We had decided to take the child back again when the second team of ambulance workers arrived. We assumed that they were the specialized Cerny medics, but they turned out to be trained to work with children and not newborns. Under their care, the baby remained stable but did not improve. When eventually the Cerny ambulance arrived and took charge, the baby turned pink again, but during these 10 minutes or so in this condition, he suffered permanent damage.
3. The 2012 film by Frigyes Fogel carried this slogan as its title: *Szabadon szülni, szabadnak születni* (http://vimeo.com/37040564, removed July 29, 2013). Comments on the film's website indicate that those who left notes consider the prosecutions against me as "show trials" in the style of the 1950s Communist regime with fabricated evidence from ill-positioned witnesses and questionable procedures.
4. See Szabad Szülés. "Flowers of Gratitude for Dr. Agnes Gereb." *YouTube*, January 28, 2018. Retrieved September 16, 2022 from https://youtu.be/U1AYJTSxgTI, and Free Gereb Agnes, "Flowers of Gratitude for Dr. Ágnes Geréb." *Facebook*, January 28, 2018. Retrieved September 16, 2022 from https://www.facebook.com/freegereb/videos/vb.167283166621117/2031765950172820/?type=2&theater.
5. Since its creation in February 2018, by June 2018, 41,806 supporters had signed

the petition: "Freedom for Agnes." *Change.org*. Retrieved 16 September 2022 from https://www.change.org/p/everyone-freedom-for-agnes.
6. Editor's note: Ágnes offered a detailed review of her activities and how she challenged established but harmful customs from early on in her medical career to helping birthing mothers, babies, the whole family, and society. See Ágnes Geréb, "Last Plea" Budapest, April 20, 2017, http://www.otthonszules.hu/last-plea-budapest-20th-april-2017.
7. "Free Gereb Agnes." Retrieved 16 September 2022 from https://www.facebook.com/freegereb/posts/pfbid021g17yYwePYGTeNECC9XnD8K8cMfE4AdjsN17EfeSXiackWvf6W7FdrdA8tHJS6GLl.

References

American College of Obstetricians and Gynecologists (ACOG). 2020. "Committee Opinion # 814. Delayed Umbilical Cord Clamping after Birth." *Obstetrics & Gynecology* 136(6): 1238–1239.

Cameron R. 2011. "Home Births on Trial after Boy Left with Brain Damage in Botched Delivery." *Radio Praha*, 17 January. Retrieved 16 September 2022 from http://www.radio.cz/en/section/curraffrs/home-births-on-trial-after-boy-left-with-brain-damage-in-botched-delivery.

Csengel, K. 2021. "Ahol erőszakkal kezdődik az élet, ott milyen lehet élni?" [How can one live in a country where life starts with violence?] Mérce.hu. https://merce.hu/2021/11/30/egy-olyan-orszagban-ahol-eroszakkal-abszurd-korulmenyek-kozott-kezdodik-az-elet-ott-milyen-lehet-elni/. November 30.

Davis-Floyd R. 2022. *Birth as an American Rite of Passage*, 3rd edn. Abingdon, Oxon: Routledge.

Daviss BA. 2005. "From Calling to Career: Keeping the Social Movement in the Professional Project." In *Mainstreaming Midwives: The Politics of Chage*, eds. Davis-Floyd R, Johnson CB, 413–445. New York: Routledge.

Deáky Z, Krász L. 2005. *Minden dolgok kezdete: A születés kultúrtörténete Magyarországon (XVI–XX. század)* [*The beginning of everything: The cultural history of birth in Hungary between the 16th and the 20th centuries*]. Budapest: Századvég.

de Jonge A, van der Goes BY, Ravelli AC, et al. 2009. "Perinatal Mortality and Morbidity in a Nationwide Cohort of 529, 688 Low-Risk Planned Home and Hospital Births." *BJOG: An International Journal of Obstetrics and Gynaecology* 116(9): 1117–1184.

DeVries R, Benoit C, van Teijlingen E, Wrede S, eds. 2001. *Birth by Design: Pregnancy, Maternity Care, and Midwifery in North America and Europe*. New York: Routledge.

En God Start i Livet [A good start to life] [Danish NGO]. 2013. "Sajtóközlemény—dr. Geréb Ágnes nemzetközi szakmai díjat kapott" [Press release: International recognition of Dr. Geréb].

Geréb Á. 2000. "About a Little Baby Girl." 6 March.

———. 2013. "The Lawsuit: Anna Ternovszky against Hungary State." Speech at Human Rights in Childbirth Conference, Eugene, Oregon, USA. April 2. http://www.humanrightsinchildbirth.com/ternovszky-vs-hungary/agnes-gereb.

Goer H. 2004. "Humanizing Birth: A Global Grassroots Movement." *Birth* 31(4): 308–314.

Goffman E. 1961. *Asylums: Essays on the Condition of the Social Situation of Mental Patients and Other Inmates*. Garden City NY: Anchor Books.

Igazságot Geréb Ágnesnek Mozgalom (IGÁM), Születésház Egyesület. 2013. "Press Release: Geréb Ágnes és az otthonszülés helyzetét továbbra sem tartja megnyugtatónak az ENSZ" [The UN considers problematic the situation of Ágnes Geréb and home birth]. 21 March.

Hope P, Breslin S, Lamont L, et al. 1998. "Fatal Shoulder Dystocia: A Review of 56 Cases Reported to the Confidential Enquiry into Stillbirths and Deaths in Infancy." *British Journal of Obstetrics and Gynaecology* 105: 1256–1261.

Janssen P, Saxell L, Page L, et al. 2009. "Outcomes of Planned Home Births with Registered Midwife Versus Planned Hospital Birth with Midwife or Physician." *Canadian Medical Association Journal* 181(6–7): 377–383.

Johnson KC, Daviss BA. 2005. "Outcomes of Planned Home Births with Certified Professional Midwives: Large Prospective Study in North America." *British Medical Journal* 330 (7505): 1416.

Magyar Közlöny. 2011. "Kormányrendelet az intézeten kívüli szülés szakmai szabályairól, feltételeiről és kizáró okairól" [Professional regulations, conditions and exclusions on giving birth outside of institutions]. *Magyar Közlöny* 35(29): 5119. http://www.complex.hu/jr/gen/hjegy_doc.cgi?docid=A1100035.KOR.

Medvegy, G. 2017. "Fogházba küldenék Geréb Ágnest" [Wanting to send Ágnes Geréb to Prison] July 21. 24.hu https://24.hu/belfold/2017/07/21/foghazba-kuldenek-gereb-agnest/

Mérce Egyesület. 1999. *Születéskalauz*. Budapest: Mérce Egyesület.

———. 2001. *Születéskalauz 2*. Budapest: Mérce Egyesület.

Nemzetközi konferencia a születésről [International Conference on Childbirth]. 1992.

Simon Z. 2014. "Orban Says He Seeks to End Liberal Democracy in Hungary." *Bloomberg*, 28 July. Retrieved 16 September 2022 from http://www.bloomberg.com/news/articles/2014-07-28/orban-says-he-seeks-to-end-liberal-democracy-in-hungary.

Tavares R. 2013. *Situation of Fundamental Rights: Standards and Practices in Hungary*. European Parliament A7-0229/2013. 2 July. Retrieved 16 September 2022 from https://www.europarl.europa.eu/doceo/document/CRE-7-2013-07-02-INT-2-454-000_EN.html?redirect.

Ternovszky, Anna. 2012. "Speech at Human Rights in Childbirth Conference." The Hague, The Netherlands.

Varró, Szilvia. 2009. "És máglyát is raknak?: Geréb Ágnes nőgyógyász, az otthon szülés hazai népszerűsítője" [Will they also prepare to burn her at the stake? Gynecologist Ágnes Geréb]. *Magyar Narancs*, 24 September, No. 39.

Wagner M. 2000. "Technology in Birth: First Do No Harm." *Midwifery Today*. Retrieved 10 December 2021 from https://www.midwiferytoday.com/web-article/technology-birth-first-no-harm/.

———. 2008. *Born in the USA: How a Broken Maternity System Must be Fixed to Put Women and Children First*. New York: Penguin.

Wiedemann T. 2021. "Nem állnak le a kismamák a hálapénzzel, mert igénylik a személyes szolgáltatást" [Pregnant women do not stop giving additional money because they want personal attention]. *Free Europe*, 12 November. Retrieved 16 September 2022 from https://www.szabadeuropa.hu/a/nem-allnak-le-a-kis-mamak-a-halapenzzel-mert-igenylik-a-szemelyes-szolgaltatast/31551864.html.

CHAPTER 9
Adopting the Midwifery Model of Care in India
Evita Fernandez

More than 40 years ago, I trained as an obstetrician. I never envisioned shifting my focus to the midwifery philosophy of care. My views have altered dramatically. I am now a fierce advocate for woman-centered respectful care for birth, and I deeply believe that adopting the midwifery collaborative model of care is the most appropriate option for my country, India.

Background and Context

India accounts for around 25 million births each year. However, 35,000 women die of pregnancy-related complications and 2.7 million babies are stillborn every year. Most of these deaths occur during childbirth and are preventable (WHO 2020). Almost 80% of all births in India occur in public health facilities where women are incentivized to give birth in these facilities with cash transfers or essential "kits" from national and state-level government programs[1] (Ministry of Health and Family Welfare 2019–21). Yet India's maternal mortality ratio (MMR)— 113/100,000 live births—remains high despite programs and incentives to improve maternal health (Ved and Dua 2005). The day of birth is the most dangerous time for mothers and babies: 46% of all maternal deaths and 40% of neonatal deaths happen during labor or in the first 24 hours after birth (Ministry of Health and Family Welfare 2015–16) (see Figure 9.1.).

There is convincing scientific evidence that maternal deaths can be prevented by the presence of a skilled birth attendant during labor,

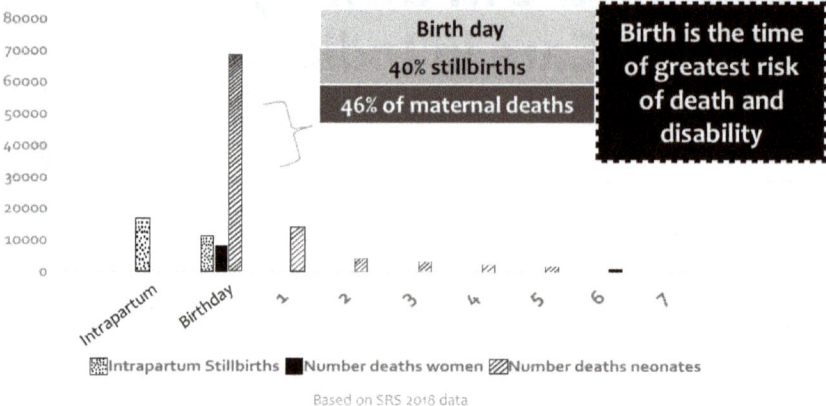

Figure 9.1. Birth days are the greatest risk to mothers and newborns. © Evita Fernandez

birth, and the immediate postpartum period (Mavalankar, Raman, and Vora 2011). However, the strongly biomedicalized birthing environments that characterize childbirth in India entail multiple unnecessary interventions, including an unacceptably high cesarean birth (CB) rate of 47.4% in private hospitals. The national cesarean rate is 21.5% of total institutional births, and the CB rate in public facilities is relatively low, at 14.3% (Ministry of Health and Family Welfare 2019–21). Nevertheless, due to obstetricians' over-medicalization of births, India faces an enormous challenge in promoting and establishing midwife-led care. Yet I have hope in the power of women's voices. World history has shown us enough examples of revolutions led by women that have caused significant changes in society; here are three such examples:

- Rosa Parks, an icon of the civil rights movement in the United States and a lifelong activist.
- Dr. Kadambini Ganguly, who succeeded in opening the doors of Calcutta Medical College for women to become doctors in India.
- Ina May Gaskin, who inspired midwives to implement humane ways of birthing and to provide women with the chance to choose the way they birth.

In India, where one of the two official languages of the Union government is English (the other is Hindi), the title "midwife" is used for various nursing cadres. It is poorly understood that midwifery is a unique profession or that the "midwife" (as defined by the International Confederation of Midwives[2]) is a highly qualified, competent, healthcare professional colleague accountable for two lives under her care. We have two distinct nursing groups:

1. Auxiliary Nurse Midwife (ANM): ANMs with an 18-month training program are now officially called Multipurpose Workers (MPWs) with a broad set of responsibilities. Some obtain additional training to manage birth and refer women with complications to higher levels of care, and some obtain additional training for the insertion of intrauterine devices. The ANM is a village-level female health worker—the first contact between the community and the health services.
2. General Nursing and Midwifery (GNM): A paramedical diploma course with a span of three years. The curriculum involves general health care, nursing, and midwifery.

In this chapter, I describe two parts of my midwifery journey: (1) the work I have done within the Fernandez Hospital in the southern city of Hyderabad, India; and (2) the consulting and advocacy work that my colleagues and I have done to help change the views and practices of midwifery across India and to introduce a professional cadre of midwives across the country. Founded in 1948, Fernandez Hospital today is a tertiary referral perinatal center of 320 beds and an annual birth rate of 10,000. Initially, my parents had set up a two-bed maternity clinic called "Stork Home," which over the years became firmly established and known as Fernandez Hospital. They handed the reins over to me in 1985.

Part I: Within the Fernandez Hospital System

As an obstetrician trained in India, I was under the mistaken impression that women needed us to help them give birth. I was at the peak of my obstetric career, riding the crest and believing I was indeed a woman-centered, sensitive, and excellent clinician. However, I was rudely awakened by two "lightbulb moments."

My First "Lightbulb Moment"

In the early 1990s, I discovered a book by Nutan Pandit called *Pregnancy: The Complete Childbirth Book* (2005). I resonated with Pandit's views about treating pregnancy as a natural, normal, physiologic event. Pregnancy, labor, and birth need to be enjoyed. I recommended the book to all the mothers who were under my care, and I encouraged pregnant women to enjoy their pregnancy, and to indulge in activities that they liked, including swimming, walking, and eating healthy foods.

In 2007, I invited Nutan Pandit to run an antenatal childbirth preparation course at Fernandez Hospital. I sought permission to join one of her classes to help understand what was being taught. To my utter horror and dismay, I discovered that our practices in the labor and birthing rooms were out of sync with Nutans's teachings. I discovered that we were horribly interventional. We were not woman-centered.

My Second Lightbulb Moment

By 2007, as noted above, Fernandez Hospital had grown into a tertiary perinatal referral center. Obstetric colleagues within the city of Hyderabad and across the state referred women with complex needs for antenatal care and delivery. Sometimes young women with multiorgan failure would arrive, and heart-wrenchingly, it was too late to save them. I began reading about maternal mortality and discovered that wherever midwifery care formed the backbone of maternity services, the ratios of maternal and infant mortality were low. Sweden, Denmark, the UK, and our neighbor, Sri Lanka, demonstrated this fact (Högberg 2004). India did not have such a unique professional cadre of midwives. In 2010, Andy Beckingham, a public health consultant from the UK, was in India, and my colleagues and I shared our dream of starting a midwifery training program with him. We had a vision in mind but lacked the understanding and the tools to make it happen. Andy returned to the UK, and several months later wrote to say that he was willing to help. He offered to devote one year of his life to this cause. He did not want any remuneration. All he wanted was to be housed and fed!

Launch of the In-House Midwifery Program at Fernandez Hospital

Andy researched the midwifery curricula of different countries. In 1974, the Indian Nursing Council (INC) had introduced a one-year, post-basic diploma course for registered nurses who wished to qualify as midwives. The curriculum had a strong nursing element and an equally strong biomedicalized approach to pregnancy, labor, and birth. A qualifying exit exam certified the nurse as a Nurse Practitioner in Midwifery. The INC believed that midwives should have a nursing background. However, this course did not attract nurses, as there was no clear career path or understanding of their role. We decided to amalgamate the curriculum of the INC with the core clinical competencies of the International Confederation of Midwives (ICM). This resulted in a two-year structured training program with 80% of the time spent in clinical training. A qualifying exit exam at the end of two years, followed by one year of preceptorship (apprenticeship), certified the trainee as a midwife. This resulted in the trainees' engagements in a comprehensive three-year journey. For ideological reasons, we opted to call them "midwives" instead of "nurse-midwives" because we wanted to establish midwifery as being separate from the nursing profession. Our objective was to aim for global standards in both training and clinical competencies achieved by the trainees. We were conscious of the fact that a new "professional entity"—the professional midwife who is trained in the midwifery model of care—was being introduced into the hospital workforce (see Figure 9.2).

It was a major challenge to create a new working relationship: to make everyone understand the role of a professional midwife, to practice and teach woman-centered care, and, most importantly, to unlearn what had been taught. However, as Paulo Coelho noted, "When you want something, all the universe conspires in helping you to achieve it"—and

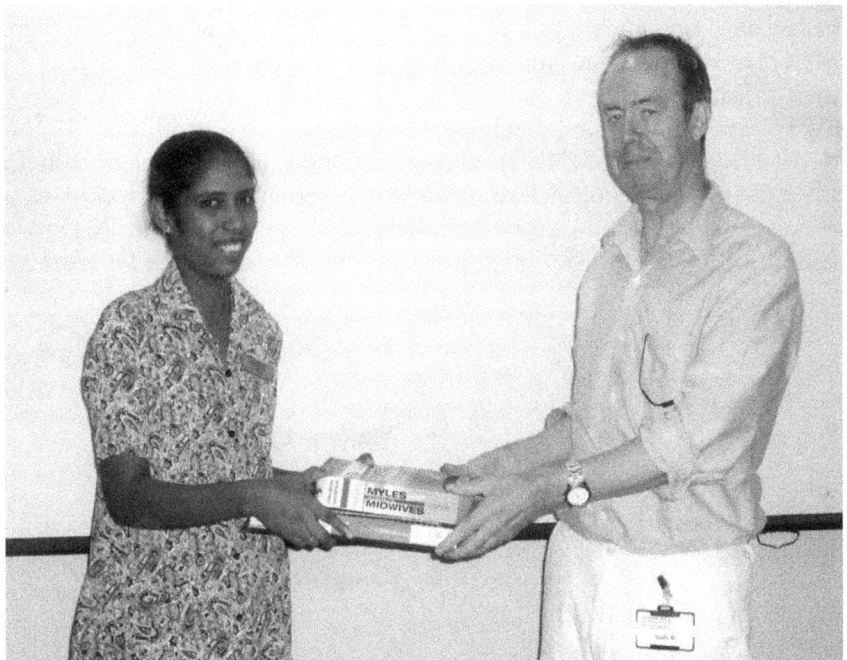

Figure 9.2. Andy with a midwife in India. © Fernandez Foundation

I believe that, in our case, it did. The program was launched on August 15, 2011 with seven very brave nurses who decided to step into the unknown. Twelve weeks into the program, I received an email from Becky Reed, a senior British midwife with more than two decades of clinical experience, offering to train the pilot group. Becky had led the highly successful Albany practice in the UK, which had achieved a 43% homebirth rate among its clients (with a very low perinatal mortality rate) before it was suddenly shut down, most likely because of that high homebirth rate. (For a description of the Albany practice in its heyday, see Reed and Walton 2009. For an analysis of its statistical outcomes, see Homer et al. 2017. For a description of its closure, see Reed and Edwards, forthcoming).

Becky came on board as the first midwifery educator for the Professional Midwifery Education and Training (PMET) Program of Fernandez Hospital. She challenged the existing infrastructure and thinking at Fernandez. She looked at the stirrups in birthing rooms and asked why those were needed. Such queries made us seriously question all aspects of our practice. The more I read and understood midwifery philosophy, the more I was convinced of the need to change. I shared blogs and research articles with my obstetric colleagues. We debated, discussed, and finally were convinced of the need to change. The change was possible because we saw the impacts of midwifery care on the women we served. My obstetric colleagues noticed that women were seeking midwives as their primary caregivers.

Following on Becky's heels were several midwives from the UK National Health Service (NHS) who volunteered time and talent to help strengthen the in-house PMET program. Fernandez Hospital owes a massive debt of gratitude to each one of these women. In 2015, we launched the PROMISE campaign with four objectives (see Figure 9.3).

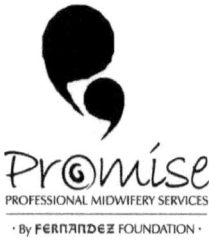

- **Make pregnancy safe**
- **Humanize birthing**
- **Train a workforce**
- **Promote midwifery**

Figure 9.3. PROMISE campaign. © Evita Fernandez

PROMISE helped to establish and endorse our commitments to midwifery, natural birth, and respectful care for every pregnant woman and her newborn. A simple feedback form introduced in 2014 helped to reinforce these radical changes in our practices. The Tables below show the questions asked (Table 9.1) and the change in the grading of excellence thereof (Table 9.2). A gradual change in the grading can be seen in Table 9.2. While mothers rated us at 81.8% in the year 2015, 2020 saw an overall 96% "excellent" ranking, thus validating the midwifery model of care at Fernandez Hospital.

By late 2021, a total of 51 midwives had gone through the course to become clinically certified, qualified midwives. Sadly, only 28 are currently working with us. Marriage and relocation to areas where they cannot pursue their trainings and careers are challenges that prevent these young professionals from continuing to work as midwives. As ob-

Table 9.1. Eight key questions addressed to mothers birthing at Fernandez Hospital with a midwife as their primary caregiver. The questions were carefully curated to gauge how the mothers felt and whether or not they had a positive birth experience. © Evita Fernandez

	A lot	Mostly	Average	A Little	None
I felt that my midwife valued me as a woman and not just as a "patient."					
I felt trust in my midwife during my labor and the birth.					
My midwife explained my options for pain relief and walking around.					
My midwife explained my options during labor and childbirth for things like which position I might give birth in.					
My midwife respected my choices about labor and birth.					
I felt that my midwife listened to me carefully.					
I felt confident that my midwife is a very skilled professional.					
I would recommend the midwives to my friends when they have their babies.					

Table 9.2. Maternal satisfaction grades. © Evita Fernandez

	Excellent	Good	Average	Poor
2020* Total sample (82)	79 (96%)	2 (3%)	1 (1%)	0 (0%)
2019 Total sample (747)	699 (94%)	45 (5.6%)	3 (0.4%)	0 (0%)
2018 Total sample (948)	883 (94%)	60 (5.5%)	5 (0.5%)	0 (0%)
2017 Total sample (1475)	1321 (89.5%)	126 (8.5%)	20 (1.3%)	8 (0.7%)
2016 Total sample (1054)	903 (85.7%)	136 (12.9%)	9 (0.9%)	6 (0.6%)
2015 Total sample (1029)	842 (81.8%)	166 (16.1%)	15 (1.5%)	6 (0.6%)

*In 2020, due to COVID lockdown, the feedbacks received from mothers were limited in numbers.

stetricians, a lot of what we were taught needed to be unlearned. We were trained to look at birth as a catastrophe waiting to happen. Nearly all laboring women were hooked onto an intravenous line "just in case" something might happen. Somewhere in our professional lives, we had forgotten that a woman's body that holds and nurtures a baby could also birth that baby, if only we obstetricians would allow her to do so, if only we had the humility and conviction to step back and watch nature unfold itself in this sacred event. We had to unlearn and open our minds to re-learning the physiology of birth. We learned to look at birth in a whole new manner, taking a 180-degree turn in our approach.

Challenges

- There was no role model for our trainees to emulate or understand a professional midwife's vital roles and responsibilities.
- Combating the age-old tradition of doctors attending every birth was a significant challenge. I had to introduce a new type of professional while facing the fears and prejudices of my obstetric colleagues.
- The solid patriarchal environment had to be cracked as the midwifery trainees empowered with evidence-based practices began to question old beliefs.

- New working relationships had to be built. Obstetricians and midwives needed to work together as colleagues with mutual respect and trust.

The Impacts of Midwifery Care at Fernandez Hospital

The positive impacts of midwifery care have been palpable. Here are the three areas that experienced them the most (see Figures 9.4, 9.5, and 9.6):

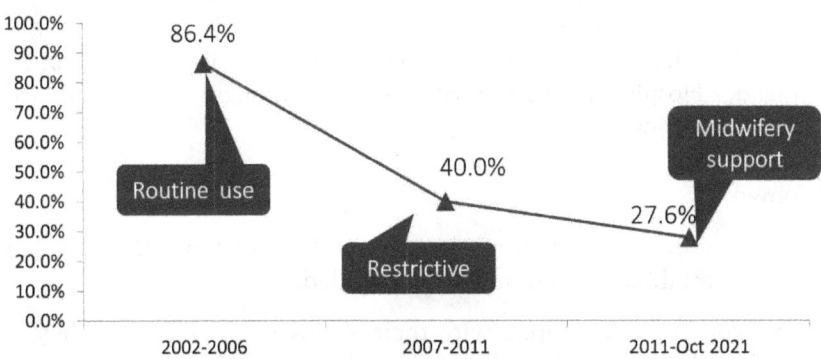

Figure 9.4. Episiotomy rates in spontaneous vaginal births from 2011 to 2021 at Fernandez Hospital. © Evita Fernandez

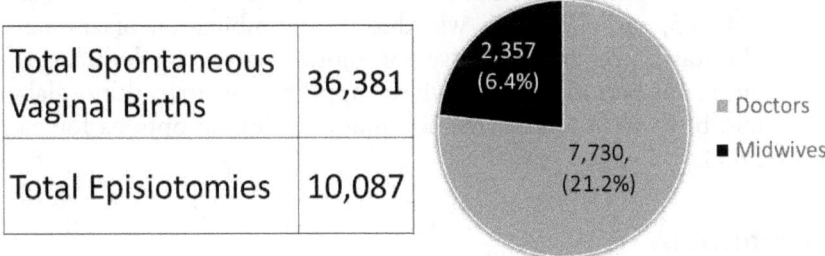

Figure 9.5. Midwife-attended births displayed a lower incidence of episiotomies compared with obstetrician-attended births. © Evita Fernandez

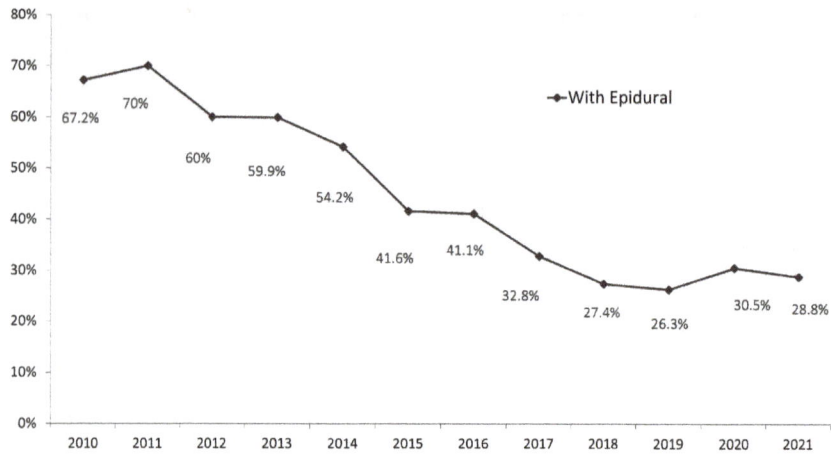

Figure 9.6. Reduction in use of epidural analgesia for vaginal births at Fernandez Hospital, due to midwifery support throughout labor and birth. © Evita Fernandez

Women

At Fernandez Hospital, from August 2011 to October 2021, 15,237 (41%) of total births were midwife-attended.

- Women were happier with their birthing experiences as they felt heard, supported, and encouraged by the continuity of care offered by the midwives (see Table 9.2 above).
- Women were supported by midwives to birth in positions of choice and felt they were involved in decision-making.

Hospital Practice

- Interventions: episiotomies and epidurals saw a decrease (Figures 9.4, 9.5, and 9.6). This was due to a combination of antenatal childbirth preparation classes, promoting natural birth during the antenatal period, and midwives supporting women during labor and birth with alternative non-pharmacological options for pain relief.

Obstetricians

The obstetricians discovered the benefits of the collaborative model of care, wherein women with complex needs were able to enjoy midwifery support. Women laboring and birthing in positions of their choice was a new concept, and some obstetricians sought permission to observe midwives working with birthing women to better understand the physiology of normal birth. This led new working relationships of mutual respect and trust. Hierarchies were very slowly beginning to erode.

How Our Practices Changed in Other Ways

Now that we understood what woman-centered care was all about, we discussed women's birth plans, encouraged them to attend childbirth preparation classes, and worked with the physiotherapy department in seeking optimal birth positions for women with musculo-skeletal dysfunction. Skin-to-skin, delayed cord clamping, healthy eating and drinking during labor, and physiologic third stage grew into default processes. We also explored non-pharmacological options for pain relief, and hydrotherapy leading to water births became a real option. Everyone worked sincerely toward minimizing separation between mother and newborn. Skin-to-skin was offered in operation theaters if a CB was warranted. The newborn was with the mother in the post-operative recovery room to initiate early breastfeeding. The baby was kept warm in a thermal blanket known as "Embrace," made of Phase-Change Material (PCM) (PCMs release/absorb sufficient energy at phase transition to provide useful heat/cooling), as post-operative recovery rooms have lower room temperatures. Younger obstetricians joined midwives and physiotherapists for workshops to learn about midwife Gail Tully's "spinning babies" method and its importance in helping avoid a CB wherever possible. ("Spinning babies" helps fetuses to put themselves into vertex, or head-first, presentation for vaginal birth.) This led to an active interest in a workshop on breech births taught by Dr. Shawn Walker.

The impacts of the in-house midwifery program include the following:

- Practices in the labor and birthing suites of Fernandez Hospital underwent radical humanistic changes.
- Antenatal outpatient clinics led independently by qualified midwives today have a waiting time of two weeks for an appointment, showing that the care provided by such midwives is highly desired.
- Dedicated clinics for VBACs (vaginal births after cesarean) and vaginal breech births led by midwives offering counseling and collaborative care have been established.
- A midwife-led birthing unit was set up in 2019 alongside the obstetric-led unit.

Part II: Advocacy and Change in India

In this section, I will share with you the ways in which we have tried to increase awareness and availability of midwifery services in the country.

The National Midwifery Task Force

In June 2016, UNICEF called for an All-India Conclave to discuss India's spiraling CB rate of 17.2% across the country. This rate may seem very low, not needing change, but it doesn't reflect the very high rates of CBs in numerous Indian hospitals in urban areas. And the current health survey for 2019–2021 records a national increase to 21.5%—clearly, this number will keep growing if we don't intervene. A mix of public health experts, obstetricians, and executives from the Ministry of Health and Family Welfare came together to seek solutions. Midwifery was considered one of the options to help reduce the CB rate. Following the conclave, the Fernandez team was invited to be on the National Midwifery Task Force (NMTF), which brought together representatives from the Ministry of Health, the Indian Nursing Council, global funding agencies, the Federation of Obstetric and Gynecological Societies of India (FOGSI), and other stakeholders from across the country. We met at regular intervals to discuss how midwifery could be rolled out and scaled up in India. As members of NMTF, we were responsible for the overall implementation of midwifery services in the country, and to ensure that the education and training of the Midwifery Educators (MEs) and Nurse Practitioner Midwives (NPMs) was in line with international best practices.

In January 2017, Ms. Inderjeet Kaur (MSc, RM, RGN), a consultant midwife at the National Health Service, UK, with more than 20 years of clinical experience, took a sabbatical from her job to join us in helping to promote and establish midwifery care in Fernandez Hospital. In 2018, she became the Director of Midwifery Services. Indie (as she is popularly known) has been a key factor influencing our commitment and progress in India's midwifery journey.

The Launch of Midwifery in Telangana State

In June 2017, the Government of Telangana State invited the Fernandez Foundation to run a midwifery training program for its first cohort of 30 registered nurses.[3] Ms. Karuna Vakati, Commissioner, Health and Family Welfare, Government of Telangana, envisioned midwifery as a vital need to help serve rural areas of the state where there was an acute shortage of doctors. She challenged us to bring respectful maternity care into public hospitals, in addition to clinical skills and competencies. UNICEF facilitated this unique tripartite venture.

The pilot cohort of 30 registered nurses was diverse in terms of age and years of clinical experience. At the very beginning, ground rules were laid for both trainers and trainees. We emphasized the need to be respectful of each other before we could offer respect to the women we served. This meant addressing each other by name or using a prefix if required. The trainees were encouraged to voice their opinions on topics being discussed and to clarify all doubts, no matter how trivial these may have appeared to them. In short, we began to build an environment of respect and trust. This approach led to sharing personal birth stories, tears, and healings of traumatic memories. The cohort felt united and decided they would be "agents of change"—a slogan they carved into their hearts.

Indie, assisted by Kate Stringer, a midwife from the UK, along with five midwives qualified from the in-house PMET program, formed the faculty for this clinically intense 18-month course. The trainers worked alongside the trainees in antenatal clinics and labor and birthing rooms, and held bedside case discussions. We also conducted workshops on respectful maternity care, obstetric emergencies, vaginal breech births, and basic life support. The trainees were well-equipped to handle emergencies. Every attempt was made to ensure that respectful, woman-centered care was the common thread through the entire program. The impact of this effort was evident in the small but vital changes that took place in the District Hospital. (The term "District Hospital" refers to a hospital at the secondary referral level responsible for a district of a defined geographical area containing a defined population. In India, the population size of a district varies from 35,000 to 30,00,000 [Ministry of Health & Family Welfare, India, 2012]). For example, more seating was arranged for pregnant women in the antenatal clinic; and initial screening was done to help segregate first bookings, term pregnancies, and women with complex needs. These arrangements helped obstetricians focus on the women who needed their care, while the midwife trainees were taught to care for the low-risk, uncomplicated pregnant women. Childbirth preparation classes were introduced for small groups of women while they were waiting for their antenatal check-ups. Advice on diet and physical activities was offered in an interactive format where the women felt safe asking questions. The security guard at the hospital's main entrance was asked to dispense with the *lathi* (a heavy stick, often of bamboo bound with iron, used in India as a weapon—especially by police to disperse a crowd or quell a riot) and to greet people with respect and a smile. Patients and visitors were not asked to remove footwear; instead, they were allowed to walk in like any of us employees did, so that form of discrimination was removed.

With the active presence of the midwifery trainers and trainees in birthing rooms, the number of normal births increased, and primary CBs decreased by 10% (Figure 9.7). This created ripples in the town of Karimnagar where the pilot group was being trained. Accredited Social Health Activists (ASHAs) accompanying mothers saw these changes and helped spread the word to other women in the community.

The ASHAs began to believe in midwives when they saw how they worked in the birthing rooms. They found that midwife-attended women were indeed having normal physiologic births and positive experiences. The midwifery trainees had a distinctive uniform of colorful shirts and dark trousers as against the nurses' white uniforms. Soon, women from a larger geographical area began to seek care at this mother and child health center because they had heard about the "trouser-and-shirt" ladies and the high level of care they gave.

The mother and child health center in Karimnagar soon attracted the curiosity of the Ministry of Health and Family Welfare, Government of India, which sent Dr. Dinesh Baswal (Joint Commissioner, Maternal Health Division) with an official team from Delhi to inspect firsthand the impacts of the program. This visiting team enjoyed an interactive discussion with the trainees, spoke with the obstetric fraternity, and even took feedback from the mothers in the hospital. UNICEF invited the Institute of Public Health (IPH) to evaluate the Telangana Midwifery Training Program. As a third-party evaluator, following a baseline and

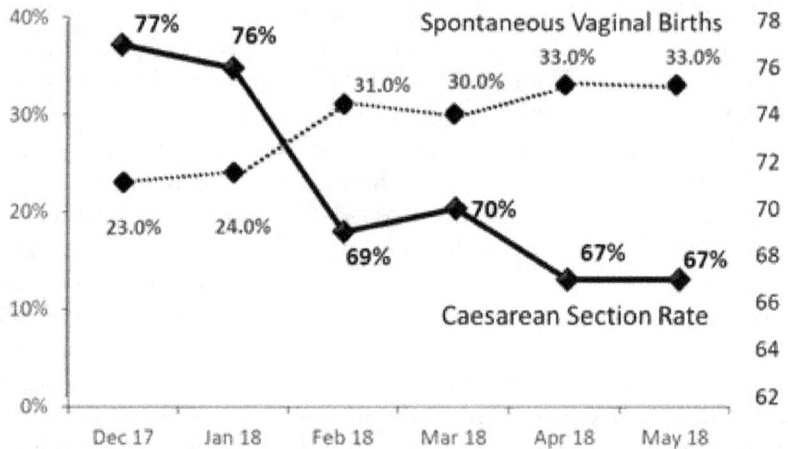

Figure 9.7. The drop in CB rates in Karimnagar between December 2017 and May 2018. © Evita Fernandez

an end line assessment, the report confirmed that there was a distinct change in the attitudes of the midwifery trainees from a medicalized nursing mentality to the humanistic midwifery model of care (Institute of Public Health, Bengaluru 2019). Apart from improvements in clinical skills, the trainees displayed respectful maternity care (see Figure 9.8). The evaluators had this to say about the training program:

> While learning knowledge and skills is the easiest part of the training, we were impressed by the changes in attitude in the trainees. While we have not observed all the trainees in action, those whom we have observed (at least 20 of the 30) are able to treat the woman with respect. They introduce themselves, ask for consent, give choices to the women, and are empathetic to their situation. This has been a major achievement, and the entire credit for this goes to the trainers who taught by practicing these concepts. The trainees observed the trainers and followed in their steps. They now have a role model and a gold standard to follow.

During the 20 weeks of preceptorship/apprenticeship following the qualifying exam, the Telangana midwives helped 1,400 women birth in their positions of choice (Figure 9.9). No woman birthed in the lithotomy position and every woman had a birth companion. The midwives set up the triage and helped streamline care at the district hospital.

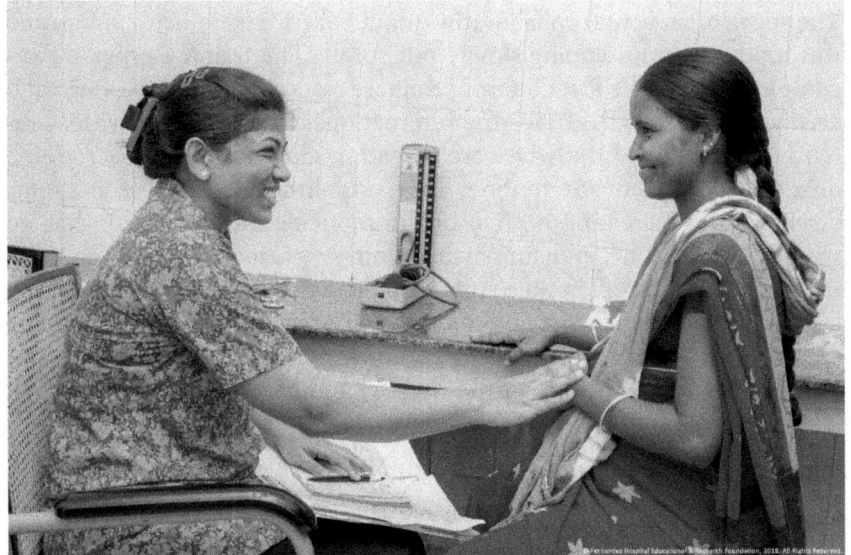

Figure 9.8. A midwife from Telangana ensures that the mother is comfortable during the antenatal check-up. © Fernandez Foundation

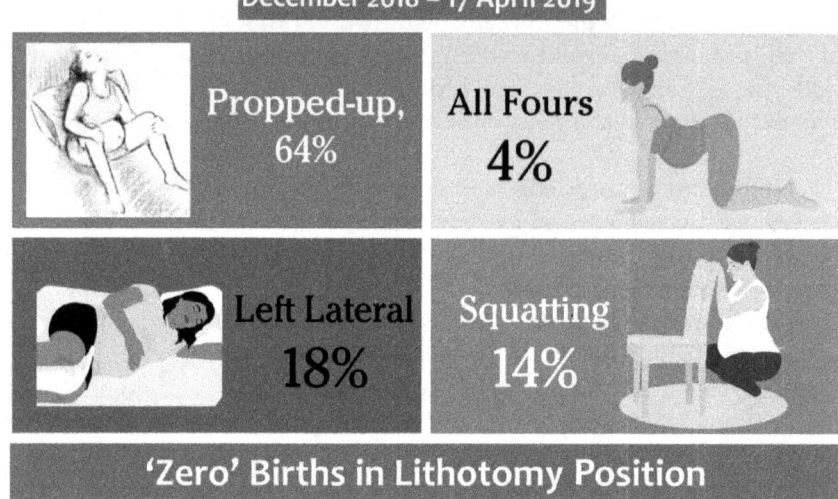

Figure 9.9. Midwife-led births and choice of birthing positions during preceptorship. © Evita Fernandez

The obstetricians in this hospital were delighted and eager to learn about alternative birthing positions. They discovered that they could focus on the women with complex needs who required their expertise. The seeds of an actual collaborative model of care were being sown, and this model was developing slowly but surely. The training program was completed, with the first cohort of trainees graduating and receiving their certificates on May 5, 2019—the International Day of the Midwife. Currently, the qualified midwives are spread in clusters of three across ten districts of Telangana State. They have established themselves as agents of change by increasing normal births, reducing CBs, ensuring that no woman births alone, and supporting women to labor and birth in positions of their choice. They also offer food and drink to the mother during labor. Telangana is the first and to date (2022) only state in India running an active midwifery education and training program for both streams of training: Nurse Practitioners in Midwifery and Midwifery Educators.

National Midwifery Guidelines: A Landmark Policy Decision

The Government of India made a landmark policy decision to roll out midwifery services to improve the quality of care and ensure respectful care to pregnant women and newborns. In December 2018, the government released the *Guidelines on Midwifery Services in India, 2018*[4] (Ministry of Health and Family Welfare 2018) at the Partners' Forum Meeting. The Ministry of Health and Family Welfare and the Indian Nursing Council jointly led a series of meetings in 2019 with various stakeholders. Representatives from the International Confederation of Midwives were also invited to help put together the curricula for the training of midwives and midwifery educators. Besides the ones we trained, India does not have midwifery educators with clinical credibility. We have tutors who can talk theory, but midwifery should be taught in an apprenticeship model that focuses on hands-on learning with an experienced midwife (see Cheyney, Davis-Floyd, and Jordan 2020 for detailed descriptions of the extreme differences between didactic and experiential learning). Thus, the trainer must have adequate clinical experience to be with the trainee in the birthing room to teach midwifery skills.

A decision was made by the Ministry of Health and Family Welfare to identify and build 14 national midwifery training institutes to help create a cohort of midwifery educators. In June 2019, the Fernandez Foundation was recognized as one of those national midwifery training institutes. In November 2019, a cohort of 30 nurses selected from five states of India was the first to begin the residential phase (24 weeks of intense clinical training) of the 18-month National Midwifery Educators Training Program at Fernandez Foundation. Selected with the help of the University of Central Lancashire as International Midwifery Educators, seven midwives from the UK formed the faculty for this program.

Unfortunately, 20 weeks into the course, the training came to a standstill because of the COVID-19 pandemic. However, on returning to their respective states, the midwifery educator trainees became involved in maternity services and the care of COVID-positive pregnant women. They shared with us how they could use some of the evidence-based practices they had learned in the 20 weeks of training. Most importantly, they were able to create small yet significant changes in childbirth practices in their respective states. The program resumed in September 2021, and we look forward to seeing these future midwifery educators fulfill India's vision of establishing midwifery care in all public health facilities.

The pandemic and the lockdowns that followed resulted in a global "pandemic" of webinars. Various platforms, with Zoom being the most popular, became vehicles for communication and teaching. The Ministry of Health and Family Welfare organized several webinars for nurses to help raise awareness of the importance of midwifery as a profession, while simultaneously outlining a clear career path. In November 2020, the Ministry of Health and Family Welfare proposed finalizing the National Nursing and Midwifery Commission Bill[5] for setting up a National Nursing and Midwifery Commission and repealing the Indian Nursing Council Act of 1947, which, at the time, combined the nursing and the midwifery courses into a single course. All stakeholders were asked to share their comments online before December 6, 2020. This was a big step that endorsed the government's commitment to help establish a separate Midwifery Council in India.

In June 2021, the Ministry of Health and Family Welfare, the Government of India, and the Indian Nursing Council jointly released a document titled *Scope of Practice for Midwifery Educator and Nurse Practitioner Midwife*. This was soon followed by an advocacy toolkit giving clear instructions on branding, and a poster design with content including the pattern and color of the midwife's uniform that should be adopted across India. These two initiatives further endorse the government's commitment to establishing midwife-led care units (MLCUs) in the public health facilities of India

Conclusion: India's Vision for Midwives

India's vision of establishing the midwifery collaborative model of care across its public hospitals will be a success only if obstetricians and midwives learn to work as professional colleagues with mutual respect and trust. The midwife must remain the primary caregiver for low-risk pregnancies, and for women with complex needs, she will work with obstetricians and other specialists to offer midwifery support. I look forward to the day when India will have enough midwives to form the backbone of its maternity services. The Fernandez Foundation considers it a privilege to be involved in this journey and will continue its PROMISE to advocate for midwifery with women, the obstetric fraternity, and policy makers.

Evita Fernandez is an obstetrician and the Chairperson of the Fernandez Foundation, Hyderabad, India. She is a Fellow of the Royal College of Obstetricians and Gynaecologists, London. She strongly believes in the need to empower women to make choices, especially regarding issues surrounding birth. Evita is a champion of natural birthing and midwifery in India. She has spearheaded the country's first Professional Midwifery Education and Training (PMET) Program. Her PROfessional

MIdwifery SErvices (PROMISE) campaign is committed to creating a national cadre of professional midwives, who are vital to the care of low-risk pregnant women. In a career spanning three decades, Evita has been at the forefront of maternal and newborn care in India.

Notes

1. The Union government runs the "Janani Suraksha Yojana," which offers a cash incentive to pregnant women in states with low institutional delivery rates (see "Janani Suraksha Yojana." *National Health Mission*. Retrieved 1 December 2021 from https://www.nhm.gov.in/index1.php?lang=1&level=3&sublinkid=841&lid=309). Various Indian states also have their own schemes. The state of Telangana offers a "KCR kit" (named after the incumbent Chief Minister) to incentivize institutional deliveries. The kit includes diapers, a mosquito net, and other such products (see "KCR Kit." *Hyderabad District*, 30 July 2022. Retrieved 1 December 2021 from https://hyderabad.telangana.gov.in/scheme/kcr-kit).
2. The International Confederation of Midwives officially defines a "midwife" as: "a person who has successfully completed a midwifery education programme that is based on the ICM Essential Competencies for Basic Midwifery Practice and the framework of the ICM Global Standards for Midwifery Education and is recognized in the country where [the midwife] is located; who has acquired the requisite qualifications to be registered and/or legally licensed to practice midwifery and use the title 'midwife'; and who demonstrates competency in the practice of midwifery." "ICM Definitions." *International Confederation of Midwives*. Retrieved 17 September 2022 from https://internationalmidwives.org/our-work/policy-and-practice/icm-definitions.html.
3. The Fernandez Foundation is a not-for-profit organization that works on several initiatives to improve the health of women and children. Fernandez Foundation is committed to taking forward its legacy of leadership in health care through excellence and compassionate service, in the spirit of inclusion and justice; being respectful of every human being and upholding their dignity at every stage of life; and adhering to values enshrined in Christian beliefs. All the institutions under the Foundation's aegis also conform to these values. The Foundation's activities encompass different areas—Healthcare, Child Development, Advocacy, Education, Innovation, and Research—focusing on ensuring respectful and equitable care and a life of dignity for women, newborns, and children. The Foundation believes that these are the rights of every woman and child. (See Fernandez Foundation homepage. Retrieved 17 September 2022 from https://www.fernandez.foundation/)
4. The first *Guidelines on Midwifery Services in India* were published by the Ministry of Health and Family Welfare in 2018 (see Ministry of Health and Family Welfare 2018).
5. The draft national nursing and midwifery commission bill 2020 for setting up a National Nursing and Midwifery Commission (see Ministry of Health and Family Welfare 2020).

References

Cheyney M, Davis-Floyd R, Jordan B (posthumously). 2020. "Authoritative Knowledge: Ways of Doing, Teaching, and Learning about Birth. A Tribute to Brigitte Jordan." *Practicing Anthropology* 43(1): 41–48.

Högberg U. 2004. "The Decline in Maternal Mortality in Sweden: The Role of Community Midwifery." *American Journal of Public Health* 94(8): 1312–1320.

Homer C, Leap M, Edwards N, Sandall J. 2017. "Midwifery Continuity of Carer in an Area of High Socio-Economic Disadvantage in London: A Retrospective Analysis of Albany Midwifery Practice Outcomes Using Routine Data (1997–2009)." *Midwifery* 48: 1–10.

Institute of Public Health, Bengaluru. 2019. "Evaluation of Midwife Training in Telangana (EMTT)." *Institute of Public Health, Bengaluru*, 22 November. Retrieved 17 September 2022 from https://iphindia.org/health-services/evaluation-of-midwife-training-in-telangana-emtt/.

Mavalankar D, Raman PS, Vora K. 2011. "Midwives of India: Missing in Action." *Midwifery* 27(5): 700–706.

Ministry of Health and Family Welfare, Government of India. 2018. *Guidelines on Midwifery Services in India 2018*. Retrieved 3 December 2021 from https://nhm.gov.in/New_Updates_2018/NHM_Components/RMNCHA/MH/Guidelines/Guidelines_on_Midwifery_Services_in_India.pdf.

Ministry of Health and Family Welfare, Government of India. 2020. "Draft the National Nursing & Midwifery Commission Bill 2020." *Ministry of Health and Family Welfare*, 5 November. Retrieved 3 December 2021 from https://main.mohfw.gov.in/newshighlights-21.

Ministry of Health and Family Welfare, Government of India. 2021. *Scope of Practice for Midwifery Educator and Nurse Practitioner Midwife*. Retrieved 17 September 2022 from https://www.indiannursingcouncil.org/uploads/pdf/1626159560175927057460ed39c8888fe.pdf.

Ministry of Health and Family Welfare, Government of India. 2015–16. "NFHS-4: National Family Health Survey 2015–16." Retrieved 17 September 2022 from http://rchiips.org/nfhs/factsheet_nfhs-4.shtml.

Ministry of Health and Family Welfare, Government of India. 2019–21. "NFHS-5: National Family Health Survey 2019–21." Retrieved 17 September 2022 from http://rchiips.org/nfhs/nfhs5.shtml.

Ministry of Health and Family Welfare, Government of India, 2012. "Indian Public Health Standards: Guidelines for District Hospitals." Retrieved 12 October 2022 from https://nhm.gov.in/images/pdf/guidelines/iphs/iphs-revised-guidlines-2012/district-hospital.pdf.

Pandit N. 2005. *Pregnancy*. New Delhi, India: Rupa Publications.

Reed B, Walton C. 2009. "The Albany Midwifery Practice." In *Birth Models That Work*, ed. Davis-Floyd R, Barclay L, Daviss BA, Tritten J, 141–158. Berkeley: University of California Press.

Reed B, Edwards N. Forthcoming. *Closure*. London: Pinter and Martin.

Ved RR, Dua AS. 2005. "Review of Women and Children's Health in India: Focus on Safe Motherhood." *NCMH Background Papers: Burden of Disease in India*, 85–111. New Delhi, India: Ministry of Health and Family Welfare.

World Health Organization. 2020. "Midwives: Central to Providing Quality Care to Mothers and Newborns during COVID-19 Pandemic and Beyond." Retrieved 12 October 2022 from https://www.who.int/india/news/photo-story/detail/midwives---central-to-providing-quality-care-to-mothers-and-newborns-during-covid-19-pandemic-and-beyond.

CHAPTER 10

"Birth with No Regret" in Turkey
The Natural Childbirth of the 21st Century

Hakan Çoker

I am an obstetrician aged 56, from İstanbul, Turkey. I will share my story of change from a semi-medicalized obstetrician to a humanistic and respectful birth supporter. I admit that this was not an easy road to travel in a country with 58% cesarean rate and a highly biomedicalized obstetric culture (Eyi and Mollamahmutoglu 2021). I hope that mine will be a story of hope for the young obstetricians with conflicted feelings about supporting women, families, and normal, physiologic birth.

I don't really remember why I chose obstetrics. In those days (the 1990s), obstetrics was a very popular specialization in Turkey, and I thought that was why I chose it. But years later, after working with prenatal psychologists and birth psychotherapists, and reading about transgenerational epigenetics, I now realize that I didn't really have a choice. My mother was a professional home and hospital midwife as was my aunt. Both of my grandmothers were village midwives who practiced for many years until they finally got their licenses via a quick education with my mother as their teacher. I didn't realize how important my family history was in choosing my career until I read about transgenerational effects.

I spent the years 1990–1994 doing my obstetric residency. We were taught that the only target was to deliver the babies in safety. "Safety" meant a healthy beating heart, good breathing, no tissue damage, both for the mother and the baby. We were so busy with "delivering" the babies that we had no idea about the psychology of the mother. The baby? Babies were unseen, invisible, not even full-fledged humans. They don't remember anything from womb life or birth, so it didn't matter how we treated them. The mothers were lonely during labor and birth.

Most were scared. But there was no culture about preparation for birth or asking for one-to-one support during the birthing process. After birth, the mothers stayed together in one room with nine other postpartum mothers. Their babies were taken away from them for most of the time and only given to them for breastfeeding. The rest of the time, the newborns stayed in bassinets in a nursery called the "Baby Room," at least ten to 20 at a time, all crying all the time. Today, with my knowledge that babies are conscious beings, I can hear them asking, "Where am I? Who are these strangers? Where is my mom? I need my mom. I am hungry. Mom left me alone. I don't trust mom." And at least once a month, one of them was found dead in their bed. This was called "cradle death" and was often seen as normal. Why did we do all this to that generation? I really don't know. I guess it was because we thought it was safer for the babies to be in the Baby Room than to be with their mothers, but now we know that it wasn't.

As birth assistants, during residency our only target was to learn more techniques, more skills, more surgeries so that we could "help" women and babies. But we never realized back then that only around 20% of pregnant women actually needed our help for deliveries or other illnesses in pregnancy, labor, and birth. The other 80% only need our support. And supporting the physiology of birth and acknowledging its psychological aspects was never taught to us—neither in our educational curriculum nor by the senior consultants. I don't blame anyone, but I still feel ashamed of myself that I never questioned what we were taught in those days.

I must also admit that the midwives who worked in our maternity unit were the same. Yes, we all know that they are supposed to be the protectors of women and the guides and guardians of normal physiologic births. But, given the heavy autocratic pressure of the doctors, midwives had no right to offer any suggestions to the women they cared for; they could only follow doctors' orders. For them too, the target was to deliver the babies in safety. Drug-free relaxation and breathing techniques, visualizations, pelvic movement techniques—these were unknown to all of us. And standard practices went unquestioned. They were all good people working really hard, but we never even considered the very real need for humanistic support for women and babies.

From 1996–2001, I worked in a small town with six midwives as the only obstetrician in a community hospital with only eight beds; we were responsible for nearly 1,000 births per year. I always trusted these midwives. In the first six months, we created our own labor and birth guidelines and applied them. We were highly standardized, yet our cesarean rate was only 15% in total, and our level of medicalization was quite low. Our maternity and neonatal mortality/morbidity met the expected standards. But still, something was missing. We still had no idea about supporting women prenatally or teaching them about drug-free comfort measures and one-to-one continuous support. Birth psychology and prenatal psychology were nowhere in our consciousness. Yes, something was indeed missing. Then, in 2003, in the span of four hours, my life changed.

I was attending an obstetric conference and I checked in a day before. While exploring the hotel, I noticed that there was a preconference workshop on Childbirth Education Classes. I sneaked in. (Later, I worked a lot with the organizer nurses in many conferences and workshops. They said they noticed my sneak-in, but they were pleased to see it.) There, for the first time in my life, I heard about Lamaze, Leboyer, Grantly Dick-Read, Active Birth, respectful birth, and more—I even participated in the prenatal exercise class. These were all new and life-changing for me; it was like a door opening to a bright future. And when I did an internet search, I found that they were already there waiting for me to explore.

My second life-changing event was a Midwifery Today Conference in Bad Wildbad, Germany, in 2004. Nearly 200 women—mostly midwives and some doulas—were present. Michel Odent and I were the only two men and the only two obstetricians at that conference. It was an honor for me to meet Odent and to listen to him. (After that, I read all his books within six months.) Most shocking to me was meeting independent professional midwives from all over the world—Gail Hart, Sally Kelly, Jan Tritten, Cornelia Enning, Elizabeth Davis, Gail Tully, and many others. I think they were also a bit in shock. Probably, in addition to Michel Odent, I was among the first obstetricians interested in their work. Every lecture was so interesting to me. Midwifery skills, water birth, spinning babies (a series of techniques invented by midwife Gail Tully in 1998 to reposition babies in utero), doula work, techniques for using the *rebozo* (shawl) for pain relief and labor support, moxibustion, relaxation techniques, and many more. The main difference between this midwifery conference and the obstetric conferences I had attended was that all speakers were talking from their hearts. From wisdom. From pure experience. It was my first conference with them but would not be the last. I attended at least six more Midwifery Today conferences, every two years, with many obstetrician and midwife colleagues accompanying me.

Yet at these conferences, I noticed that the midwives often talked about how often obstetricians didn't listen to them, but at the same time, they were talking about themselves as a "tribe." This concept of us/

them didn't feel good. Maternity care is teamwork. During the closing ceremony, I (loudly) voiced this opinion. In the birthing world, teamwork is important, by which I mean that midwives, obstetricians, doulas, nurses, and birth psychologists (see below) should work together.

And at all of them, I met and got to know the anthropologist Robbie Davis-Floyd, our three-volume Book Series lead editor. When they heard me present my model of "Birth with No Regret," she and Canadian midwife Betty-Anne Daviss asked me to contribute a chapter to their coedited collection *Birthing Models on the Human Rights Frontier: Speaking Truth to Power* (Daviss and Davis-Floyd 2021) which I did (Çoker, Karabekir, and Varlık 2021), along with the other two members of my "Birth with No Regret" team, midwife and doula Serpil Varlık, and birth psychologist Neşe Karabekir.

Still, it took me four years to digest all the information I now had. I searched for workshops in the United Kingdom and the United States. I discovered "HypnoBirthing: The Mongan Method" in the UK. Thus in 2007, I found myself sitting together with 30 women (midwives, nurses, and hypnosis practitioners). I was the only male and the only obstetrician present, and I felt deeply that I was questioned by everyone participating in the course: "What is he doing here?" It was a third life-changing event for me. My language changed in one day. No more negative words in my medical language like "patient," "pain," "bursting the amniotic sac," and so on. On the third day of this course, I asked the teacher if I could borrow some of the books for the night. That night I finished four books and wrote summaries of them. (Of course, later I ordered all of these for my library.) The most interesting one was *The Secret Life of the Unborn Child* by Thomas Verny (1982). This was my first contact with the world of pre- and perinatal psychology. Yes, preborn babies can hear, can remember, can learn, and can feel in the womb. And the most important thing I learned was that they can remember their births so clearly that they need a gentle, humanistic, and respectful welcome.

After this 2007 course, within six months I stopped cutting the cord immediately, my episiotomy rate went down from 100% to 15%, and skin-to-skin contact immediately after birth went up to 100%. For the first time in my life, I deeply understood the importance of active, shared decision-making, and I gained deep respect for serving pregnant women. At the age of 43, after 19 years of my obstetric life, I was changing. That was a good feeling, because by then I could really feel and understand why I chose obstetrics.

I had become very enthusiastic about learning. After taking the HypnoBirthing class, I got my Lamaze certification within six months. One year later, I invited the teacher of the HypnoBirthing class, Gilbert Sherry, and organized a HypnoBirthing Course in Turkey, which was attended by 40 people. Half of them were midwifery teachers and nurses. Most of them are pioneer teachers teaching respectful births. By coincidence, one of the participants was Janet Balaskas, the founder of Active Birth. I invited her to come back to Turkey to teach an Active Birth Course and she agreed to come and to support me. So, as you can imagine, three months later she returned to Turkey. And since then, we have held around six Active Birth courses in Turkey with her. So, Turkey started meeting the best pioneers of the world in childbirth education and respectful births.

Four years after I sneaked into that Childbirth Education workshop, I was ready to open childbirth classes for my families. From 2008 on, I have been teaching monthly childbirth education classes, all adjusted to Turkish culture. The more I read about physiology and psychology, the more I changed my practices. And the more I taught these families, the better I understood them. At the same time, I started writing in Turkish about evidence-based obstetrics, the importance of humanistic natural births, birth support, privacy in birth, and a respectful environment in labor and delivery rooms. In those days, I was the only one in Turkey writing about natural births. People started writing to me and coming to my classes from different cities.

In 2009, after I took a course on water birth, my teaching colleague Laurence Issele Arslan became pregnant and wanted a home water birth. I warned her that it would be my first water birth. She said, "I trust first in my body and then in you, let's do it!" So began my attendance at water births. I wrote to Barbara Harper (the international speaker and expert on water births) to ask her for advice. Even though she didn't know me at all, she helped me a lot with good advice and by sending me many papers to read. Today, when I think about all the pioneers of respectful births whom I have met, I notice that they are all humble and ready to help anyone working to humanize births. They never hesitated to share their knowledge, articles, and books. They were always as supportive as they could possibly be. Thus, here I need to thank them all for what they changed and supported in my professional life. And it is a bit ironic, but yes, I learned many medical issues from many doctors. But when the subject was a natural, respectful, and humanistic approach, with the exception of Michel Odent, none of those I learned from were obstetricians—they were all midwives, nurses, doulas, psychotherapists, and anthropologists such as Robbie. So then I understood that one of my future goals had to be to support other obstetricians who are trying to take a humanistic approach to their families, because I know how lonely many of them are in taking that approach, as some of them have described in other chapters in this volume.

Returning to Laurence's story, yes, we ordered the pool. Of course, as an obstetrician attending my first water birth, I carried almost all the delivery room instruments to the house, including a vacuum extractor. The midwife was with me, and the ambulance waited in front of the house "just in case" something might go wrong. To tell the truth, practically it was a hospital-like home water birth. Luckily everything went beautifully and there were no problems at all. In addition to helping me learn how to attend a water birth, this birth also made me understand the importance of privacy in labor. It was a two-story house. We noticed that when Laurence was upstairs alone with her husband, the contractions were more frequent and regular. But when she came downstairs and we were all together, her labor slowed down. Even though we were not strangers, we were affecting the physiology of this labor.

Another lesson I learned from this birth was that no obstetrician can pretend to be a midwife, at least not me. It was the first time in my life staying in the room with a woman giving birth throughout much of her labor and birth as a homebirth midwife would do. But it was not easy for me. I felt that I should *do something*. I again came to respect midwives for their patience and support in every birth. After that I said to myself, "If I continue with private professional life, I will always have a private midwife with me in every birth." Two years later, I got to live this experience again. This time Laurence was pregnant with twins, and she again wanted a home water birth. Yes, we did it. She really enjoyed challenging me!

The Birth of the "Birth with No Regret" Team

In 2010, I met Neşe Karabekir, a psychodramatist who was also working with pregnant women and babies. Even though I was teaching childbirth education, I always felt that something was missing in my classes. When Neşe and I met, we noticed that we were both passionate about women and births, and about respectful welcomings for newborns. We started working creatively together. We combined not only our professional work, but also our private lives: we got married. Over the course of six months, we created many psychodramatic roleplays for the course, and we opened the Istanbul Birth Academy, where we started with childbirth education classes, breastfeeding and newborn care courses, yoga classes, and psychological support. We also started taking care of the families together. I decided to offer this team support to all my clients as an obligation. That's how the "Birth with No Regret Team" was born.

But we started having problems with some of our couples. To them, the birth psychologist was an entirely new concept. Even though we didn't charge any money for the psychologist's participation in birth, and very little for the preparatory sessions, some couples didn't like the idea of working with a psychologist or even a midwife. In Turkey's new healthcare system, the "Doctor as God" concept had been politically implemented and midwives had already lost their important role, as the culture taught that the doctors do everything more safely. Because the fee of the team is added to the doctor's fee, some found the teamwork expensive. We had to make a big decision. After months of discussion, we decided to accept only couples who wanted the whole team and the whole philosophy. At that point, our "Birth with No Regret" team fully emerged. We lost nearly 40% of our couples. Today, however, many more come to us because they want the complete holistic approach.

It took a lot of discussion to name the team and the philosophy; we debated about whether we should put a negative term like "no regret" at the front of a potentially magical birth experience. But the reality, in this modern world with its technocratic birth services (Davis-Floyd 2001, 2018, 2022; see also the Series Overview, this volume) is that women often end up with many regrets after their birth experiences. Some regrets are so obvious that the women can name and understand them, but many other regrets get buried in the cells of women's bodies and unconscious minds. Even the separation of a newborn baby from the mother in the name of routine care can be traumatic. Turkish women have so many regrets about their births, yet most of them are preventable with good care and conscious, informed decision-making. This is why an 18-hour childbirth education class, which includes videos and plenty of time for questions and answers, is obligatory under our model, so that both practitioners and parents speak the same language of birth and can understand each other's decisions and choices.

In our teamwork model of "Birth with No Regret," three professionals work together. An obstetrician is responsible for routine examinations and birth. A midwife, who also acts as a doula, provides essential one-to-one support during labor and birth. The birth psychologist starts working with the couple after they complete the childbirth education course. The aim is to get information about the couple: who are they, what are their needs, their life philosophies, any fears about labor and birth, any transgenerational issues that might affect their birthing process, their preferences around labor and birth. Not only the couple but also the grandmothers are invited for sessions. In a culture like Turkey's, grandmothers (meaning the mothers or the grandmothers of the pregnant women) expect to take active roles in couples' decision-making, going to the hospital at the beginning of labor and staying there throughout labor and birth. Because most of the couples want to keep their privacy, these sessions have great importance. The grandmothers get information from an expert, narrate their birth stories (often for the first time in their lives), receive information about transgenerational issues, and come to understand why they usually should not be present at their daughters' or granddaughters' births. These sessions may also restore the mother-daughter relationship if it was previously broken.

The birth psychologist does not limit her work to these sessions. When labor starts, she comes to the hospital and makes sure that everyone involved is protected and cared for during birth. Her first priority is to support the couple, and, especially in complicated labors, she also supports the birthing team. We call her "the mother of the birth and birth team."

To briefly summarize how this model works, "Birth with No Regret" begins with a labor that starts on its own (unless there is some strong medical indication for induction), in which the natural hormones are actively secreted under optimum conditions. It is a birth with as few interventions as possible, in which the laboring women are free to eat and drink at will and to adopt any positions they wish, and where the babies meet their mothers with uninterrupted skin-to-skin contact immediately after birth. The three professionals taking care of the mother—an obstetrician, a midwife, and a birth psychotherapist—have equal levels of autonomy. Beyond a healthy mother and a healthy newborn, the overall goal is that no one present at the birth has any regrets about any aspect of the labor, birth, and postpartum process.

Birth with No Regret is MotherBaby-Friendly. It respects all six Lamaze Care Practices and implements all 12 Steps of the *International Childbirth Initiative* (ICI): *12 Steps to Safe and Respectful MotherBaby-Family Maternity Care* (found at www.icichildbirth.org; see also Lalonde et al. 2019 and Lalonde's chapter in this volume),[1] and the World Health Organization's 2018 "WHO Recommendations: Intrapartum Care for a Positive Childbirth Experience." In my opinion, it is the natural childbirth of the 21st century.

We developed this model in a conscious and deliberate manner in the belief that birth with no regret will create a future with no regret. Its characteristics include the following:

1. It is based in teamwork. Again, the team consists of the doctor, midwife, and birth psychologist.

2. All work starts in the first half of the pregnancy.
3. The family fully participates in our 18-hour education program of physical and psychological preparation.
4. After completing this program, our families participate actively in all decisions.
5. Labor starts by itself unless there is a medical indication for induction.
6. Women act freely on their instincts.
7. They labor and give birth actively in whatever positions they prefer.
8. The mothers are strengthened and empowered by their birth experiences.
9. The fathers take active roles in the birth by fully supporting the mothers.
10. The babies experience not the rupture of separation but convergence via immediate and uninterrupted skin-to-skin contact with their mothers after birth.
11. The babies start life with confidence.
12. Birth with No Regret does not refuse interventions nor epidural analgesia, but they are not used routinely, only when truly felt necessary.
13. If a cesarean is needed, we use what we call the "Mother/Father/Baby-Friendly Cesarean." The mother is awake, the father is present, the baby is immediately placed on the mother's chest after birth for skin-to-skin contact, bonding, and breastfeeding, and they are never separated again.

Spreading the Model and the Wisdom and Experience that Underlie It

After two years of experience in using our model, our work started to be preferred by many couples. In the world of technocratic births, women and families need humanistic, supportive birth professionals. So again, it was time for us to make another decision. Either we would keep the knowledge to ourselves or spread it throughout the country. Keeping it to ourselves meant more money for us; spreading it meant more people in the country having access to our model and the knowledge and wisdom that underlie it. We chose the second option and decided to offer courses about our model. In our first course, there were 30 people—obstetricians, midwives, nurses, psychologists, doulas, and physiotherapists. Our dream was coming true: many professionals of different types taking the same course and sitting next to each other in equality—the beginning of new birth teams. And it really worked! They have all become pioneers of humanistic births in Turkey.

This course takes nine months to finish with nine modules. It is a standardized international childbirth education course based on the best available evidence. It includes self-development, energy therapies, acupressure techniques, newborn and breastfeeding information, doula training, drug-free relaxation techniques, and much more. After completing the modules, the course participants watch how we teach and how we describe our experiences of the ways couples change during and after their childbirth education classes. And then they open their own group education courses (four different days, three-hour lessons, minimum 12 hours). We don't watch them during their lessons, but after each lesson they teach, they get a one-hour debriefing session, which means that they tell us what they did in the lesson and about any problems that arose, and we help them work through those problems. In this way, we can standardize the course for every graduate to retain the integrity of the courses. We know what they teach, which words they use, which films they show, and so on. It is not helpful to supervise them while they teach, because being watched is stressful, and, since these courses are now offered all over the country, it is practically impossible to watch them all. After finishing the course, participants attend four births; after every birth they again get a de-briefing session with us, during which we help them work through any issues, problems, or conflicts that arose. With the help of these de-briefing sessions, they become standardized in our model, by which I mean that they learn to speak the same language and to serve women without judgment or criticism.

This big decision that we collectively made also gave birth to a new profession: birth psychologist. We know there are prenatal, perinatal, and postnatal psychologists in the world working for mothers.[2] But Neşe is the first psychologist we know of to work with couples prenatally and also to guide them through their births (Karabekir 2016). With her experience as a basis, we have been able to start training other psychologists and therapists to also become birth psychologists. After childbirth education and doula training, they continue with birth psychologist modules and supervisions. And now there are quite a number of them in Turkey—70. Their work truly forms the foundation for the work of the entire team and the parents' work to birth their baby. We believe that the support of the birth psychologist is a major factor in the high satisfaction rates we achieve—including our own.

Between 2012 and 2022, 25 groups (550 people from different professions) have taken the course and spread the wisdom of humanistic birth around the country. They all post about their experiences on their social media sites. Some have carried the knowledge to universities and midwifery students. Some have opened their own practices based on our model. Some have become highly sought-after midwives and doulas.

"Too Good to Be True": The Problems Begin

When I was on my own as an individual, there were no problems. Even after we developed and implemented our teamwork model, there were no problems. We were often invited to speak at midwifery conferences and to organize childbirth education conferences. When writing in social media about the rights of women and babies, about evidence-based childbirth care, and about supporting women with midwives and doulas, we still experienced no problems. We were even invited to speak to the Ministry of Health Mother-Friendly Hospital Committee. In those days, before the creation of the *International Childbirth Initiative (ICI): 12 Steps to Safe and Respectful MotherBaby-Family Maternity Care* in 2018 (see Lalonde et al. 2019 and Lalonde's chapter in this volume), I was the official Turkish representative of the *International MotherBaby Childbirth Initiative* (IMBCI)*: 10 Steps to Optimal MotherBaby Maternity Services*. In our talks with the members of the Board of the International MotherBaby Childbirth Organization (IMBCO)—the group that created the IMBCI, we had nice discussions about the 10 Steps of this precursor to the ICI. (See Davis-Floyd 2022b for the stories of the developments of the IMBCI and the ICI). In the end, we had our national 10 Steps for the Mother-Friendly Hospitals of Turkey, which means that these hospitals have single rooms for each labor and birth, are more respectful of the physiology and psychology of birth, and perform fewer interventions and cesareans. On paper, we already have 80 Mother-Friendly Hospitals in Turkey, but the truth is that they still have a long way to go to be real Mother-Friendly Hospitals. The hospitals that cannot achieve that designation either don't have suitable maternity wards or have very high cesarean rates, or both.

After the first year of training, we encouraged our graduates and new students to make connections with other obstetricians to help them to educate their patients and to support them during labor and birth. There was an obstetricians' Facebook page and anyone could become a member. So most of the students became members and started participating in the discussions. One day the obstetricians on this Facebook page noticed that there were midwives and doulas in the group. Because these obs didn't like what the midwives and doulas were writing, without any warning they blocked all non-obstetricians. Of course, I criticized that move, and there I was noticed. The discussions targeted me for teaching doula classes to non-healthcare professionals; for blaming other obstetricians for not treating women humanistically; for making birth into a business and making too much money from it; and for exaggerating the baby's awareness (turning off the spotlights, not cutting the cord immediately, respecting the "golden hour" with skin-to-skin contact, and so on). Not using the spotlights during birth is "show business." Babies do not remember. Bonding and the "golden hour" have no importance. Delayed cord-cutting has no importance for the baby. (Now it is done all over Turkey in every hospital.) Episiotomy is necessary and good. I was the "charlatan." I was stealing couples' money through "useless" childbirth education. I was teaching unacceptable human rights in childbirth. (Now these human rights are taught around the country.) I had no right to teach childbirth education classes because I had no university degree. I had no right to train doulas; they were useless and dangerous—they could not teach couples the right hospital rules. They were (derogatorily) calling us "natural birthers."

These were very tiring days, but I had been expecting all these critiques. I read Grantly Dick-Read's *Birth without Fear* (1942) twice. I remember pages of him describing being attacked by his colleagues. I saw that nothing had changed since then. I actually felt honored by these attacks; they were proof that I had made these obstetricians think, and also opportunities to spread the humanistic approach to birth among obstetricians. Thus, I used each attack as an opportunity to write about evidence-based birth, women's preferences, informed consent, humanistic and respectful birthing environments, delayed cord clamping, the safety of non-interventionist, Mother-Friendly approaches, and Mother-Baby-Friendly Cesareans. The more I wrote respectfully in responding to their concerns, the more obstetricians started being interested not only in what I wrote but also in how I wrote. Later many came to our courses secretly, saying that they had been affected by my respectful answers, even though I was still being viciously attacked by other obs.

These attacks lasted for around four years. As noted above, their advantage for me was that the obs who attacked me started questioning the interventions they consistently performed. Yes, Turkey still has a 58% cesarean rate and that remains unacceptable. Yes, interventions are really high—mainly routine episiotomies, inductions, position restrictions, cutting the cord immediately, no skin-to-skin after birth, no one-to-one continuous labor support. But due to the malpractice laws, being sued was their main concern, and they were really scared about that.

After Mother-Friendly Hospitals started spreading all over Turkey, and after some FIGO (International Federation of Gynecology and Obstetrics) and ACOG (American College of Obstetricians and Gynecologists) publications—and especially the WHO 2018 recommendations mentioned above—the attacks on me slowed down. Yet our practices of teaching women about their human rights in childbirth, making lists of their birth preferences, questioning the system, and looking for one-to-one doula support are still being criticized.

Then a new group of attacks began. Our graduates were in action, were preferred by many mothers, and were becoming more powerful. Turkish obs see doulas as threats against their routine practices. They believe that it is all because of doulas that families ask questions about obs' practices, question or resist routine interventions, and pay a great deal of attention to the first hour after the baby is born and uninterrupted skin-to-skin contact immediately after birth. Turkish obstetricians in general still think that doulas are "ignorant" and "dangerous." They don't understand that doulas are the women who are in love with their support for women giving birth, who left other careers to become doulas, who respect midwives and doctors and are trained to understand their fears about birth and to support them to deal with those fears, and to support the laboring woman and her partner.

Some Turkish midwives and midwifery associations also say that doulas and doula trainings must be banned. These midwives too were angry with me because I was training doulas. They said that doulas are dangerous for the system and for midwifery, that they have no place in labor and birthing rooms, and that to support women is a midwife's job. I really feel very sorry when they talk like that. Midwives should be the first to support women's rights to make their own childbirth choices. Every woman has the right to choose where and how to give birth and with whom. But some midwives see doulas as threats to their profession. Because I train doulas, about half of the midwives in Turkey do not like me and often attack me.

Such attacks may not be that important to an obstetrician who knows his path and has the courage to follow it. Many of the obstetricians and midwives who come to our courses really want to change their practices, but either hospital policies don't let them or the families they serve don't understand the importance of their humanistic teamwork approach. To the ones in such situations who feel really stuck, I say that you are not alone. Dick-Read lived that in the 1940s, and in this contemporary world there are many like you, fighting against the system for the rights of women and babies. Examples of such system-fighters can be found in other chapters in this book.

Yet in practice, as other chapters in this volume also show, it is not easy to fight against a huge health industry on your own. Supporting natural births needs time, patience, and respect. Yes, we do support our students wherever they have problems; sometimes they are traumatized by certain births. Sometimes their freedom to support women is taken away from them. Sometimes they witness obstetric violence and feel powerless to stop it. And sometimes their ideal of "wonderful humanistic births" is not well understood well by the family and our students feel unsuccessful in their efforts to apply a humanistic approach. Sometimes obstetricians who want to make changes cannot change even one simple routine in their hospitals.

Conclusion

Being responsible for births is not easy. But there we are. We choose this and with our own will we keep on going. Once we step out of the "responsibility hat" saying that "I am responsible for everything, so I have to control everything," attending births becomes much easier. We cease the efforts at controlling labor that led us to perform multiple interventions, and we let go of the lithotomy position that gives us control over the birth. Instead, we must understand that we are the supporters and messengers. Yes, we do help women to give birth, but we should not decide *how* they will birth. We also need to understand that preborn and newly born babies are conscious beings with souls, and can remember how they were welcomed—or not—into this world, which means that the baby as well as the mother needs to be respected. Every woman has her own inner wisdom and the right to choose her place of birth, her birth attendants, and how she labors and gives birth. In other words, we obstetricians cannot truly control births, and there is never a guarantee in any birth. Yet the more we trust and support the woman and her birth process, the more easily and physiologically that birth will unfold, and the greater will be the psychological satisfaction for the mother, her birth partner, the baby, and the birth team.

Of course, there is always risk in birth and the possibility of being sued for negative birth outcomes. Yet, as noted above, the greater the confidence and trust that the woman and her partner have in the birth team, the less likely they will be to sue them. Here I share what I have done to protect myself from lawsuits:

1. Asked the families to participate in our 18-hour childbirth education class;
2. Supported them with a professional private midwife who knows the family;

3. Asked them to have sessions with a birth psychologist to check themselves as parents-to-be;
4. Asked the birth psychotherapist to be in action during the birth to support the family and the birthing team;
5. And called this the "Birth with No Regret Team."

Do the results satisfy us? Yes, definitely yes—see Table 10.1.

Table 10.1. Our "Birth with No Regret" Statistics on 450 Births (2010–2021). © Hakan Çoker

	%
Cesarean (All are MotherBaby-Friendly Cesareans, in which the atmosphere is respectful, the sheets are lowered so the mother can watch the birth, the baby is passed directly to the mother immediately after birth, and breastfeeding can begin while the mother is being sutured.)	12–15%
Enema / Continuous EFM / IV	0
Epidural	5%
Labor induction (42 week postdate/EMR (early membrane rupture) + 24 hours)	10%
Pitocin during labor (augmentation)	4%
Physiologic cord clamping (after 1–15 minutes)	95%
Episiotomy (3rd degree tear 1, 4th degree tear: 0)	8%
Vacuum extraction	4%
Bonding (60 min–2 hours)	95%
Fathers' participation and bonding	100%
Mortality/morbidity	0
Postpartum depression	0
NICU (congenital infection, SGA [small for gestational age], breathing problems)	1%

Yet more important than these statistics are the satisfaction and joy we experience in every birth. Birth with No Regret does not mean easy and short births. Of course, we see those too, but more important is the satisfaction every family feels, no matter what the outcome of the birth turns out to be. Because except for real emergencies, the team never decides about anything in labor and birth; the family does and is supported to do so. This is active decision-making and has been proven to be one of the main factors generating satisfaction in birth (Hodnett 2002). The other three factors are personal expectations, the amount of the support provided by caregivers, and the quality of the caregiver-patient relationship (ibid.). After careful research, Ellen Hodnett concluded that the primary factors in the psychological outcome of a birth are the attitudes and ideologies of the caregivers. Thus it is no wonder that our model of Birth with No Regret works so very well.

If you are reading this book as an obstetrician, it means that the system does not satisfy you, just as it doesn't satisfy many other obstetricians in the world—as clearly shown in other chapters in this volume. When I read the works of pioneers like Grantly Dick-Read, Frédérick Leboyer, and Michel Odent, I felt that I was not alone. You too are not alone, as obstetricians who believe in women's and babies' childbirth rights to humanistic treatment are growing in number and supporting each other (see, for examples, Davis-Floyd and Georges 2023). Let's work together for our future;[3] you can reach me at the email address in my bio below.

We also have an NGO association called "Hand to Hand for Birth Association." I conclude this chapter with this association's "4R motto":

- Respect for newborn
- Respect for mother
- Respect for childbirth
- Respect for birth teams

Hakan Çoker is an obstetrician/gynecologist. After working in various hospitals in his home country of Turkey, Hakan decided to become an advocate for natural births, childbirth education, and continuous birth support. He became a Lamaze Certified Childbirth Educator, HypnoBirthing Practitioner, and Active Birth Trainer, and is co-creator of the Birth with No Regret model in which the obstetrician, midwife, and birth psychologist work together. In 2010, he and psychologist Neşe Karabekir founded the İstanbul Birth Academy. Since then he has been a teacher for Birth with No Regret teams, childbirth education classes, doula trainings, and birth psychologist trainings. He is the country representative for the *International Childbirth Initiative (ICI): 12 Steps to Safe and Respectful MotherBaby-Family Maternity Care*, found at www.icichildbirth.org. He is also the founder of the Hand to Hand for Birth Association. He is author of *Natural Birth in 100 Questions* and editor for the Turkish translations of Michel Odent's books *The Caesarean* (2004) and *The Scientification of Love* (2014); *HypnoBirthing: The Mongan Method* by Marry Mongan (2016); *Birthing from Within* by Pam England and Rob Horowitz (1998); and *Mindful HypnoBirthing* by Sophie Fletcher (2017). Email: hakancoker@icloud.com.

Notes

1. These 6 Lamaze practices, found at Lamaze Healthy Birth Practices, include:
   (1) Let labor begin on its own
   (2) Walk, move, change positions
   (3) Continuous labor support
   (4) Avoid routine interventions
   (5) Avoid giving birth on your back and follow your urges to push
   (6) Keep parent and baby together
   The *International Childbirth Initiative* (ICI)*: 12 Steps to Safe and Respectful MotherBaby-Family Maternity Care* homepage. Retrieved 17 September 2022 from www.icichildbirth.org.
2. Birth Psychology and The Association for Prenatal and Perinatal Psychology and Health homepage. Retrieved 17 September 2022 from https://birthpsychology.com/.
3. You can sign on to become a supporter and implementer of the *International Childbirth Initiative* (ICI)*: 12 Steps to Safe and Respectful MotherBaby-Family Maternity Care* at www.icichildbirth.org.

References

Çoker H, Karabekir N, Varlık S. 2021. "'Birth with No Regret' in Turkey." In *Birthing Models on the Human Rights Frontier: Speaking Truth to Power*, ed. Daviss BA, Davis-Floyd R, 347–350. Abingdon, Oxon: Routledge.

Davis-Floyd R. 2001. "The Technocratic, Humanistic, and Holistic Paradigms of Childbirth." *International Journal of Gynecology & Obstetrics* 75, Supplement No. 1: S5–S23.

———. 2018. "The Technocratic, Humanistic, and Holistic Paradigms of Birth and Health Care." In *Ways of Knowing about Birth: Mothers, Midwives, Medicine, and Birth Activism*, ed. Davis-Floyd R, 3–44. Long Grove IL: Waveland Press.

———. 2022a. *Birth as an American Rite of Passage*, 3rd ed. Abingdon, Oxon: Routledge.

———. 2022b. "The International Childbirth Initiative: An Applied Anthropologist's Account of Developing Global Guidelines." In *Anthropologies of Global Maternal and Reproductive Health: From Policy Spaces to Sites of Practice*, ed. Wallace LJ, MacDonald MM, Storeng LT, 239–248. Cham, Switzerland: Springer Nature.

Davis-Floyd R, Georges N. 2023. "The Paradigm Shifts of Humanistic and Holistic Obstetricians: The 'Good Guys and Girls' of Brazil." In *Obstetric Violence and Systemic Disparities: Can Obstetrics Be Humanized and Decolonized?*, eds. Davis-Floyd R, Premkumar A, Chapter 9. New York: Berghahn Books.

Daviss BA, Davis-Floyd R, eds. 2021. *Birthing Models on the Human Rights Frontier: Speaking Truth to Power*. Abingdon, Oxon: Routledge.

Dick-Read G. 1942. *Childbirth without Fear: The Principles and Practice of Natural Childbirth*. London: Heinemann Medical Books.

England P, Horowitz R. 1998. *Birthing from Within*. Albuquerque NM: Partera Press.

Eyi EGY, Mollamahmutoglu L. 2021. "An Analysis of the High Cesarean Section Rates in Turkey by Robson Classification." *Journal of Maternal-Fetal and Neonatal Medicine* 34(16): 2682–2692.

Fletcher S. 2017. *Mindful HypnoBirthing*, London: Ebury Publishing.

Hodnett ED. 2002. "Pain and Women's Satisfaction with the Experience of Childbirth: A Systematic Review. *American Journal of Obstetrics and Gynecology* 186(5): S160–172.

Karabekir N. 2016. "Using Psychodrama in Childbirth Education and Birth Psychotherapy: Birth with No Regret." *Journal of Pre- and Perinatal Psychology and Health* 30(3): 34–43.

Lalonde A, Herschderfer K, Pascali Bonaro D, et al. 2019. "The International Childbirth Initiative: 12 Steps to Safe and Respectful MotherBaby-Family Maternity Care." *International Journal of Gynecology and Obstetrics* 146: 65–73.

Mongan MF. 2016. *HypnoBirthing*. Deerfield Beach FL: Health Communications.

Odent M. 2004. *The Caesarean*. London: Free Association Books.

———. 2014. *The Scientification of Love*. London: Free Association Books.

Verny T. 1982. *The Secret Life of the Unborn Child: How You Can Prepare Your Baby for a Happy, Healthy Life*. New York: Dell Publishing.

World Health Organization (WHO). 2018. "WHO Recommendations: Intrapartum Care for a Positive Childbirth Experience." WHO, 7 February. Retrieved 24 January 2022 from https://www.who.int/publications/i/item/9789241550215.

CHAPTER 11

Attempting to Maintain a Positive Awareness about Vaginal Breech Birth in Australia

Andrew Bisits

Introduction: Learning about Vaginal Breech Birth

Globally, around 3–5% of childbearers have babies who are in the breech (bottom-first) position (Hofmeyr, Hannah, and Lawrie 2015). In Australia, Canada, New Zealand, and the United States over the past 30 to 40 years, there has been a near-complete disappearance of vaginal breech birth (VBB) as a legitimate option for women with a breech presentation at term.[1] Other countries, particularly in Scandinavia and Europe, have maintained VBB as a supported and responsible option for these women. In this chapter, I describe how and what I have learnt about vaginal breech births over the years and refer to the many ambient pressures that have added to my learning. My descriptions of this learning about VBBs aim to inform, teach, and give confidence to all obstetricians and midwives so that they too can become safe breech birth practitioners.

My full-time career in obstetrics commenced in 1984 in a small District Hospital in Western Sydney. There, I was fortunate to learn some of the skills required for the safe conduct of vaginal breech birth and breech birth in general. Since that time, there have been several trends and emphases that have significantly influenced the practice of obstetrics and in particular the practices around breech births. I summarize these trends as follows:

- Increasing medical insurance costs arising from increased medicolegal case payouts. These have resulted in a climate of anxiety, fear, and a defensive mindset in the practices of obstetrics and midwifery, and have affected individual practitioners, hospitals, and health departments around the world. All obstetric practice is guided by the worst-case scenario with the central question: "If there is a bad outcome as a result of my practice, can I show that I have undertaken correct steps to have prevented it?" This negative mindset remains prominent in current obstetric practice.

- The emphasis on evidence-based medicine. Obstetrics has responded to this emphasis more than other specialties because of the perception in wider biomedical circles that obstetric practice was driven more by anecdote, authority, and opinion rather than by acceptable scientific evidence. This was clearly articulated with the publication of *Effective Care in Pregnancy and Childbirth* (Enkin, Kierse, and Chalmers 1989). According to this seminal publication, the debates and questions around VBB demanded rigorous evaluation in adequately powered randomized control trials.
- Fuelled by "evidence" and dominated by the language and mindset of statistics, the above two trends occurred within a growing climate of risk and fear. "Risk" became the dominant mood and mindset around childbirth.
- Information available via the internet led to the "democratization" of highly specialized knowledge, which up to that time was mostly contained in hard-to-access specialized textbooks or journals.
- The emphasis on client/patient involvement in decision-making around clinical care.
- Gender political developments aiming to undo the paternalistic approaches so common in obstetric practice up to the late 20th century.

In the climate of these influences, I have pursued an interest in breech birth and continue to do so (see also the chapter by André Lalonde, this volume). It has been a fascinating and rich journey. As previously noted, my first exposure to VBBs occurred in 1984 in a small but busy District Hospital in Western Sydney. During that year, despite my very junior status, I was given a reasonable amount of responsibility in the obstetrics and gynecology department. There was not a single ultrasound machine in this hospital, so we had to refer women who wanted or needed an ultrasound to a larger hospital located 15 minutes away from the District Hospital by car. Breech babies therefore would arrive unexpectedly. If a breech presentation was detected prior to labor, then the standard advice was for the woman to proceed with a vaginal birth. Often an epidural was recommended; however, these were administered less frequently compared to current practice. The women were instructed to birth in a lithotomy position with their legs elevated in stirrups. Continuous electronic monitoring of the baby's heart during labor was not always done. There was little or no discussion about the risks of a vaginal breech birth compared to birth by cesarean. The senior obstetricians (obs) in the department—the final arbiters of appropriate practice—were confident and matter-of-fact about their practices. Midwives commanded no such authority, even though a good number of them were more experienced than some of the obs, and particularly the ob trainees. Their role was more that of an obstetric nurse. Yet at the time, I learnt just as much from the midwifery staff as I did from the senior obstetricians, and I found this aspect of the learning very enjoyable. (It was also a very good ego-taming experience for me!)

The main principles around breech birth were to first encourage the woman to push out as much of the baby's body as she could. Then once we could see the shoulder blades of the baby, we would grasp the baby at the hips and rotate the baby 90 degrees one way and then 180 degrees the other way—a technique called "Lovset's maneuver." This maneuver facilitated the birth of the shoulders and arms. After this, we were instructed to routinely apply forceps to the head to control the speed of the delivery and thereby minimize any major decompression forces, which in turn was meant to minimize the possibility of any major blood vessels tearing in the baby's brain. I was told that breech vaginal delivery on the part of the obstetrician was an "art." I did observe an occasion where a senior obstetrician hurriedly tried to deliver a breech baby's leg and unintentionally fractured the baby's femur. Thus the main lesson for me was *patience*.

However, my key learning at this time was the need to work in a complementary way with midwives. Because I enjoyed this aspect of practice so much, I decided to specialize in obstetrics. In that year, 1984, the medicolegal aspect of obstetrics started to become a greater concern. Obstetric complications leading to longer term problems for babies were often followed by substantial payouts, and these lawsuits seemed to be increasing, following the lead of the United States. More and more, Australian obstetricians felt the need to practice defensively—to over-investigate and over-intervene to protect themselves.

In the following year, I moved to a bigger hospital in Liverpool, Southwestern Sydney, which was also in a lower socioeconomic area with a higher proportion of immigrant women. As in the smaller District Hospital, all the senior obstetricians were men. There were several very experienced senior midwives from whom I learnt a great deal. They would let you know very directly if they had concerns about your practices. I remember that when I started to work at the larger hospital, one of them specifically said, "Dr. Bisits, I hope you are going to be kind to the women who birth in our hospital!" At that time, the cesarean rate in that hospital was only 9%. VBBs were still an acceptable and encouraged part of obstetric practice. One senior obstetrician stated to me, "Doc, vaginal breech births are as safe as houses, if you look after them properly." The principles of the conduct of vaginal breech were very similar to those of the District Hospital: women would birth in stirrups; they would push the baby out until the shoulder blades emerged; at that stage you did the Lovset's maneuver referred to above; once the arms were birthed, you were instructed to let the baby's body hang over the edge of the bed in order to help the head flex and deliver. After waiting a short while, either forceps were applied to the head, or hands were used to further flex and deliver the head. There was one induced breech birth during which no electronic fetal monitoring was done. There was some mechanical difficulty in delivering the baby, which was eventually done by the midwife and not by the attending obstetrician. Sadly, the baby could not be resuscitated. Current practice recommendations are that breech babies should have continuous electronic heart monitoring during labor. The outcome of that birth suggests that this is a reasonable recommendation.

Overall, during that time I became more confident with VBBs, due to the confidence and competence of the senior obstetricians and midwives. The senior obstetrician who used to call me "Doc" (never by my first name) and had told me that breech vaginal births were "as safe as houses" also referred to a quality called "obstetric courage." At first, I dismissed this as a slightly arrogant, "macho"-based quality. However, I have come to think he meant that obstetricians need to develop a level of "steel" to deal with some of the difficult situations they are faced with. He further said that we need to rein in the level of "drama" that had increasingly become a feature of childbirth. The senior midwife, who worked closely with this obstetrician, told me that that the Latin translation of obstetrics (*obstare* or *ob-stare*) was "to stand by." In addition, she said, "Remember, Dr. Biscuits (a common nickname for me), that what we do to these women during childbirth stays with them for the rest of their life." These words of wisdom have stayed with me and have been a fundamental part of my approach to women who choose to birth their breech babies vaginally.

In 1987, I moved to Newcastle, two hours north of Sydney. There in the tertiary hospital that was closely linked with the relatively new Newcastle Medical School, I completed my formal training as an obstetrician and gynecologist. Newcastle became the first regional center in

New South Wales to have a tertiary level hospital, including a neonatal intensive care unit that could care for very preterm babies. This medical school was the first in Australia to adopt new teaching methods—in particular problem-based learning, following the model from McMaster University in Hamilton, Ontario, Canada. The Newcastle Medical School had been established in 1979 to develop new and fresh methods of education for doctors, and this approach influenced the mindset of biomedical practice in that town. An important part of the new medical course on Clinical Epidemiology was a module called "Critical Reasoning." The emphasis here was a thorough grounding in the evolving area of evidence-based medicine, which included a rigorous approach to the critical appraisal of evidence based on the work of David L. Sackett, R. Brian Haynes, and Peter Tugwell (1985) and of William Silverman (1985). I completed the course in Clinical Epidemiology and therefore was strongly influenced by the emphasis on using evidence to guide clinical decisions.

When the seminal textbook *Effective Care in Pregnancy and Childbirth* (Enkin, Kierse, and Chalmers 1989) was published, I greeted this book enthusiastically, and, along with a senior midwife, purchased the two hefty volumes. (We shared the cost because it was so expensive.) This book became the foundation of evidence-based medicine, and eventually led to the current Cochrane Collaboration—an international not-for-profit organization that aims to make up-to-date, accurate information about the effects of healthcare readily available worldwide.[2] The book was a summary and synthesis of the most rigorous evidence in maternity care that could be used to justify clinical practice. This textbook was the first to use meta-analysis as a form of evidence synthesis, which until that time had mostly been a narrative and qualitative exercise. In this book, there was a whole chapter devoted to mode of birth for the breech baby at term. Two smaller randomized trials had been conducted, and these pointed to a slightly increased risk of severe adverse neonatal outcomes for the neonate; however, because of the small numbers, the conclusions were not definitive (see Collea, Chin, and Quilligan 1980; Gimovsky et al. 1983). The chapter concluded with the recommendation that more research in the form of adequately powered randomized controlled trials needed to be done to offer more solid evidence on which to base clinical decisions. At the same time, the frequency of VBBs was clearly decreasing in Australia and elsewhere in both private and public obstetric practices. I wrote a clinical commentary for my specialist exam on this subject and came to conclusions similar to those in the above-mentioned textbook. In this commentary, I wrote about the role of "formal decision analysis" as a way of helping women come to decisions about mode of birth when there is a breech baby at term. I made extensive reference to Harold Sox—a physician from California who had written a book called *Medical Decision Making* (1988). The main thrust of this approach was to incorporate the patient's values and preferences in coming to an agreed decision about any aspect of clinical care.

Along with a few of my senior colleagues, I became increasingly concerned about the drift toward an excessive number of cesareans in obstetrics, particularly for breech births. I felt at the time that the reasoning around these decisions and trends was fear-based and negative, and therefore we needed a more positive and reasoned approach. In the area of vaginal breech birth, I saw the need to better understand the mechanics of these births along with better support for the normal process and maximizing safety. The advice in textbooks—including very eminent textbooks—was quite limited. Instead, I found it most useful to speak with experienced obstetricians. I also became interested in discussing risks with women in relation to decisions around mode of birth. I became frustrated with what I saw as a simplistic approach to managing the decision-making, which seemed to amount to "I'm scared, you're scared, let's do a cesarean section."

During this time, I worked more closely with midwives in women's clinical care. In Newcastle, there was already a strong emphasis on midwifery, and the midwives were quite assertive. Several midwives had established themselves as independent practitioners, which was quite revolutionary at the time, and was viewed with great apprehension by various obstetricians. These midwives taught me an enormous amount about childbirth. They helped me to understand the primary and pivotal role of midwifery in a woman's pregnancy, birth, and postnatal period. As I started to think more about vaginal breech birth, they gave me the contact details for New Zealand midwife Maggie Banks. I had read her book *Breech Birth, Woman Wise* (1998). Via emails, I discussed with her women adopting positions other than lithotomy for the births of breech babies. I commented to Maggie that obstetricians seemed to be psychologically locked into the lithotomy position. She agreed with this, politely. I therefore looked for the evidence behind other birthing positions at the critical time of pushing. If more gravity could be used, then upright positions could be more efficient ways to birth the breech baby—and hopefully to minimize hypoxia (fetal oxygen lack), which occurred more frequently in newborns after vaginal breech births.

A midwife who worked in our unit had developed and marketed a birth stool (see Boenigk 2021). I had seen a report of such a stool used in a birthing unit in Germany with encouraging results. I had attended a breech birth with this midwife, in which the woman was known to have a baby greater than 4 kg; she had previously birthed bigger babies. This was an instructive occasion for me, during which I simply sat and watched the birth unfold; the midwife was the primary accoucheur. The woman birthed in an almost-standing position, leaning forward against a wall. The midwife did need to help one of the baby's arms out. She also performed some additional flexion of the head with her hands. The baby was in good condition and weighed 4.3 kilograms (around 9½ pounds). Surprisingly, my main learning from this birth was simply the need to be quiet at births. (I had commenced a discussion with the husband whilst the woman was laboring; I was then told sternly by the midwife to keep quiet because the woman needed a quiet space to continue with the birth.) It was also instructive to watch the midwife confidently deal with the birth of a bigger baby. Her manipulations of the baby were minimal yet effective.

Since that time (1997), I have encouraged women to use the birth stool for vaginal breech births. The stool favors the efficient descent of the baby's body and encourages maximal expulsive efforts from the woman. It has also resulted in a limited need for significant manipulations of the arms or the head. Since using this birth stool, I have not had to use forceps at all for the birth of the after-coming head. I have noted that in most VBBs in our hospital, especially in the births of multips (women who have already given birth), the baby's head is born within three minutes of the buttocks being born.

Most women find the use of the birth stool acceptable, and if they favor another position at the time of the birth, then the position is changed. With the use of the birth stool, the birth of the head tends to require more manual help compared to the hands and knees position, which opens the pelvis to its maximum diameter and is ideal both for breech births and for shoulder dystocia (stuck shoulder) (see Bruner et al. 1998). My colleagues and I have summarized our experiences with these vaginal breech births, 95% of which were in an upright position, in an article (Borbolla et al. 2014).

During my time in Newcastle, the critical event that influenced all practice around vaginal breech births was the publication of the International Term Breech Trial (Hannah et al. 2000). Our hospital had agreed to participate in this trial; however, I had significant reservations and expressed these directly to the first author, Dr. Mary Hannah. Among these reservations was my concern that it would be difficult to standardize care with the involvement of so many hospitals around the world. The conduct of the trial involving so many centers with so many variations in practice (despite the best efforts of the trial authors to prescribe appropriate standards of practice) would lend itself to a bias against the safety of vaginal breech birth. In the end, although our hospital had agreed to participate, not one woman agreed to participate in the trial. The investigators stopped the trial after the second interim analysis showed an unacceptable excess of adverse events in the vaginal breech arm of the trial. The results were then rigorously analyzed and published later that year in *The Lancet* (Hannah et al. 2000). The key result was that in countries such as the United States, Australia, Canada, and the UK, the frequency of some more serious short-term outcomes was 5% in the planned vaginal breech arm of the study; in the planned cesarean section arm, this number was 1%. Due to these findings, most hospitals and countries that had been allowing VBBs suddenly stopped doing them or decreased them significantly. There have been few other trials in clinical medicine that have had such a dramatic and sudden impact.

However, it was clear that despite these results, many women still wanted to be supported to have a vaginal breech birth. In Australia at the time, there was a crisis about medical indemnity insurance when the chief underwriter of the main medical defense association, Health Insurance Holdings (HIH), collapsed. This had been the largest corporate collapse in Australia's history. The collapse was attributed to poor corporate governance management, poor risk management, and a lack of oversight, along with corrupt behaviors. Up to that time, obstetricians in private practice had faced increasing premium charges for their medical defenses. After the collapse of HIH and the medical defense organizations, it seemed that there would be no medical insurance available for private obstetricians. The then-government therefore offered financial support to obstetricians so they could afford the medical defense premiums; thereby a new medical defense organization was established. In the public discourse around these issues, obstetrics was described as one of the riskier specialties in clinical medicine. It was little surprise that in this fragile environment, the Term Breech Trial had such a profound effect on reducing the frequency of vaginal breech births to almost zero in Australia.

The international Term Breech Trial and its results were claimed as a critical triumph for evidence-based medicine (Lumley 2000). Here was a clear clinical question that needed to be resolved: namely, the safest mode of birth for a breech presenting baby at term. Every effort was made to design the trial carefully, with careful attention to sample size, standardization of procedures and protocols, and rigorous data collection. Both short- and long-term outcomes were collected for both mother and baby in the conduct of the trial. Adequate funding was obtained for the study from a Canadian government research body. It was anticipated confidently that the results of the trial would have a significant impact on clinical practice. Interim analyses were planned and conducted. Having done all of this, a clear result was achieved, and this indeed did influence clinical practice. Because of this "triumph," there was remarkably little discussion or debate about the results for the first two years after the study was published. This lack of discussion is reflected in the limited number of letters and comments that were forwarded to *The Lancet* three months after the study was published (Ponzone and Sismondi 2001). The American College of Obstetricians and Gynecologists (ACOG 2006) deemed that planned vaginal breech birth may no longer be an appropriate standard of care. Thus, I experienced further pressure to cease offering the possibility of VBB, or at least to strongly dissuade women from attempting it. Nevertheless, in Newcastle we continued to offer vaginal breech birth because our outcomes seemed to be better than those reported in the Term Breech Trial, and there were still women with a breech baby at term who wanted to pursue a VBB even after considering the results of the trial.

Therefore, I concentrated on thinking about ways of optimizing the safety of VBBs to continue to achieve better results than those of the Term Breech Trial. One area of concern was the increasing number of cesareans that were done for breech, especially if the woman was in advanced labor, fully dilated, and pushing. This resulted in quite difficult cesarean births, which had become increasingly hazardous for both the mother and the baby. In a regional center in New South Wales, such a cesarean was performed and resulted in a post-operative abdominal hemorrhage where there was delayed recognition of its seriousness, and this delayed recognition eventually led to the woman's death. This cesarean had been performed at a very advanced stage of labor on a woman who had birthed her two previous children vaginally. There were several other reports from around the world where women who were good candidates for a VBB died as a result of planned or semi-planned cesareans. Such reports gave me further impetus to consider ways of optimizing safety in vaginal breech births. The key components to this approach over the years became: (1) provide adequate information for the woman to make an informed decision; (2) provide an understanding about the mechanics of breech birth; (3) individualize risk counseling around mode of birth; (4) promote a responsible confidence about VBB when the woman was deemed a good candidate for it; (5) adopt a systematic approach for dealing with problems that can arise during VBBs; and (6) have a senior skilled midwife and obstetrician present during the labor and birth.

In 2006, two events gave me further impetus to pursue the above approaches. One of these events was the publication of the PREMODA study of 6,000 breech births in France and Belgium (Goffinet et al. 2006). In contrast to the results of the Term Breech Trail, the authors of the PREMODA study concluded that: "In places where planned vaginal delivery is a common practice and when strict criteria are met before and during labor, planned vaginal delivery of singleton fetuses in breech presentation at term remains a safe option that can be offered to women" (Goffinet et al. 2006:1002). The results of this study were presented at a small international meeting in Vancouver about breech birth. This meeting was designed to facilitate responsible and critical discussions of the Term Breech Trial results and to consider ways to improve the safety of vaginal breech birth. By that time, several detailed critiques of the Term Breech Trial had appeared; the essence of these was to acknowledge that the trial did report an increased frequency of risks with VBB, and also to acknowledge that there were unintended biases in the conduct of the study that contributed to its results. One such critique from Marek Glezerman (2006) catalogued a detailed number of biases in the study that he considered so significant that he called for the conclusions of the Term Breech Trial to be formally withdrawn (they were not). It is critical to also note other limitations in the trial, such as the facts that the neonatal deaths that occurred did not meet the inclusion criteria for the trial itself, and that secondary analyses demonstrated that obstetricians' discomfort with attending vaginal breech births in the Term Breech Trial played key roles in adverse outcomes (Su 2003). According to Canadian midwife Betty-Anne Davis and myself (Daviss and Bisits 2021:149):

> Several explanations of what this study did and didn't prove have been published in reputable medical journals (Glezerman 2006; Menticoglou 2006; Daviss, Johnson and Lalonde 2010; Lawson 2012). In the end, there is general consensus that undue weight was applied to initial bad fetal and neonatal outcomes recorded as early as the first five minutes of life, and categorized as "serious" injury, but which then quickly disappeared. When the follow-up study at two years revealed that the apparent greater number of these bad outcomes among the babies born vaginally had disappeared, the final conclusions of the Term Breech Trial were that planned cesarean section for breech "is not associated with a reduction in risk of death or neuro-developmental delay in children at two years of age" (Whyte et al. 2004:871).

In other words, these later, more careful considerations of the evidence showed no additional long-term harm to breech than head-down babies when skillfully attended, as did the PREMODA study cited above.

Breech babies born vaginally do commonly have lower early Apgar scores due to cord compression during delivery, yet these differences vanish quickly soon after birth (Daviss and Bisits 2021).

The international meeting held in Vancouver in 2006 was a very stimulating occasion where there was critical thinking about many of the issues related to term VBB. In particular, several midwives present were very experienced with normal vaginal breech births. They gave very detailed descriptions of the mechanics of breech birth; these were far more informative than any of the descriptions in standard obstetric textbooks. Among these midwives were Jane Evans from the UK, Anne Frye from the United States, and Betty-Anne Daviss from Canada. In her textbook on holistic midwifery, Anne Frye (2005) provides a comprehensive description of normal and abnormal breech birth mechanics that is far superior to that in any obstetric textbook. The discussions of such knowledge among obstetricians, midwives, and women themselves led to very fruitful conclusions and possibilities to improve the care of women and babies during vaginal breech labors and births. (For descriptions of how best to attend vaginal breech births,[3] see Frye 2005; Daviss and Bisits 2021.) Since that 2006 meeting in Vancouver, there have been four other such meetings over the years, and each time there has been a healthy mix of midwives, obstetricians, physiotherapists, and lay women. The increasing use of video clips of their vaginal breech births generously donated by mothers has led to much better education around their conducts. This sharing of experiences in various breech birth centers around the world, in particular Frankfurt, Germany (see Daviss and Bisits 2021), Newcastle Hospital in Sydney, Australia, the Netherlands, the Scandinavian countries, Canada, and France has led to constructive considerations of factors that can promote the safety of VBBs. This information-sharing has led to a better internationally agreed-upon understanding of the mechanics of breech birth. In addition, these discussions have promoted important research initiatives to further clarify broader questions about VBB and the challenges that it poses.

The international discussions and collaborations described above have ensured that research into vaginal breech birth will continue. At this time of writing (January 2022), another randomized trial around optimizing breech birth is being developed in the UK, and several excellent observational and qualitative studies have appeared in the obstetric literature about the issues surrounding VBB and the Term Breech Trial.[4] In the United States, George Washington University has promoted a Vaginal Breech Initiative (Marko et al. 2019), while the Hellen Diller Medical Center at the University of California San Francisco has been offering singleton vaginal breech deliveries for the past 40 years (see Flanagan et al. 1987; Laros, Flanagan, and Kilpatrick 1995; Hopkins et al. 2007).

In Australia, a group of obstetricians, midwives, and general practitioners have developed and run a breech birth course called "Becoming a Breech Expert" (BABE). This course, held two to three times a year, teaches the important learnings from the various international collaborations and conferences on breech birth. The course also utilizes several of the excellent video clips of VBBs that are now widely available on various closed websites. The use of higher-fidelity plastic mother and baby models allows much more effective teaching around the practical skills necessary for the safe conduct of vaginal breech birth. The course also presents the views of consumers who have had to make decisions around breech birth amidst the many pressures they faced from family, friends, and the media. Finally, a session is dedicated to discussing breech birth and its attendant risks with women. This is done in the form of a role-play; a consistent script guides the discussion, and then there is the opportunity for participants to ask questions. We have found the feedback about this course to be almost universally positive. Several institutions have requested that we conduct these courses at their hospitals, and where possible, we do so.

At the hospital where I currently work, there is a weekly breech clinic to which women with a breech presentation at term are referred. We always advise an ultrasound to assess the growth of the baby. Should this be normal along with the amniotic fluid volume, then we enthusiastically encourage and offer external cephalic version (turning the baby in utero to a head-down position). If this is not successful, then we discuss mode of birth. This discussion consists of demonstrating the mechanics of breech birth in both cesareans and vaginal births, then outlining the logistics of care, and finally considering the comparative risks of planned vaginal breech birth and planned elective cesarean birth. The women consider this information and read the Royal College of Obstetricians and Gynaecologists (RCOG) guidelines (Impey et al. 2017), our hospital guidelines, and the Society of Obstetricians and Gynecologists of Canada (SOGC) guidelines on breech birth (Kotaska and Mentigoclou 2019). I also encourage women to visit the Breech without Borders website because of the excellent descriptions, demonstrations, and videos of breech births available there. The women and their partners consider this information and then call me about their decision regarding mode of birth; the majority of women I care for whose babies are breech choose a cesarean birth. Yet as I am writing this chapter in January 2022, currently four of the women I am caring for have decided that they will attempt a vaginal breech birth.

Conclusion: Suggestions for Optimizing the Safety of Vaginal Breech Births

In conclusion, I offer you the following thoughts and suggestions about optimizing the safety of vaginal breech births:

1. All obstetricians and midwives, whether or not they feel comfortable with vaginal breech birth, need to acknowledge that the care of the women having VBBs is a necessary skill.
2. If any institution is to offer vaginal breech birth, then its practitioners must develop collective confidence around it.
3. Obstetricians and midwives need to have a tight and constructive framework of cooperation around the care of women with breech babies.
4. Hospitals offering VBBs need to hold regular training sessions in which obstetricians, midwives, and labor and delivery nurses participate.
5. All maternity care providers should attend one of the dedicated courses on VBBs. These include the BABE course in Australia, the Breech without Borders course (held in the United States and internationally), Shawn Walker's Breech Study days (UK), and the one-to-two day course offered by Betty-Anne Daviss and Ken Johnson (held in North America and internationally).[5]
6. They need to have clear guidelines regarding appropriate care during VBBs.
7. All practitioners need to agree on the normal parameters around a normal vaginal breech birth and to recognize the abnormal.
8. All practitioners need to be able to deal with the delays in the first and second stages of labor that sometimes occur during VBBs, with ready recourse to cesarean where appropriate. Cesarean is advised for slow progress in the active first stage (defined as starting at 6 cm of cervical dilation). In Australia, we use 0.5 cm cervical dilation per hour over a 6-hour period as our standard, which is more stringent than in France and Belgium, where VBB practitioners allow 7 hours from 5 to 10 cm (Goffinet et al. 2006), or in Frankfurt, where 17–18% of women attempting VBB took more than 10 hours to dilate from 5 to 10 cm (Louwen et al. 2017). A passive second stage without

active pushing may last up to 90 minutes, allowing the breech to descend well into the pelvis. We recommend cesarean when the buttocks have not birthed after an hour of active pushing (Kotaska et al. 2009), although others in other countries do not follow this protocol, giving laboring women more time to push (see Louwen et al. 2017; Daviss and Johnson 2021).

9. At the expulsive phase of birth, we recommend that all practitioners at any institution agree in advance on the signs of deviation from the cardinal movements from the birth of the buttocks to the birth of the head (Daviss 2014; Louwen et al. 2017) and consider how delays and timelines will be used (Daviss and Johnson 2021).
10. If delay is recognized after the buttocks are born, all birth practitioners need to diagnose and deal with the cause of the delay (most frequently the baby's arms are obstructing the descent of the body and head [i.e., nuchal arms]).
11. Practitioners need to be able to encourage and help a woman change position and to work with her in different positions for the vaginal birth of her breech baby, including sitting on a birth stool, hands and knees (again, the position that opens the pelvis to its maximum diameter), or squatting. In all of these positions, it is possible to deal with abnormalities and delays. The key to learning about the benefits of these various positions is rehearsal with a pelvic model and a model of a baby.
12. When a woman is laboring to accomplish a vaginal breech birth, the birth room must be kept quiet and calm, and the number of staff in the room needs to be monitored carefully so that the presence of too many people does not impede her capacity to birth.

Andrew Bisits is Director of Obstetrics at the Royal Hospital for Women, Sydney, Australia—a tertiary academic hospital that oversees 4,000 births per year. In Newcastle, he served as Director of Obstetrics for eight years. Dr. Bisits has been in full-time obstetric practice for 30 years and has long had a strong interest in breech birth. In the research arena, he has a strong leaning toward epidemiology and biostatistics. In the clinical arena, he has participated in several initiatives to promote normal birth through helping establish primary midwifery care programs for pregnant women. Dr. Bisits has a conjoint associate professorial position with the University of New South Wales and is on the Australian board of ALSO (Advanced Life Support in Obstetrics).

Notes

1. Preterm breech babies are usually delivered via cesarean due to associations with a higher frequency of adverse perinatal outcomes, inclusive of perinatal death, during a vaginal birth (Ciblis, Karrison, and Brown 1994; Robertson et al. 1995). However, during the periviable period (22–25 weeks), route of delivery for a breech-presenting baby has not been associated with a difference in perinatal outcomes (ACOG 2017).
2. See Cochrane homepage. Retrieved 17 September 2022 from www.cochrane.org.
3. The book *Re-Thinking the Physiology of Vaginal Breech Birth* by Betty-Anne Daviss—a manual that includes detailed descriptions and photos of appropriate techniques—is available to buy online. "Bringing Back Vaginal Breech Birth." *Understanding Birth Better*. Retrieved 17 September 2022 from https://understandingbirthbetter.com/section.php?ID=25&Lang=En&Nav=Section.
4. See, for examples, Giuliani et al. 2002; Alarab et al. 2004; Kotaska 2004; Hopkins et al. 2007; Albrechtsen 2010; Azria 2012; Demirci 2012; Toivonen et al. 2014; Vlemmix et al. 2014; Kessler, Moster, and Albrechtsen 2015; Catling et al. 2016a, 2016b; Petrovksa et al. 2016, 2017; Louwen et al. 2017.
5. To access these latter courses, write to Betty-Anne Daviss at bettyannedaviss@gmail.com and/or to Ken Johnson at ken47johnson@gmail.com

References

ACOG. 2006. "Mode of Term Singleton Breech Delivery. ACOG Committee Opinion #340." *American College of Obstetricians and Gynecologists*. Found at: Mode of Term Singleton Breech Delivery | ACOG. Accessed February 9, 2022.

———. 2017. "Obstetric Care Consensus No. 6: Periviable Birth." *Obstetrics & Gynecology* 130: e187–e199.

Alarab M, Regan C, O'Connell MP, Keane DP, O'Herlihy C, Foley ME. 2004. "Singleton Vaginal Breech Delivery at Term: Still a Safe Option." *Obstetrics & Gynecology* 103(3): 407–412.

Albrechtsen S. 2010. "Vaginal Delivery in Breech Presentation." *Tidsskr Nor Laegeforen* 130(6): 589.

Azria E, Le Meaux JP, Khoshnood B, et al. PREMODA Study Group. 2012. "Factors Associated with Adverse Perinatal Outcomes for Term Breech Fetuses with Planned Vaginal Delivery." *American Journal of Obstetrics and Gynecology* 207(4): 285.e1–9.

Banks M. 1998. *Breech Birth, Woman Wise*. Hamilton NZ: Birthspirit Books.

Boenigk M. 2021. "BirthRite Birthing Seat." *Brithrite*. Retrieved 18 September 2022 from birthrite.com.au.

Borbolla FA, Bagust A, Bisits A, et al. 2014. "Lessons to be Learnt in Managing the Breech Presentation at Term: An 11-Year Single-Centre Retrospective Study." *Australia New Zealand Journal of Obstetrics and Gynaecology* 54(4): 333–339.

Bruner JP, Drummond SB, Meenan AL, Gaskin IM. 1998. "All-Fours Maneuver for Reducing Shoulder Dystocia during Labor." *Journal of Reproductive Medicine* 43(5): 439–443.

Catling C, Petrovska K, Watts N, Bisits A, Homer CS. 2016a. "Barriers and Facilitators for Vaginal Breech Births in Australia: Clinician's Experiences." *Women and Birth* 29(2): 138–143.

———. 2016b. "Care During the Decision-Making Phase for Women Who Want a Vaginal Breech Birth: Experiences from the Field." *Midwifery* 34: 111–116.

Cibils LA, Karrison T, Brown L. 1994. "Factors Influencing Neonatal Outcomes in the Very-Low-Birth-Weight Fetus (< 1500 Grams) with a Breech Presentation." *American Journal of Obstetrics and Gynecology* 171(1): 35–42.

Collea JV, Chein C, Quilligan EJ. 1980. "The Randomized Management of Term Frank Breech Presentation: A Study of 208 Cases." *American Journal of Obstetrics and Gynecology* 137(2): 235–244.

Daviss BA. 2014. *Re-Thinking the Physiology of Vaginal Breech Birth: Evidence-Based Guide to Upright Delivery*. Ottawa, Ontario: Informed Descent Publishing. Available at: www.understanding birthbetter.com.

Daviss BA, Bisits A. 2021. "Bringing Back Breech: Dismantling Hierarchies and Re-skilling Practitioners." In *Birthing Models on the Human Rights Frontier: Speaking Truth to Power*, ed. Daviss BA, Davis-Floyd R, 145–183. Abingdon, Oxon: Routledge.

Daviss BA, Johnson KC. 2021. "Upright Breech Birth: New Video Research Risks Reviving Friedman's Curse." *Birth* 49: 11–15.

Daviss BA, Johnson K, Lalonde A. 2010. "Evolving Evidence since the Term Breech Trial: Canadian Response, European Dissent, and Potential Solutions. *Journal of Obstetrics and Gynaecology Canada* 32(3): 217–224.

Demirci O, Tuğrul AS, Turgut A, et al. 2012. "Pregnancy Outcomes by Mode of Delivery among Breech Births." *Archives of Gynecology and Obstetrics* 285(2): 297–303.

Enkin M, Kierse MJC, Chalmers I. 1989. *Effective Care in Pregnancy and Childbirth*. Oxford UK: Oxford University Press.

Flanagan TA, Mulchahey KM, Korenbrot CC, et al. 1987. "Management of Term Breech Presentation." *American Journal of Obstetrics and Gynecology* 156(6): 1492–1502.

Frye A. 2005. *Holistic Midwifery: A Comprehensive Textbook for Midwives in Homebirth Practice*. Volume 2: *Care During Labor and Birth*. Portland OR: Labrys Press.

Furedi F. 2002. *Culture of Fear: Risk Taking and the Morality of Low Expectation*. New York: Continuum.

Gimovsky ML, Wallace RL, Schifrin BS, Paul RH. 1983. "Randomized Management of the Nonfrank Breech Presentation at Term: A Preliminary Report." *American Journal of Obstetrics & Gynecology* 146: 34–40.

Giuliani A, Schöll WM, Basver A, Tamussino KF. 2002. "Mode of Delivery and Outcome of 699 Term Singleton Breech Deliveries at a Single Center." *American Journal of Obstetrics & Gynecology* 187(6): 1694–1698.

Glezerman M. 2006. "Five Years to the Term Breech Trial: The Rise and Fall of a Randomized Controlled Trial." *American Journal of Obstetrics and Gynecology* 194(1): 20–25.

Goffinet F, Carayol M, Foidart JM, et al., PREMODA Study Group. 2006. "Is Planned Vaginal Delivery for Breech Presentation at Term Still an Option? Results of an

Observational Prospective Survey in France and Belgium." *American Journal of Obstetrics and Gynecology* 194(4): 1002–1011.

Hannah ME, Hannah WJ, Hewson SA, Hodnett ED, Saigal S, Willan AR for the Term Breech Trial Collaboration Group. 2000. "Planned Caesarean Section versus Planned Vaginal Birth for Breech Presentation at Term: A Randomised Multicentre Trial." *The Lancet* 356: 1375–1383.

Hofmeyr GJ, Hannah M, Lawrie TA. 2015. "Planned Caesarean Section for Term Breech Delivery." *Cochrane Database of Systematic Reviews* 7 (7): CD000166.

Hopkins LM, Esakoff T, Noah MS, et al. 2007. "Outcomes Associated with Cesarean Section versus Vaginal Breech Delivery at a University Hospital." *Journal of Perinatology* 27(3): 141–146.

Impey LWM, Murphy DJ, Griffiths M, Penna LK on behalf of the Royal College of Obstetricians and Gynaecologists. 2017. "Management of Breech Presentation: Green-Top Guideline No. 20b." *British Journal of Obstetrics and Gynaecology* 124: e151–e177.

Kessler J, Moster D, Albrechtsen S. 2015. "Intrapartum Monitoring with Cardiotocography and ST-Waveform Analysis in Breech Presentation: An Observational Study." *British Journal of Obstetrics and Gynaecology* 22(4): 528–535.

Kotaska A. 2004. "Inappropriate Use of Randomised Trials to Evaluate Complex Phenomena: Case Study of Vaginal Breech Delivery." *British Medical Journal* 329(7479): 1385.

Kotaska A, Menticoglu S. 2019. "SOGC Clinical Practice Guideline No. 384—Management of Breech Presentation at Term." *Journal of Obstetrics and Gynaecology Canada* 41(8):1193–205.

Laros RK Jr, Flanagan TA, Kilpatrick SJ. 1995. "Management of Term Breech Presentation: A Protocol of External Cephalic Version and Selective Trial of Labor." *American Journal of Obstetrics and Gynecology* 172(6): 1916–23

Lawson GW. 2012. "The Term Breech Trial Ten Years On: *Primum Non Nocere?*" *Birth* 39(1): 3–9.

Louwen F, Daviss BA, Johnson KC, Reitter A. 2017. "Does Breech Delivery in an Upright Position Instead of on the Back Improve Outcomes and Avoid Cesareans?" *International Journal of Gynaecology and Obstetrics* 136(2): 151–161.

Lumley J. 2000. "Any Room Left for Disagreement about Assisting Breech Births at Term?" *Lancet* 356(9239): 1369–1370.

Marko KI, Gimovsky AC, Madkour A, et al. 2019. "Current Experience with the Vaginal Breech Initiative at the George Washington University Hospital." *Obstetrics & Gynecology* 133: 53S–51S.

Menticoglou S. 2006. "Why Vaginal Breech Delivery Should Still Be Offered." *Journal of Obstetrics and Gynaecology Canada* 28(5): 380–385.

Ponzone R, Sismondi P. 2001. "Term Breech Trial." *The Lancet* 357(9251): 226–227; author reply 227–228.

Petrovska K, Watts NP, Catling C, et al. 2016. "Supporting Women Planning a Vaginal Breech Birth: An International Survey." *Birth* 43(4): 353–357.

———. 2017. "'Stress, Anger, Fear and Injustice': An International Qualitative Survey of Women's Experiences Planning a Vaginal Breech Birth." *Midwifery* 44: 41–47.

Robertson PA, Foran CM, Croughan-Minihane MS, Kilpatrick SJ. 1995. "Head Entrapment and Neonatal Outcome by Mode of Delivery in Breech Deliveries from Twenty-Four to Twenty-Seven Weeks of Gestation." *American Journal of Obstetrics and Gynecology* 173(4): 1171–1176.

Sackett DL, Haynes RB, Tugwell P. 1985. *Clinical Epidemiology: A Basic Science for Clinical Medicine*. New York: Little, Brown and Company.

Silverman WA. 1985. *Human Experimentation: A Guided Step into the Unknown*. Oxford: Oxford University Press.

Sox HC. 1988. *Medical Decision Making*. Stoneham MA: Butterworth Publishers.

Su M, McLeod L, Ross S, Willan A, et al., Term Breech Trial Collaborative Group. 2003. "Factors Associated with Adverse Perinatal Outcome in the Term Breech Trial." *American Journal of Obstetrics and Gynecology* 189(3): 740–745.

Toivonen E, Palomäki O, Huhtala H, Uotila J. 2014. "Maternal Experiences of Vaginal Breech Delivery." *Birth* 41(4): 316–322.

Vlemmix F, Bergenhenegouwen L, Schaaf JM, et al. 2014. "Term Breech Deliveries in the Netherlands: Did the Increased Cesarean Rate Affect Neonatal Outcome? A Population-Based Cohort Study." *Acta Obstetricia et Gynecologica Scandivica* 93(9): 888–896.

Whyte H, Hannah ME, Saigal S, et al. 2004. "Outcomes of Children at 2 Years after Planned Cesarean Birth versus Planned Vaginal Birth for Breech Presentation at Term: The International Randomized Term Breech Trial." *American Journal of Obstetrics and Gynecology* 191(3): 864–871.

CHAPTER 12

Mixing Modalities in My Technocratic/Humanistic Obstetric Practice
Ideology and Rationales

Marco Gianotti

Introduction

Thoughts on Being a Technocratic/Humanistic Obstetrician: My Ideology, Practice, and Rationales

Regarding terminology, in this chapter I draw on Robbie Davis-Floyd's explications of "the technocratic, humanistic, and holistic paradigms of birth and health care" as delineated in the Series Overview at the beginning of this volume, and ground my ideology and my practice in both the technocratic and humanistic models, with the occasional incorporation of holistic modalities. Although the practice of technocratic biomedicine in and of itself has become much more trying during the COVID-19 pandemic, I have found that it is still very possible to integrate more humanistic (and sometimes holistic) measures of practice into a care plan for patients seeking such a balance. Yet the incorporation of humanistic, and even holistic, patterns of care into technocratic practice has been made more difficult during the pandemic (see Davis-Floyd, Gutschow, and Schwartz 2020; Gutschow and Davis-Floyd 2021). As these authors have shown, patient care has been severely restricted by limited access to caregivers and, in many hospitals, to their partners and other family members, just at the time when they need these loved ones most.

While not all humanistic and holistic methods will always be acceptable to even the most open-minded obstetrician (ob), there can be a justifiable balance that allows for a birth care plan that satisfies the patient's goals and desires as well as those of the ob. Much of this goes back to how the physician was trained and the beliefs and perceptions that a doctor both internalizes during training and develops over time. The practice of obstetrics presents a particular opportunity to incorporate doula support in hospitals, along with other humanistic and holistic modalities. My experience has shown that this can be done safely and with excellent clinical outcomes, even during a pandemic.

Adapting to a Rapidly Changing Landscape: A Traditionalist's Approach to Obstetrics and Gynecology in a New Millennium

Long before the advent of the COVID-19 pandemic, the practice of biomedicine, and of obstetrics, had been rapidly changing with the arrival of computer technology, the internet, and the patient's ensuing ability to readily access medical information at the touch of a keyboard or smartphone. Whether it's an individual's own post or multiple interactions through specifically themed message boards, there is no doubt that many individuals are turning to the internet (more specifically, social media) to obtain their medical information. With the advent of lockdowns attributable to the pandemic and the push to work from home, this became even more prevalent, as people are now connected to their devices almost continuously. Some may see this as positive (and indeed to some degree it may be), but we must also exercise prudence when approaching online information.

In my home office, I keep my father's original leatherbound 1970 *Encyclopedia Britannica* as a reminder of what our "Google" used to be. The information contained therein was our "go to" for writing papers and book reports throughout the years. Furthermore, this encyclopedia was kept current by the addition of yearly volumes entitled *Book of the Year*, which not only made corrections to previous versions, but also contained updates on current events pertaining to that specific year. The information was cited with bibliographies and source notes, all of which were verifiable. The problem with this type of information was that it was somewhat expensive and required ongoing payments in order to remain current, lest it become a historical document as opposed to a current source of verified information. Certainly not everyone had the ability to have this type of information at their fingertips.

Having information at the touch (or swipe) of a smart device or computer has indeed revolutionized information technology, but this revolution has come at a cost, specifically when it comes to medical and health information. While there are many verifiable and trustworthy online sources that individuals can access with questions about their health, there are many more that remain sources of questionable information or even outright misinformation. Message boards and discussion groups have become places where, in some instances, individuals freely dispense medical information without having the professional knowledge (or degree) to do so. And this may lead to great harm and the rapid or "viral" spread of misinformation.

Biomedical professionals often joke about the term "Dr. Google." Whether one sees this as good or bad, it very much remains a reality. There is not one of us (myself included) who has not specifically opened Google to quickly look up some bit of medical information, even just out of sheer curiosity to see what result the behemoth search engine would come up with. While a trained medical professional can sift through the mountains of links that show up, this can be daunting for a lay person, especially when seeking specific biomedical information. Professional groups such as ACOG (American College of Obstetrics and Gynecology) produce a myriad of patient-centered handouts each year that, while informative, seldom seemed to be picked up and used by patients. I don't recall the last time I was asked a question related to such a pamphlet or handout. It is easy to slip down a rabbit hole of data, out of which one can emerge even more confused than they were before they started.

In my own practice, I noticed a change in where patients obtain their information simply by asking the question, "How did you hear about my practice?" I always ask my new patients this question as part of our introductions, and I feel it's an important one. When I started my private practice 24 years ago, 99% of the time the answer was "by word of mouth." This has changed rapidly over the past few years, as now, at least half of my patients have heard of me via various search engines and even more so through social media message boards such as moms' or pregnancy groups. Certainly, most potential patients google the doctor they have been referred to (even if by word of mouth) before they call to schedule their first visit.

This transition to the heavy use of social media and medical platforms as information sources means that patients come to their first visit armed with a good amount of information (both holistic and technocratic) about the condition that prompted the visit. Not only are patients now familiar with where their physician obtained their training and board certifications, but they also know the physician's practice style and philosophy when it comes to treating specific conditions, even before they meet them, and depending on what is on their website. This is a beneficial use of technology; it helps patients come to their visits more prepared with specific questions and/or concerns, which streamlines the visit. The patients' advance familiarity with the doctor's practice style can help to solidify the patient-doctor relationship. Alternatively, it may steer a patient away from a caregiver who may not share the same ideals the patient is seeking in their care. Many physicians have even taken to posting short bios about themselves, their families, and what they enjoy doing during their off time. This type of familiarization became even more important during the ongoing COVID-19 pandemic when patients often feel especially separated from their providers.

The use of such information technology can pose some difficulties as well. Patients may come to their visit armed with both valid and invalid information, which can sometimes make the initial visit a difficult one for both provider and patient. Keeping an open mind and avoiding personal bias as it relates to what the patient has obtained online is crucial in nurturing the incipient relationship. The old cliché is still true: we all know too well that "first impressions are everything." As a provider, keeping an open mind and being somewhat flexible are especially critical when encountering a patient for the very first time. Patients are understandably nervous and anxious about not only meeting a new provider, but also about how that provider will react to their concerns, particularly regarding more holistically oriented subjects such as accepting the use of a doula or a birth plan.

The traditional technocratic way for an ob to meet new patients was to have them already gowned and lying on the table in the exam room. Yet, in a more humanistic approach, I have found that meeting new patients in my office before going to the exam room helps them know a little bit more about me before I walk in to meet them and vice versa. Sure, diplomas on the wall are important, but even more so are the pictures, family photos, and knick-knacks that inhabit my office space. Patients are much more at ease sitting and meeting me in the office in their street clothes and first discussing their history before entering an exam room and changing into a gown. Additionally, the office provides a space where I can place a patient who is going through a difficult moment. Whether it is discussing a miscarriage, a cancer diagnosis, or an abnormal ultrasound finding, this space takes the patient away from the bustle of the clinical area and allows them privacy and quiet.

I always encourage my patients to come to our visits with a list of questions regarding the issues they want to address. I realize that most biomedical physicians groan inside when a patient pulls out a paper with a list of questions or turns to the notes section of their smartphone, but I find lists to be quite helpful. They help to keep patients focused on their concerns, which keeps the conversation on topic without the patients having to search for or remember their questions. Many questions that revolve around more humanistic and holistic approaches, such as incorporating birth plans and doulas, can be more streamlined this way, and addressed in a manner that allows greater patient and provider satisfaction.

In sum, the advent of the internet has provided us with the tools of limitless healthcare information. It has also, unfortunately, simultaneously become a haven of healthcare misinformation. As providers, we must be diligent and empathetic while helping patients navigate through the massive amounts of information they are encountering. Doing so with care and professionalism will allow both traditionalist technocratic and innovative humanistic and holistic approaches to flourish in this new world.

Technocratic Graduate Obstetric Training and the Humanistic Approach to Private Practice: A Blending of Ideologies

I completed my formal graduate training in obstetrics and gynecology in the summer of 1997—just before residency programs began to undergo a fundamental change from the very traditionalist biomedical training that had been the norm since the dawn of such training programs. Beginning in internship (now called first-year residency), unrestricted work hours and heavy caseloads were normative, and it was expected that residents would perform under these conditions. Training was very "patient-centered," consisting of heavy operative schedules to maximize learning during a relatively short training period; indeed, the amounts of on-call and work hours were taxing. Residents were just supposed to comply, no matter how exhausted they became. Since that time, training has shifted to a more "doctor-centered" model; there are now strict regulations and limitations on the number of calls a given resident is allowed to take and on the amount of time spent on direct patient care. Mandatory rest periods have been worked into residents' schedules to avoid the fatigue that often resulted in errors in judgment and, in turn, patient harm (see Accreditation Council for Graduate Medical Education 2020). The unintended consequences of this change, however, may be fewer clinical situations and training opportunities experienced by each intern/resident, as the length of the training program has not changed in many years, and there is no possible way to include the same amount of training into a four-year program when restrictions on the amount of time spent training are in effect. Subspecialty training has arisen in an attempt to compensate for some of these shortfalls, adding an additional one to three years of training; however, many obstetric subspecialists (such as perinatologists) participate in more of a consultant role, as opposed to delivering direct care the way generalists do. Whether these changes are good or bad in terms of overall outcomes is beyond the scope of this chapter. Nevertheless, there has been one topic that bridges both models of training and has carried over into my own private practice—namely, the incorporation of more humanistic modalities into the practice of women's health care, and more specifically, into obstetrics.

During my third year of residency training, another resident and I were approached by our department chair with the task of evaluating many of the processes we were performing to determine if the cost was really justified and whether the procedures (some of them seemingly an unnecessary burden to the patient) were likely to really change the care outcomes. For example, if a patient presents to labor and delivery and undergoes a precipitous delivery before an IV can be started, does she really need the IV at all? Why not give oxytocin intramuscularly—or not at all if she is doing well—immediately after she delivers? Do women with hypertensive disorders of pregnancy of varying degrees (which typically require delivery for resolution) really have to stay in a hospital bed until they deliver, regardless of gestational age? Could they not be in a home environment with outpatient monitoring or even home healthcare visits?

Bear in mind, the idea of something more humanistic like a "birth plan" was wholly out of anyone's thoughts during my training, but these simple questions, which were really on the cutting edge at that time, were the starting ideas in which technocratic and humanistic care would begin to blend in my practice into a more "hands-off" approach. At the time, this mode of thinking was received with mixed emotions by both residents and professors (attending physicians). After all, we were used to taking care of patients using more invasive approaches such as internal fetal heartrate leads (i.e., fetal scalp electrodes), intrauterine pressure catheters, and even scalp Ph measurements (a now-obsolete modality) for fetal assessment. The idea of minimal intervention before and after delivery was a difficult one for most of us to incorporate into practice. Nonetheless, it was this novel approach that began to pave the way for the incorporation of more humanistic modalities in obstetric health care; we just didn't realize it at the time. A few of the professors were particularly upset at these novel approaches, arguing that they weren't based on scientific research and therefore had no place in our training program. However, over a relatively short period of time, these humanistic changes came to be more accepted. And while they were not fully holistic measures per se—meaning that they did not, in Davis-Floyd's terms, incorporate mind/body integration, energy, and spirit into the treatment process—they did lead to an opening of ideas that would eventually lead me to create a blended approach to obstetric care in my private practice.

Private Practice and the Humanistic and Holistic Models in Obstetrics: Can the Three Go Hand in Hand?

When I began my private practice in 1997 in The Woodlands, Texas, the idea of incorporating any kind of holistic ideology into obstetric care was not even remotely in my thinking. Although those early ideas of a more humanistic, hands-off approach had come with me as part of my training, I was focused on providing the best possible care to the patients of our community and those surrounding us while growing my practice. I had never heard of a "birth plan" and had no idea what the word "doula" meant. In fact, it was a good number of years before a greater appreciation of humanistically based approaches began to take shape and become integrated into my obstetric practice.

Regarding this integration of humanistic practices into my delivery of obstetric care, there have been two main approaches that I have developed over time. One approach involves the use of birth plans and support personnel, such as partners and doulas; the other involves actual care decisions and labor/delivery management based on patients' desires and preferences—an important tenet of the humanistic model as Davis-Floyd defines it (please see the Series Overview at the beginning of this volume). I will admit that the incorporation of these non-traditional modalities for myself as a private practitioner did not occur overnight. Instead, as the years passed, I began to see and experience different levels of humanistic and sometimes holistic approaches, most of which were introduced to me by my patients. Some of these I readily incorporated into practice, such as the use of doulas and birth plans, while others I still counsel against, such as trial of labor after a cesarean (TOLAC) based on the TOLAC guidelines outlined by ACOG (2017). I believe that this balanced approach has helped me to safely incorporate a measure of holistic medical care into what I consider to be a very traditional private practice.

Birth Plans

The "birth plan" has become quite popular in recent years. In its simplest form, a birth plan is a document expressing the parents' particular desires for the birth experience once labor begins. These plans are typically simple and reasonable in their scope; for example, requesting delaying the use of Pitocin, avoidance of a continuous IV, and only intermittent, not continuous, fetal monitoring, should the situation allow. A reassuring fetal heart rate pattern and the absence of untoward medical conditions such as maternal fever or elevated blood pressures are examples of prerequisites that would allow such intermittent monitoring. On the other hand, some plans can be extremely detailed, addressing not only desires regarding the birth itself, but also what lighting the room should have and what music will be played.

The proliferation of social media sites and message boards alluded to earlier has allowed the creation of a sort of database of various birth plans (both straightforward and complex), many of which can be filled out in PDF format and printed out for the family, providers, and delivery centers involved. The idea of a birth plan is to give patients a clear way of communicating their desires and decision-making when it comes to the actual process of their impending labor and delivery. Over the last few years, I have seen an uptick in the utilization of birth plans in our community, and I do support this humanistic method of informed decision-making with the patient. Such plans make patients more comfortable, knowing that their desires are communicated clearly to the healthcare team and anyone else involved; this is good for patients and their families, and can be helpful to the care team.

However, as previously noted, birth plans can also be somewhat cumbersome and restrictive, which is why many obs cringe when they see a patient who presents such a plan. In my own practice, I typically see one of two scenarios when patients discuss or ask about birth plans: (1) "*Should* I have a birth plan, and what should be included in it or excluded from it?" and (2) "I *have* a birth plan that I would like you to review to let me know if you have any issues with it." Although certainly not a requirement for labor and delivery, I do encourage patients to take their time and do their research while formulating a birth plan. At times, given all the information available online, this can become overwhelming, and, I believe, almost detrimental to what the patient is trying to achieve, as it can create undue stress and anxiety with the whole process, which, in my opinion, undermines the whole purpose of the plan. Childbirth is a beautiful and natural process that often requires little (if any) intervention by caregivers; thus, when guiding patients about making choices about what should or should not be in their plan, I strongly encourage them to "keep it simple." In short, a bigger birth plan is not a better birth plan. Creating a plan that respects the parents' wishes while not trying to over-control the labor and delivery process is the key element, and one that I strongly encourage.

Those who come with a birth plan already prepared, or who have already experienced childbirth with a birth plan, typically have a very specific and detailed plan for their ideal birth experience. However, having a very regimented plan can also create a negative experience when every expectation is not met; thus, expectations of what can and cannot be achieved during delivery must be clearly discussed and defined ahead of time, and also during the labor process as salient issues emerge. Although I do not actively encourage every patient to come up with a specific birth plan, I am always supportive of my patients' wishes and desires for their ideal birth. Thus, I always spend at least one visit (sometimes several) ahead of the delivery carefully reviewing the desires expressed on the plan one by one, and consider with each step how these desires can be achieved. During this process, I also discuss the feasibility of the request: is it possible within reason and within the protocols and other constraints of the hospital environment? Most importantly, when our discussion is completed, I tell the patient that the most important thing is to always keep an open mind and to be flexible to changes that may occur. While my goal is to meet every expectation, the process of laboring and delivering is its own entity and each labor can be quite different, even for the same mother. Being open-minded about expectations and what can be achieved is critical to having a fulfilling labor and delivery experience, even if things don't go quite as planned.

Thankfully, and by a large margin, I can accommodate most couples' desires without any issues, and a mutual decision can be made going forward to the delivery about what expectations can be met. I feel that the word "expectations" is important, as many issues that may arise during labor and birth can be resolved even before the issue comes up when expectations are discussed well before the birth.

Humanizing Labor and Delivery Care: Nutrition during Labor, the Use of Doulas, and the Roles of Nurses

According to Davis-Floyd (2018a, 2022), a basic tenet of the humanistic paradigm of birth and health care (see also the Series Overview at the beginning of this volume) is a "balance between the needs of the individual and the needs of the institution." Many birth plans request the omission of an IV, which keeps the patient tethered to an IV pole; in a humanistic balance between the needs of the patient and those of the caregivers, a saline lock can be inserted, allowing physicians and nurses immediate IV access should it be needed for an emergency. For those mothers who request ambulation during labor, hospital protocols have been developed to allow the nurses to perform intermittent monitoring, which allows the safe assessment of fetal wellbeing and at the same time allows the laboring patient the ability to move freely—another example of the humanistic balance between the needs of the patient and those of the caregivers and the institution. More recently, Bluetooth technology has been incorporated into fetal monitoring; a small, flat, low-profile device is placed on the maternal abdomen, which sends a continuous signal back to the nurse—which appears on a centralized monitoring system (as well as on my cellphone)—who can thereby monitor the fetus while giving the mother even more freedom and time to ambulate in-between cervical checks normally performed by the labor nurse to assess dilation and the progress of labor. Birthing balls, "peanut balls," and squat bars for laboring and for the delivery itself have become mainstays on the labor unit in my hospital, demonstrating its movement toward more humanistic forms of practice, and can be utilized at any time the patient desires, or at the suggestion of the nursing staff if a patient is unfamiliar with these "soft" technologies and the upright positions they facilitate. Using dim lighting and music helps with rest and pain control; most patients who wish to listen to music during labor come well prepared with preplanned play lists and Bluetooth speakers for comfortable listening. The holistic modality of aromatherapy, in the form of topical oils, atomizers, and diffusers can safely be utilized in the hospital setting. Even dietary restrictions have changed dramatically over recent years, with many obs and nurses allowing clear liquids such as broth, juices, popsicles, and Jell-O to be consumed during labor. These offer much better relief to thirst and hunger than the proverbial ice chips, which for decades were the only thing offered (and that sparingly). Although critiques of standard obstetric procedures such as those of series editor Robbie Davis-Floyd (2003, 2018a, 2018b, 2022) insist that laboring women should be allowed to eat actual foods if they wish, my hospital and I have not gone that far into "deeply humanistic" practice (Davis-Floyd 2018a, 2022; see also the Series Overview in this volume), due to our perceptions of the danger of aspiration should the need for general anesthesia arise. Despite our concerns, meta-analytic data would suggest that the risk for aspiration pneumonia isn't as high as we were taught (see Ciardulli et al. 2017). Despite ACOG recommendations for a clear liquid diet only, more commentaries from maternal-fetal medicine specialists (MFMs) are suggesting that we should allow laboring women to eat as they please (see Sperling, Dehlke, and Sebai 2016). Although this does remain a controversial topic, we continue to learn more with increasing data and research and to adjust accordingly.

The humanistic use of a birth doula has also become much more common in hospital labor and delivery units, especially over the last few years, as the birth doula provides physical, emotional, and informational support to women during the birth process. While not yet mainstream, I have seen an uptick in the incorporation of doulas in our practice. (Most of our patients have private insurance and approximately 20% have Medicaid, but I do not have any stratified data on the use of doulas in each group.) I am supportive of my patients using them, but as discussed earlier, I prefer to review the parents' desires and expectations of what role the doula will play well ahead of the delivery itself, ideally with the doula present, especially since biomedical care providers have never actually meet the doula before labor begins. Knowing in advance how much of a role the doula will play and to what degree is not only important for myself as the obstetrician, but also for the nursing staff involved in the care of the patient. Most of the information we receive about the doula and her practice style/preferences, however, is obtained via the patient until the time of labor.

In fact, the role of the nurse is important for all aspects of the birth plan. Labor nurses are at the bedside off and on during the process of labor, whereas I am not; as such, they are a critical part of the process of discussing what the patients' desires are and how these can be met while keeping the patient and her baby safe. These discussions are carried out shortly after admission so that there is ample time to discuss any questions and/or concerns. The main points that I discuss with my patients with regard to the use of a doula are those of decision-making during issues that may arise during labor and how large a role the doula may play in those decisions. Shared decision-making—another basic tenet of the humanistic model—is critical during labor, but I feel that such decisions should be made between the patient and the family/advocates who are present, along with the caregivers (nurses/doctors) involved. Doulas should, of course, be a part of the decision-making process, but mainly in a supportive role. There may be situations that arise during labor that require an intervention the doula may not agree with or support. This can create undue confusion for the patient and an undermining of patients' confidence in their hospital practitioners. This is why it is so important to discuss the use of a doula and to what degree she will be involved with the patient well ahead of labor. Over the years, I have had positive experiences with doulas during labor and delivery and am very supportive of my patients who utilize them. They constitute helpful sources of support and tirelessly encourage patients throughout potentially long labors. I strongly believe that these good relationships have arisen from honest discussions with patients and their families early in their prenatal care, and that, again, the doula should be a part of those discussions in person during the prenatal visits.

In my opinion, what may lead to a negative experience during birth depends largely upon how flexible and open-minded patients are willing to be. Those patients who have very regimented plans that become almost a checklist of what must happen and in what order during labor and delivery tend to end up having more negative experiences. It is human nature to have negative feelings when expectations can't be met (see Davis-Floyd 2022). To one degree or another, labor and delivery present a unique challenge to every birth plan that can possibly be conceived. While we know so much about the process of labor and delivery, we know so much less about how that process will unfold. It is unpredictable and, not infrequently, things can change for the worse for mother and baby in just a few moments or seconds of time. This can make decision-making difficult for the patient when time is short and things are moving rapidly and not according to plan. Alternatively, non-emergent situations such as the labor not progressing as well as we would hope also occur; and while my patients are not placed on any type of particular labor curve or timeline, these situations may necessitate interventions that were not a part of the original birth plan. This can lead to mothers feeling defeated or as if they have "failed" to have the birth experience they had originally planned for (again, see Davis-Floyd 2022). This is precisely why it is so important to discuss a plan well ahead of labor—the sooner during prenatal care, the better. As noted above, this gives ample time for the patient who may come up with questions about her birth plan to discuss them with me as well as with the staff who will be caring for her. Most of this discussion takes place in advance during office visits due to the unpredictability of when labor will occur and how rapidly it will progress. Unfortunately, there is simply no way for the labor nurse to interact with the patient in advance of labor.

In summary, an inclusive humanistic and sometimes even holistic model can be incorporated into a busy labor and delivery unit, while keeping safety and excellent clinical outcomes a priority. For this model to work, discussions between myself and the patient must begin early in the prenatal process, allowing time for additional questions that may arise as the pregnancy progresses. Clinical scenarios can change, which may lead to changes in the ability to accommodate certain aspects of the birth plan. Additionally, active involvement of nursing staff and other caregivers (such as doulas) is critical during the labor and delivery process, and success depends upon open and honest communications between the patient and these caregivers. In my practice, the person best suited to coordinate these discussions with everyone involved is myself, which is why I actively discuss these plans (as well as their potential limitations) at length, in an effort to achieve a desirable outcome for the patient and her family.

Access to Health Care and Patient Support during the COVID-19 Pandemic: Lessons Learned

As we have come to know all too well, the COVID-19 pandemic has had a profound and significantly negative impact on access to and delivery of health care to patients in general. This was especially notable at the beginning of the pandemic, when there was understandably a great deal of fear and panic surrounding the virus. As hospitals were scrambling for PPE (personal protective equipment) and the general public was fighting for toilet paper, our practice was struggling with the decision of what to do in the coming weeks to "stop the spread." We had already heard that many practices in our area were simply shutting down for the time being, which to me was inconceivable, even considering the potential impacts of this virus. The idea of not being present and available for my patients never crossed my mind. My clinical staff and I discussed but quickly dismissed the idea of not performing well-woman visits and just seeing ob patients as needed. While many patients cancelled appointments because they were uncomfortable entering public spaces, many wanted to keep their visits with us as scheduled. We quickly made the decision to adopt safe practices such as temperature screening, implementing medical grade mask use for our staff, and mandating social distancing in our waiting areas and break room. Patients who felt more comfortable waiting outside would be called in when I was ready to see them. Those who did not want to keep their appointments were still allowed refills on their prescriptions (within reason), and we triaged questions on the phone just as always. If a COVID-positive ob patient absolutely had to be seen—for example, a high-risk diabetic or hypertensive patient who needed weekly fetal testing or, without care, would risk untoward consequences to herself or her fetus—we made specific and safe arrangements to allow her care to continue. I saw such patients at the very end of the day when other patients and staff members had left, with only myself and a voluntary assistant present, both of us wearing appropriate PPE. At the end of the visit, professional cleaners would clean the room and any areas the patient had accessed. This system allowed us to appropriately continue to care for patients affected by the virus. In short, we never closed, and we never stopped, and looking back, for the sake of our patients I am very thankful that we came to that decision.

I think back over the years on how many times during a routine visit I detected a breast lump or received reports with abnormal cells on a pap test and what the consequences of that would have been had the patient had waited an additional year. From the beginning of 2021, when asking my patients about their previous mammogram, the better part of 50% stated that they missed their annual mammogram in 2020 because of COVID-19. The potential negative consequences of this are staggering and unfortunately, as a result, we are seeing these very scenarios each week.

These consequences are not limited to medical issues, but also involve profound mental issues. One situation that struck me was a patient—a paramedic—who presented to me with a miscarriage at the very beginning of the pandemic. She had seen another obstetrician during what was supposed to be her initial ob visit and ultrasound. Her husband was not allowed to attend the visit (due to that ob's COVID-19 restrictions) and was therefore on video chat with his wife when they learned that their baby did not have a heartbeat. I cannot imagine the anguish she felt at that moment, alone with strangers, nor the helplessness her husband must have felt not being able to be with her to comfort and support her in person. Because I welcomed them both, this couple came to our office the next day, where we were able to safely see them and to answer their questions before coming up with an appropriate treatment plan for compassionately dealing with the loss of her pregnancy. Patients should and must always have advocates; this can be done safely and humanely, even during a deadly pandemic.

Throughout the pandemic, access to care for my obstetric patients was no different than before. With the implementation of the safety measures described above, I continued caring for my ob patients without interruption. We allowed limited family/support to be present at each visit (especially ultrasound visits), so that they could continue to be an active part of the patient's decision-making process and most importantly, the patient's advocate.

For labor and delivery, the hospital in which I work initially allowed only one family member or support person, such as a doula, to be present throughout the process, thereby forcing the pregnant patient to choose, usually between her partner and her doula. Later this policy was changed to allow two support people, then changed back when the Delta variant reached our community. Health screening was carried out upon hospital admission, including rapid COVID screening, and all appropriate precautions were taken during the labor and delivery process. For patients who were COVID positive, appropriate adjustments and additional safety precautions were taken without sacrificing the patient's labor and delivery experience. One nurse was typically assigned to a COVID+ laboring mother to limit patient-provider interactions. PPE was readily available, and the number of staff in attendance at the actual delivery was limited to only the very most essential to perform the necessary tasks at hand. The PPE included the disposable gowns, shoe and head covers, and N95 masks that were typically used. The laboring mother's family member/partner who was present (who, along with the patient, typically just wore a mask) continued to be actively involved as they had been in the past. Should the need for a cesarean arise, one of our three labor and delivery operating rooms was specifically dedicated to COVID+ patients, with all necessary equipment and supplies readily available.

During the postpartum period, nothing changed as well. Breastfeeding continued as normal and lactation consultants visited the patient as needed. Although there was some discussion about possible maternal-neonatal viral transmission at the beginning of the pandemic, and unlike in many other hospitals around the country (see Davis-Floyd, Gutschow, and Schwartz 2020; Gutschow and Davis-Floyd 2021), in my hospital, the newborns of COVID+ mothers were not separated from their families (unless the mother was too ill to care for her baby). It is often argued how important the "golden hour" is after childbirth, and in my opinion, this hour should remain golden, even during a pandemic.

Obstetrics, Humanistic and Holistic Practice, and COVID-19: Final Thoughts

There was one moment during the pandemic that struck me the most. It was near the very beginning, when there was much uncertainty around what to do or how to move forward for any of us. A patient for whom I had cared for many years had come in for her wellness visit, and we struck up a normal conversation, which then drifted toward how her year had been and how her family and friends had been dealing with the pandemic. As we came to the end of our visit, she said, "Thank you, Dr. G." I asked her why she was thanking me, and she simply stated "Thank you for being here for us. A lot of other doctors have just closed up, and we don't even get a call back when we try and contact them. As patients, we need to be able to see our doctors, even during these times. We are so very thankful you are here." Her simple statement was profound, and for many days afterward I thought deeply about what she said. I had never been thanked before simply for "being present."

Caregivers need to be there for their patients, even during pandemics. Period. Many obs and other practitioners switched to telemedicine due to the pandemic (see Gutschow and Davis-Floyd 2021). Telemedicine is a wonderful tool, but it is limited and can only go so far in the full and proper treatment of patients. At some point, a patient must be seen and examined, and a video chat doesn't achieve this, no matter how hard clinicians try to justify its use. During the pandemic, to some degree, we came to a moment in health care where it was acceptable for a provider to say, "I can't see you in person because it's just too dangerous." As a healthcare provider for almost 28 years now, I wholeheartedly disagree with this type of thinking. We can and must treat all our patients as we always have, even during a terrible pandemic; this can be safely achieved without a loss of humanistic compassion and caring and with excellent clinical outcomes.

Imagine what our patients must think if we as frontline providers are too afraid to meet them and care for them in person, as we always have since the dawn of health care. The COVID-19 pandemic will likely not be the last crisis we face as providers, and it may very well not be the last pandemic we see during our lifetimes. But we can be heartened by the lessons we have learned from COVID-19 and move forward, keeping the patients we treat first and foremost, and caring for them in the professional and unfailing manner that we would like to see for ourselves and for our own loved ones.

Marco Gianotti is a board-certified obstetrician/gynecologist who has practiced in The Woodlands, Texas for the past 25 years. In addition to primary/general care for women, his practice includes high-risk obstetric care as well as minimally invasive gynecologic surgery with the Davinci robotic surgical system. He is Medical Director for the Honduras Medical Mission of his parish, providing medical and dental care to several remote mountain villages on the northern coast of Honduras. He is married to his college sweetheart Barbara, and has two children, Annalisa and Gianluigi.

References

Accreditation Council for Graduate Medical Education. 2020. *ACGME Program Requirements for Graduate Medical Education in Obstetrics and Gynecology*. Retrieved 20 September 2022 from https://www.acgme.org/globalassets/PFAssets/ProgramRequirements/220_ObstetricsAndGynecology_2020.pdf?ver=2020-06-29-162338-630&ver=2020-06-29-162338-630}.

American College of Obstetricians and Gynecologists (ACOG). 2017. "ACOG Committee Opinion on Planned Home Birth, No. 697." *Obstetrics & Gynecology* 129(4): e117–e122.

Ciardulli A, Saccone G, Anastasio H, Berghella V. 2017. "Less-Restrictive Food Intake during Labor in Low-Risk Singleton Pregnancies." *Obstetrics & Gynecology* 129(3): 473–480.

Davis-Floyd R. 2003. *Birth as an American Rite of Passage*, 2nd edn. Berkeley: University of California Press.

Davis-Floyd R. 2018a. "The Technocratic, Humanistic, and Holistic Paradigms of Birth and Health Care." In *Ways of Knowing about Birth: Mothers, Midwives, Medicine, and Birth Activism*, Davis-Floyd R and Colleagues, 3–44. Long Grove IL: Waveland Press.

Davis-Floyd R. 2018b. "The Rituals of Hospital Birth." In *Ways of Knowing about Birth: Mothers, Midwives, Medicine, and Birth Activism*, Davis-Floyd R and Colleagues, 45–70. Long Grove IL: Waveland Press.

Davis-Floyd R. 2022. *Birth as an American Rite of Passage*, 3rd edn. Abingdon, Oxon: Routledge.

Davis-Floyd R, Gutschow K, Schwartz DA. 2020. "Pregnancy, Birth, and the COVID-19 Pandemic in the United States." *Medical Anthropology* 39(5): 413–427.

Gutschow K, Davis-Floyd R. 2021. "The Impacts of COVID-19 on US Maternity Care Practitioners: A Follow-Up Study." *Frontiers in Sociology* 6(655401): 1–18.

Sperling JD, Dehlke JD, Sebai BM. 2016. "Restriction of Oral Intake during Labor: Whither Are We Bound?" *American Journal of Obstetrics and Gynecology* 214(5): 592–596.

CHAPTER 13

How an Obstetrician Promoted Respectful Care in Canada and in the World

André Lalonde

Introduction

Born and raised in a small rural town in Ontario, Canada, I was influenced by our country family doctor to think about a medical career. After medical school, during my internship I decided to specialize in obstetrics and gynecology because I cared deeply about women's health. I entered practice at McGill University's Royal Victoria Hospital and in Hôpital Général La Salle, a Montreal community hospital, as Chief of Service, where I decided to make changes in the day-to-day practice of maternity services and to humanize the practices surrounding labor and delivery.

During my training in maternity care (1969–1973), I observed that women did not have the power to discuss and question the physicians who treated them. My personal experience during the birth of our first son had a great influence on the future of my career and on my desire to humanize birth. During his birth, I could not be present in the labor room for most of the time. I was not permitted to hold my newborn son at delivery and was told repeatedly that I was not "sterile," and thus was not granted access to my child. My wife was also separated from our son, and we only saw him through the nursery window. No one talked to us about breastfeeding.

During my training at Royal Victoria Hospital, I also observed that the nurse-midwives (mostly from Europe) who acted as nurses in our labor ward had a great attitude and techniques to support laboring women. (They couldn't act as midwives because at that time, midwifery was still illegal in Canada.) Many nurses had similar great attitudes, yet were under the control of physicians and were rarely consulted on care changes. As soon as I completed my specialty training in obstetrics and gynecology (ob/gyn) in 1973, I became Chief in a community hospital for the Department of Obstetrics and Gynecology, and practiced and taught at the Royal Victoria University Hospital in 1974. In a meeting at the community hospital with doctors and nurses, I asked whether we could change current obstetric practice. I received positive support to look at how labor and delivery care was provided to women. I also started to engage the women whom I followed in labor and delivery through a committee to advise me on changes that would make maternity services more women-friendly.

Encountering difficulties in making changes at the hospital for a few years, I then decided to run for the medical position on the hospital board, and within two years became the President of the hospital board. In that position, I convinced the hospital staff that our maternity services needed much improvement and modernization. Different labor and delivery positions were unknown to the staff at that time. I worked with nurses and doctors to remove certain impediments to childbirth support, such as the absence of the father during labor and delivery, putting babies in bassinets immediately after birth, and using a nursery during the hospital stay. I met resistance from nursery personnel, including pediatricians who would not permit access to women directly in the nursery and were quite dogmatic in their approaches. However, the nurses in postpartum and labor and delivery care were enthusiastic to consider changes.

I started by having regular scientific sessions with nurses and doctors every Thursday morning to review medical issues and introduce my proposed changes. It was the first time in my region and in Canada where scientific meetings allowed all nurses and doctors to participate at the same time. Our initial step was to remove the signs that did not allow fathers in delivery rooms and prohibited taking pictures or recordings of the birth. With the Head Nurse of labor and delivery, we began to look at birthing in different countries, and noted great variations in how care was provided. The Women's Committee was critical in creating pressure on the hospital to implement changes. An important decision was to buy a birthing bed that would allow women to labor and deliver in the same room; the bed was purchased by donations from me and my ob/gyn partners. At first this birthing room was restricted to low-risk women, but soon all women, irrespective of their medical conditions, were allowed to labor and give birth in that room. Even my anesthetist colleagues stated that if an epidural was needed, they could administer it within the birthing room.

I introduced a lecture on birthing positions during labor and delivery that would lead women to adopt a position of their choice. We also started a program to allow women to be active and out of their beds during labor, as well as to nourish and hydrate themselves with light food and juices/water. Dramatic changes occurred in the birth process according to the many wishes expressed by women, such as the presence and active participation of fathers/partners, holding their newborns immediately at birth, and breastfeeding on the delivery bed. Soon this unique birthing room became so popular that demand exceeded its capacity. With the board, I then prepared a request to our government to convert our labor rooms into five single birthing rooms, which we obtained in record time. Meanwhile, we also developed hospital-based prenatal classes that were conducted by our nurses and doctors to better prepare future mothers for a more positive birthing experience.

During that time, we had a serious conflict with the medical/nursing nursery personnel. Having received information that a university hospital permitted access to mothers in their high-risk neonatal unit, I went to visit that hospital with our hospital Chief of Nursing and the Head Nurse of our delivery and postpartum unit. Upon returning, we tried again to give women access to the nursery but received a flat refusal. I decided that the only way was to force entry into the nursery for the women who had their babies in our hospital. I advised the nursery staff that we would enter with or without their permission. On the given day, I arrived with approximately 12 postpartum women to be met at the door by the nursery personnel who advised us we were illegal; I asked them to move aside, and each mother went to her newborn. Of course, a report was sent to the board, which then fully supported the desires of women to be with their newborns.

Vaginal Breech Delivery

Even after a Canadian study on breech delivery favored cesarean birth (Hannah et al. 2000), my obstetrician group continued to accompany women who wanted vaginal breech delivery, and still does. We had a very good protocol that allowed more than 70% of women with breech presentations to have normal vaginal deliveries with no untoward effects on the newborns. At the university hospital, only a few of us offered vaginal breech delivery. A few other hospitals in Quebec also had a similar experience. When I was teaching obstetric residents, I insisted on key axioms for breech delivery: do not induce labor; do not interfere with the presentation until the woman has delivered the baby up to the umbilicus; then support and gently rotate the breech baby for shoulder delivery, then followed by head delivery. In following these protocols, very few breech deliveries required forceps to assist the delivery (see also the chapter on vaginal breech deliveries by Andrew Bisits, this volume).

VBAC (Vaginal Birth after Cesarean)

Around 1978, my two partners and I became the first to offer VBACs in Montreal and possibly Canada. How did I decide to begin assisting VBACs? A woman in my practice was scheduled for a cesarean based on the now-outdated belief that "Once a cesarean, always a cesarean." She arrived at the hospital in labor at about 6 cm and I quickly came to the hospital, ready to perform a cesarean. The staff had prepared her for the operation, and she was on the operating table when I arrived. I asked the anesthetist to delay the start so that I could examine the woman before we began. To my surprise, she was fully dilated and the fetal head was at the vulva. I asked her if she preferred that we try vaginal delivery and she agreed. She then pushed three to four times and delivered spontaneously with minimal help. We put the baby on the mother's chest, and she cried from happiness while stroking the baby. We observed her carefully in the immediate postpartum period to ensure that the uterine scar was stable. The next day, I asked my secretary to look at the world literature on vaginal delivery after a previous cesarean. To my great surprise, she found that at the time, France was the only high-income country routinely letting women with previous cesareans have VBACs.

I developed a protocol with my colleagues, and we began to offer VBACs. Since this was a unique practice in Canada, we committed to be in the labor room from early labor on, and had the anesthetist in the labor ward if needed. When we reached 100 successful VBACs, we became more relaxed; we had induced only one woman, and we maintained our policy not to induce a woman with a previous cesarean scar. Unfortunately, many hospitals in Canada began to induce women planning VBACs with prostaglandins, and that led to many uterine ruptures with serious consequences for mothers and newborns (see Lydon-Rochelle et al. 2001[1]).

Antenatal Birth Plans

We instituted a systematic effort to encourage women to prepare their birth plans outlining their preferences for labor/delivery positions and their wishes. These were signed by the attending ob and made part of these women's hospital records on admission. If the woman's regular ob was not in attendance, the one on call could quickly review the woman's preferences. I received a few requests that were unusual for me, but I managed to accommodate them—for instance, when a woman wanted to deliver standing up, we accommodated her to do so. Finally, we prepared a development plan for an all-birthing room maternity ward that would allow women to have their labor, delivery, and postpartum care in one room instead of the traditional labor room, delivery room, postpartum room, and nursery. I intensively lobbied the government of Quebec, and we were approved in 1989 to construct 45 such rooms to accommodate up to 3,000 birthing people each year.

During the same time, I abolished the Family Planning Committee at the community hospital, which had been charged to approve women requesting tubal ligations. I had noticed that there was no committee to approve requests for vasectomies! At the university hospital, along with a consultation with the department Chief, there was a mathematical formula for approval of female sterilizations: a woman's age multiplied by the number of children had to add up to at least 100. (This was common practice in the 1970s and 1980s in the United States as well; see May 1995). Of course I was quite opposed to such a rule, which took years to eliminate.

By the late 1980s, I was ready to propose and implement changes across Canada with the Society of Obstetricians and Gynecologists of Canada (SOGC). I was recruited in 1990 to be the CEO of SOGC and accepted. I was then ideally placed to introduce many guidelines that would promote more humanistic and holistic approaches to birthing. This approach included care during pregnancy and childbirth that entailed many of the changes made in my community hospital. Other guidelines I introduced included vaginal breech deliveries; VBACs; rural obstetrics; breastfeeding support; the promotion of single-room labor, birthing, and postpartum care; and risk management to reduce complications. In 1996, my colleagues and I published a guideline and a book called *Healthy Beginnings* (SOGC [1998, 2000] 2005), which promoted physiologic births with an emphasis on the empowerment of women. It became a huge success for thousands of women and set the stage for the promotion of non-intervention during labor and birth (see SOGC et al. 2008; Lalonde 2009).

In 1999, I wrote an Editorial in the June edition of the *Journal of Obstetrics and Gynaecology of Canada* on defining women's health, in which I said: "Women's Health involves women's emotional, social, cultural, spiritual, and physical well-being and is determined by the social, political and economic context of women's lives as well as biology. In defining women's health, we recognize the validity of women's life experience and women's own beliefs about and experience of health" (Lalonde 1999:639). This was and is a strong belief that remains at the center of my career.

Midwifery in Canada

During the late 1980s, I served as an advisor to the governments of Ontario and Quebec to create professional recognition of midwives. Direct-entry (non-nurse) midwifery was legalized in Ontario, Quebec, and Alberta by 1994. At the same time, under my guidance the SOGC produced a policy statement on midwifery and home births. In early 2000, Dr. Ken Milne and I developed the MORE^{OB} risk management program, in which nurses, midwives, and doctors create unique interprofessional hospital committees to launch the program, which has led to better maternity care in Canada and has also reduced medico-legal problems (see Ruiter and Cameron 2021 for full descriptions of these programs). A central goal of the program is to encourage the three professions—nursing, midwifery, and obstetrics—to work as equals and to break down traditional silos and hierarchies. During that time, doctors, nurses, midwives, pediatricians, healthcare system experts, and I participated in the development of the Canadian Federal Government National Guideline *Family Centered Maternity and Newborn Care*, first published in 2000 and regularly updated ever since (Public Health Agency of Canada 2017). As the consultant for this National Guideline, I made sure that the essential guidelines on care as well as single-room maternity care were incorporated into standard policy guidance.

As CEO of SOGC, I began international work in Uganda, Guatemala, and Haiti. We created partnerships with local obstetric and midwifery associations to increase their capacity to make changes for the wellness of women, especially by reducing maternal morbidity and mortality. In 2005, I traveled to Papua New Guinea (PNG) as a volunteer at Vunapope Hospital, East New Britain, for three months, where I was the only obstetrician in a midsized hospital with few resources to take care of laboring women. Nevertheless, I was able to offer best practices to the women of PNG. For example, we had only penicillin and Kanamycin; I gave increased dosages to treat massive sepsis. I also modified the use of digoxin for heart failure, to great success.

I was fortunate to have done a one-year rotating internship, and it came to great use. I felt humbled by the courage of the sick women and how grateful they were to me. Given the security problems in PNG, the women told me to always wear my white uniform, and I could rest assured that no one would threaten me, and if they did, the women would take care of the situation. Even though it was a Catholic hospital run by nuns, when I asked the Catholic nun in charge of the pharmacy for contraceptives, I was amazed to see full cupboards of contraceptives! Sensing my wonder, the nun said, "In Rome they practice as Romans, here we practice for the women of the country." I was so impressed by these nuns from Europe, who had been there for years. With the help of local staff, they kept that hospital sparkling clean despite the daily ash clouds from the volcano. My work there was exhilarating and a firsthand experience of obstetric practice in a low-resource country that encouraged me to organize international projects for the members of SOGC, and later to become involved with the International Federation of Obstetricians and Gynecologists (FIGO, its acronym in French) in promoting exchange programs in low-resource countries.

In 2006, FIGO nominated me to chair its Safe Motherhood Newborn Health (SMNH) Committee. In 1995, I had joined the International Safe Motherhood Committee, which was very active in low-resource countries in creating partnerships to reduce complications in maternity care. Under my chairmanship of the FIGO SMNH committee, my colleagues and I developed guidelines on the prevention and treatment of postpartum hemorrhage, labor positions, the management of the second stage of labor, and human resources for health care in the low-resource world (Health Canada 2006; Stone and Lalonde 2008; FIGO SNMH Committee 2012). In 2014, I led the committee to develop a seminal FIGO guideline and policy statement on "Mother-Baby Friendly Birthing Facilities" (International Federation of Gynecology and Obstetrics, International Confederation of Midwives, White Ribbon Alliance, International Pediatric Association, World Health Organization 2015). Our initiative was comprised of 10 Steps to becoming a Mother-Baby Friendly Hospital; however we struggled to find financial support to implement these 10 Steps worldwide. In 2016, I met the Board members of the International MotherBaby Childbirth Organization (IMBCO), who had developed their own initiative in 2008, called the *International MotherBaby Childbirth Initiative (IMBCI): 10 Steps to Optimal MotherBaby Maternity Services*. The IMBCO Board, chaired by Debra Pascali Bonaro, had recruited several hospitals to implement these 10 steps. We decided to discuss how we could combine our efforts to offer better care for birthing women, and in 2018, together we created the *International Childbirth Initiative (ICI): 12 Steps to Safe and Respectful MotherBaby-Family Maternity Care*. At my request, we added "Family" to the title of this initiative (Lalonde 2020), which was wordsmithed in great part by our series and volume lead editor Robbie Davis-Floyd. (For histories of the creations of the IMBCI and the ICI, see Davis-Floyd et al. 2011; Davis-Floyd 2018, 2022).

The ICI was launched at the 2018 FIGO World Congress in Brazil; the then-President of FIGO, Dr. Carlos Fuchtner from Bolivia, made it the Presidential Initiative for the next three years. We received endorsements from the Harvard T.H. Chan School of Public Health, the International Pediatrics Association, the International Confederation of Midwives, the International Council of Nurses, the White Ribbon Alliance, FIGO, SOGC, DONA International, Lamaze International, the American College of Nurse-Midwives, and more than 15 other organizations. I became the Chair of the ICI and worked closely with my Co-Chair Debra Pascali Bonaro—a pioneering doula practitioner and trainer. The ICI's first Executive Director, who played a critical role in developing the framework and preparing the implementation process was Kathy Herschderfer, a midwife based in the Netherlands and the former CEO of the International Confederation of Midwives (see Lalonde et al. 2019; Lalonde 2020).

As of January 2022, the ICI committee members include:

- Carlos Fuchtner MD, ob/gyn, Bolivia, President of FIGO 2018–2021
- Myself, André Lalonde MD, ob/gyn, Chair, FIGO ICI Working Group, Canada
- Kathy Herschderfer RM, Netherlands, Executive Director (former)
- Debra Pascali Bonaro LCCE, US, Co-Chair
- Suellen Miller CNM, PhD, US
- Claudia Hanson MD, PhD, ob/gyn, Sweden
- Doug McMillan MD, pediatrician, International Pediatric Association (IPA) representative, Canada
- William Keenan MD, pediatrician, IPA representative, US
- Michelle Skaer Therrien, ex officio member, ICI Executive Director (current)
- Maria Fernanda Escobar MD, ob/gyn, Colombia
- Soo Downe, RM, PhD, UK

The *International Childbirth Initiative* (ICI) and the MotherBaby-Family Maternity Care Model

The ICI acknowledges and welcomes the ongoing development of care models that have shifted the traditional biomedical model of care to a value-based, humanistic model grounded in partnership between provider and user and in which the health needs and expectations of the care recipient, as well as the desired health outcomes, are the driving forces behind decision-making and quality measurements. This is especially applicable to maternal and newborn care in the context of woman-centered care, where there is a natural link to the full scope of care provided by midwives and other maternal and newborn health care providers. These models overlap in principles and aims, and mainly differ in their emphasis on the recipient of care: woman, newborn, child, person, client, patient, family, etc. Embodiment of this concept of *recipient-centered care* is found in the core statements from a large number of maternity healthcare professionals' organizations, including the international organizations representing midwives, obstetricians, pediatricians, and family doctors.

The creators of the ICI chose to place the MotherBaby-Family unit as the care recipient in the center of care provision. This model was inspired by and adapted from the *Canadian Family-Centred Maternity and Newborn Care: National Guidelines*, which state that this model of care is a complex, multidimensional, dynamic process of providing safe, skilled, and individualized care responsive to the physical, emotional, psychosocial, and spiritual needs of the woman, the newborn, and the family.

The Foundational Principles of the ICI

The following Principles are the foundation of the *International Childbirth Initiative* (ICI): *12 Steps to Safe and Respectful MotherBaby-Family Maternity Care*. They reflect the merging of the visions and principles from the founding initiatives—the IMBCI and the FIGO Initiative—integrating the characteristics of the MotherBaby-Family care model and aligned with relevant international recommendations and current evidence. These Principles are taken directly from the text of the ICI.[2]

Advocating Rights and Access to Care

- Women's and children's rights are human rights and must be ensured in all settings and circumstances, including humanitarian and conflict settings. Every woman and newborn, regardless of background, social and educational status, citizenship, age, and health status has the right to access well-staffed and equipped and free or fairly priced maternal and newborn health services that provide quality care from skilled attendants. Higher rates of maternal and newborn mortality and morbidity resulting from inadequate access to essential care services and poor quality of care are unacceptable.

Ensuring Respectful Maternity Care

- Consideration, respect, and compassion for every woman and newborn should be the foundation of all maternity care, even in the event of complications.
- Every MotherBaby should be protected from disrespectful or violent practices of any kind, as well as from infringements on their right to privacy.

Protecting the MotherBaby-Family Triad

- "MotherBaby-Family" refers to an integral unit during pre-conception, pregnancy, birth, and infancy influencing the health of one another. Within this triad, the MotherBaby dyad remains recognized as one unit, as the care of one significantly impacts the other. The addition of *Family* to this unit conveys the importance of husbands, partners, and the social and/or community family structure in which a child in conceived, born, and raised, and emphasizes that maternal care activities and systems need to fulfill the needs of the MotherBaby-Family triad in order to achieve the full potential of safe and respectful maternity care.
- Throughout the entire continuum of maternity care, the MotherBaby-Family should be actively engaged in care provision, aspiring to share decision-making, with the woman ultimately being the decision maker.

For the short version of the ICI 12 Steps, see Figure 13.1.

ICI Implementation

Today the ICI is being implemented in 70 hospitals across 30 countries, with many new sites inquiring to join as news of the Initiative spreads. The ICI is unique in that while there have been many advocates for respectful maternity care, the ICI is demonstrating and documenting the implementation of respectful care at hospitals around the world. A hospital wishing to embark on ICI implementation needs to first create a multidisciplinary committee in order to apply to the ICI Committee.

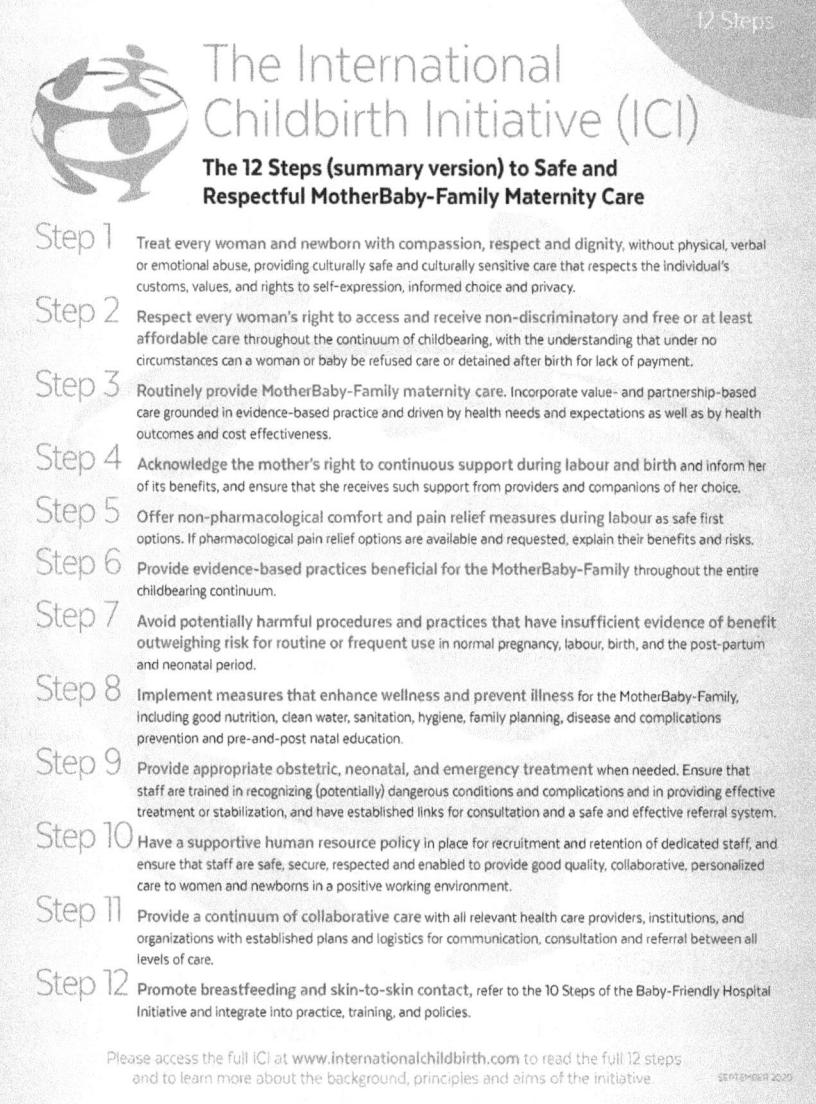

Figure 13.1. *The International Childbirth Initiative* (ICI): *12 Steps* (summary version) *to Safe and Respectful MotherBaby-Family Maternity Care.*

(To join us and to implement the ICI, go to our website www.icichildbirth.org and fill out the form with your contact information.) This Committee is founded on the principle of breaking down hierarchies and, for implementation in a particular facility, must include a lay person from the community as a full member to represent women's and families' voices. Once the ICI Committee reviews the application and accepts it, tools are shared that are intended to help a hospital evaluate its practices and strengthen them in areas as needed; the committee agrees to use three standard surveys (mother, father or companion, labor and delivery staff) to evaluate how the facility provides care and how the women and the father/partner evaluate the care they receive. Once a significant number of birthing women and their families complete the questionnaires (available in three official languages—English, French, and Spanish), the hospital or facility committee presents the results to all their staff, and they develop an action plan to address areas where they wish to see change.

With a presence on six continents, we hope to continue to register hospitals and other birthing facilities in all parts of the world to embark on significant change leading to a decrease in obstetric violence and unconsented procedures (for multiple descriptions and analyses of these, see Volume III of this series [Davis-Floyd and Premkumar 2023]), and to deliver respectful care to all women. With the help of FIGO, IMBCO, and our many sponsors, we are disseminating the ICI as a template for all healthcare personnel involved in maternity care to follow. To date (October 2022), the countries with facilities that have applied include Austria, Brazil, Canada, Chile, Colombia, Fiji, India, Indonesia, Kenya, Mongolia, Papua New Guinea, the Philippines, Rwanda, the Solomon Islands, Trinidad, Turkey, Uganda, and the United States. Countries that are initiating implementation (applications in progress) include Argentina, Australia, Burkina Faso, China, the Czech Republic, Germany, Honduras, Mexico, Nigeria, and Uruguay.

Accepted Facilities

The facilities recognized as ICI partners to date are listed in Table 13.1.

Conclusion

Many factors had a positive influence leading to my career devoted to women's health and in particular to a humanistic approach to maternity care. I owe my career to the many women who trusted the care and advice I provided. I continuously learned from them and found inspiration from listening to their concerns and working to address them. For my mother's influence and that of the many teachers and colleagues in

Table 13.1. Facility partners in the ICI network (as of October 2022). © André Lalonde and Michelle Therrien

Country	Facility Name	Contact Person
Austria	Landeskrankenhaus Feldbach- Fürstenfeld	Dr. Elisabeth Hammerlindl
Brazil	Sophia Feldman Hospital	Edson de Borges Souza
Canada	Brome Mississquoi Hospital	Sophie Perreault
Chile	Hospital Clínico Dra. Eloísa Díaz La Florida	Susan Diaz Aileen Catalan Ronny Valenzuela Rodriguez
Colombia	Fundación Valle del Lili	Dr. Maria Escobar Dr. Juan Manuel Burgos
Colombia	Clinica Imbanaco	Dr. Jairo Enrique Guerrero
Fiji	Colonial War Memorial Hospital	Dr. Kelera Sakumeni
Fiji	Lautoka Hospital	Amanda Noovao Hill Dr. Vasitia Cati
Fiji	Labasa Hospital	Dr. Inosi Voce
India	The Sanctum, Natural Birth Center	Dr. Vijaya Krishnan
India	Mahatma Gandhi Institute Sevagram	Dr. Poonam Shivkumar Dr. Shuchi Jain
India	NKP Salve, Nagpur	Dr. Anuja Bhalerao
India	Pravara Medical College Loni	Dr. VB Bangal
India	Gandhi Medical College Sultania Zanana Hospital	Dr. Aruna Kumar Dr. Shabana Sultan
India	Government College Hyderabad	Dr. Janaki
India	All India Institute of Medical Sciences	Ansari Nagar Aparna Sharma
India	Government Medical College Thrissur	Dr. Resmy
India	Atal Bihari Vajpayee Institute of Medical Sciences & Dr. Ram Manohar Lohia Hospital	Dr. Ashok Kumar
India	Government College Raipur	Dr. Tripti Nagaria
India	KGMU LKO Government College	Dr. Amita Pandey

(continued)

Table 13.1. Continued

Country	Facility Name	Contact Person
India	RIIMS Ranchi	Dr. Anubha
India	AIIMS Gorakhpur	Dr. Preeti Priyadarshani
India	Aastrika Midwifery Center	Janhavi Nilekani PhD
India	Fernandez Hospital	Dr. Evita Fernandez
Indonesia	Bumi Sehat Birthing Center	Robin Lim
Kenya	Rongo Subcounty Hospital	Wycliffe Omwanda
Kenya	Lwala Community Alliance	Wycliffe Omwanda
Mongolia	Gurvan Gal General Hospital	Ganchimeng Togoobaatar
Mongolia	Amgalan Maternity Hospital	Ganchimeng Togoobaatar
Mongolia	National Center for Mothers, Newborns and Women II	
Papua New Guinea	Vanimo Hospital	Geita Morea
Papua New Guinea	Madang Provincial Hospital	Paula Ao
Papua New Guinea	Goroka Hospital	Paula Ao
Philippines	Cumpio Midwife Clinic/Mercy in Action	Vicki Penwell
Philippines	Tison Mercy Birthing Home/Mercy in Action	Vicki Penwell
Philippines	Midwives Way Birth Center/Mercy in Action	Vicki Penwell
Solomon Islands	National Referral Hospital	Leeanne Panisi
Trinidad	Mamatoto Birth Center	Debrah Lewis
Turkey	Acıbadem Taksim Hospital	Dr. Hakan Çoker Ms. Sila Duru
Uruguay	Centro Hospitalario Pereira Rossell	Leonel Briozzo
United States	The Birth Place	Jennie Joseph
United States	National Perinatal Task Force [provider network]	Jennie Joseph

Canada and around the world, I owe them my appreciation and gratitude for whatever success I reached. To colleagues and staff at hospitals, organizations, and institutions, I pay my respects, because without them I could not have accomplished what I have.

André B. Lalonde is an international women's health specialist and Professor of Obstetrics and Gynecology at McGill University, Ottawa, Canada. He has been responsible for the development and implementation of several maternal and newborn care risk management programs that are currently being implemented across Canada, including MORE[OB] and Advances in Labor and Risk Management (ALARM). He has been instrumental in integrating the ALARM International program in over 20 low-resource countries as a method to address maternal mortality and morbidity and to strengthen obstetric and gynecological societies. He was previously President of the FIGO Safe Motherhood and Newborn Health Committee and is current Chair of the International Childbirth Initiative (ICI) (see www.icichildbirth.org).

Dr. Lalonde has received many awards for his career in promoting women's health, notably from the Royal College of Obstetricians and Gynaecologists in the UK, the Society of Obstetricians and Gynaecologists of Canada, the American College of Obstetricians and Gynecologists, Japan, Uganda, France, Argentina, and many more. He also received the Queen Elizabeth II Jubilee Medal, and the Presidential Award from Burkina Faso. Dr. Lalonde is an international lecturer on postpartum hemorrhage, mortality, mother-baby friendly birthing facilities, risk management in obstetrics, and innovative integrated mother-newborn care.

Notes

1. This study (Lydon-Rochelle at al. 2001), which was published in the United States, clearly showed, and the author firmly stated, that artificially inducing or augmenting labor with prostaglandins increases the risk of uterine rupture during trials of labor, so the obvious conclusion was: "Do not artificially induce or augment labor for a VBAC." Yet because US obstetricians couldn't imagine *not* artificially inducing or augmenting labor, the Editorial that accompanied this study in the *New England Journal of Medicine* (Greene 2001) instead focused on the danger of uterine rupture and strongly recommended that VBACs should only be attempted in tertiary-level hospitals with anesthesiologists on call 24/7. Thus VBACs disappeared as an option in community hospitals around the United States. For me, this study simply confirmed my pre-existing protocol not to induce labor for VBACs.

2. International Childbirth Initiative homepage. Retrieved 22 September 2022 from www.ICIchildbirth.org.

References

Davis-Floyd R. 2018. "Creating the International MotherBaby Childbirth Initiative (IMBCI): Anthropologically Informed Activism." In *Ways of Knowing about Birth: Mothers, Midwives, Medicine, and Birth Activism* by Davis-Floyd R, 389–396. Long Grove IL: Waveland Press.

———. 2022. "An Applied Anthropologist's Account of the Developing Global Guidelines." In *Anthropologies of Global Maternal and Reproductive Health: From Policy Spaces to Sites of Practice*, ed. Wallace LJ, MacDonald MM, Storeng KT, 179–198. Cham, Switzerland: Springer.

Davis-Floyd R, Pascali Bonaro D, Sagady-Leslie M, Vadeboncoeur H, Davies R, Ponce de Leon RG. 2011. "The International MotherBaby Childbirth Initiative: Working to Achieve Optimal Maternity Care Worldwide." *International Journal of Childbirth* 1(3): 196–212.

Davis-Floyd R, Premkumar A, eds. 2023. *Obstetric Violence and Systemic Disparities: Can Obstetrics Be Humanized and Decolonized?* New York: Berghahn Books.

FIGO Safe Motherhood and Newborn Health (SMNH) Committee. 2012. "Management of the Second Stage of Labor: FIGO Guidelines." *International Journal of Gynecology and Obstetrics* 119: 111–116.

Greene M. 2001. "Editorial: Vaginal Delivery after Cesarean Section: Is the Risk Acceptable?" *New England Journal of Medicine* 345: 54–55.

Hannah ME, Hannah WJ, Hewson SA, Hodnett ED, Saigal S, Willan AR for the Term Breech Trial Collaboration Group. 2000. "Planned Caesarean Section versus Planned Vaginal Birth for Breech Presentation at Term: A Randomised Multicentre Trial." *The Lancet* 356: 1375–1383.

Health Canada. 2006. *Family Centered Maternity Care and Newborn Care National Guidelines*. Ottawa ON: Health Canada.

International Federation of Gynecology and Obstetrics, International Confederation of Midwives, White Ribbon Alliance, International Pediatric Association, World Health Organization. 2015. "FIGO Guidelines: Mother-Baby Friendly Birthing Facilities." *International Journal of Gynecology and Obstetrics* 128: 95–99.

Lalonde A. 1999. "Editorial: What Is Women's Health?" *Journal of Obstetrics and Gynaecology Canada* 21(7): 639–640.

———. 2009. "Guest Editorial. Vaginal Breech Delivery Guidelines: The Time Has Come." *Journal of Obstetrics and Gynaecology Canada* 31(6): 483–484.

———. 2020. Special Editorial. "FIGO Collaboration for Safe and Respectful Maternity Care." *International Journal of Gynecology and Obstetrics* 52(3): 285–287.

Lalonde A, Herschderfer K, Pascali Bonaro D, et al. 2019. "FIGO Statement: *The International Childbirth Initiative: 12 Steps to Safe and Respectful MotherBaby–Family Maternity Care*." *International Journal of Gynecology and Obstetrics* 146(1): 65–73.

Lydon-Rochelle M, Holt VL, Easterling TR, Martin DP. 2001. "Risk of Uterine Rupture during Labor among Women with a Prior Cesarean Delivery." *New England Journal of Medicine* 345: 3–8.

May ET. 1995. *Barren in the Promised Land: Childless Americans and the Pursuit of Happiness*. Cambridge MA: Harvard University Press.

Public Health Agency of Canada. 2017. *Family Centered Maternity and Newborn Care*. Ottawa ON: Public Health Agency of Canada.

Ruiter JA, Cameron C. 2021. "Birth Models that Nurture Cooperation between Traditionally Competitive Professionals: Pizza and Other Keys to Disarmament." In *Birthing Models on the Human Rights Frontier: Speaking Truth to Power*, ed. Daviss BA, Davis-Floyd R, 327–346. Abingdon, Oxon: Routledge.

SOGC. (1998, 2000) 2005. *Healthy Beginnings*, 3rd edn. Canada: Society of Obstetricians and Gynecologists of Canada.

SOGC, AWHONN, CAM, CFPC, SRPC. 2008. "Joint Policy Statement on Normal Childbirth." *Journal of Obstetrics and Gynaecology Canada* 30(12): 1163–1165.

Stone W, Lalonde A. 2008. "Human Resources for Health in Low Resource World: Collaborative Practice and Task Shifting in Maternal and Neonatal Care." *International Journal of Gynecology and Obstetrics* 105(1): 74–76

CONCLUSIONS

What Have We Learned from Obstetricians?

Robbie Davis-Floyd and Ashish Premkumar

In these Conclusions, we consider what we have learned from our obstetrician authors about their trainings, practices, fears, and transformations. We also present many of the theoretical concepts and frameworks, both anthropological and otherwise, that these obstetricians—some of whom are also anthropologists—have found most useful to employ in presenting and analyzing their own autoethnographic thoughts and experiences. We begin with these, noting that they also contain many of the lessons that can be learned from these chapters. (Unless otherwise indicated, the quotations that we include below are taken directly from their respective chapters, and all italics and parenthetical references in those quotations are from the original chapters.)

The Theoretical Concepts and Frameworks Employed by Our Obstetrician Authors and the Lessons That Can Be Learned from Them

Obstetrician Scott Moses, author of Chapter 1, felt himself "transformed" by his studies with a colleague who was one of the pioneers in the field of "narrative ethics" (Hunter 1991). Inspired by her work, Scott developed a talk for medical students designed, in Scott's words, "to begin to understand the fragility and vulnerability of the patient going through the process [of abortion]." That talk became greatly enriched when he included another colleague whose views on abortion were completely different from his (she chose not to do them, whereas he had made the opposite choice), generating rich narratives and dialogues among the presenters and the students.

As an undergraduate, Scott studied both pre-med and "pre-rabbi," stating that "I felt very lucky to be able to weave the two disciplines and cultures of study." Later, like all US medical students, he took a first-year Medical Ethics course, which was considered a "distraction" by most of his fellow students, but which Scott found both fascinating and helpful: "Throughout medical school, ethics served as a frame for me to integrate subjects like biochemistry and anatomy. Ethics and the medical humanities created lenses through which to view my study of the 'hard sciences.'" Once he finished medical school and entered residency:

> This ... integration into the new world of the professional healer encouraged me to truly appreciate the power and precariousness of liminality—of being "betwixt and between" (Turner 1969). Arnold Van Gennep's description in *The Rites of Passage* (1960) of the phases of "separation, transition, and integration" gave me words and concepts that helpfully elucidated my trajectory through medical education and my transformation into professionalism.

After completing his residency in ob/gyn (obstetrics/gynecology), Scott "enrolled in two different ethics programs, one focusing on clinical ethics and one more dedicated to the medical humanities." He learned how to assist in ethics consultations in the hospital, and he "also studied great thinkers in philosophy, sociology, anthropology, religion, and literature, attempting to gain some grasp of the textual canon of ethics and medical humanities." Scott was moved by Dr. Willie Parker's (2017):

> synthesis of religion and medicine. His use of the word *conversion* to becoming an abortion provider resonates deeply as I think about my own experiences. ... Using a religious lens to guide my practice while preserving and celebrating the autonomy and humanity of the patient can be a tightrope walk. Dr. Parker has been a role model in helping me to keep my balance.

Once he made this "conversion," Scott experienced "cognitive dissonance between the emotional complexity of this lifecycle event and the relative simplicity of the surgical treatment." The book *You're the Only One I've Told: The Stories behind Abortion* by Dr. Meera Shah (2020) helped Scott "fine-tune" his thinking on abortion. Shah (2020:12) wrote, "We can simultaneously believe that there is a potential life growing inside a uterus *and* trust the person carrying the pregnancy to do what is right for them in their own lives." This sentence cogently articulated Scott's own understanding. Yet ultimately, "the language of Heschel (1945:156) speaks to me, comforts me, and inspires me most of all":

> Prayer is no panacea, no substitute for action. It is, rather, like a beam thrown from a flashlight before us into the darkness. It is in this light that we who grope, stumble, and climb, discover where we stand, what surrounds us, and the course which we should choose. Prayer makes visible the right and reveals the false. In its radiance we behold the worth of our efforts, the range of our hopes, and the meaning of our deeds.

For Scott, "the humility of meditative prayer 'makes visible the right.' At this point in my life and in my career, I indeed have 'discovered where I stand,' and performing abortions firmly gives 'meaning to my deeds' because I feel better participating than not, and because I now understand that it is the right thing for me to do."

The authors of Chapter 2, anthropologists Rebecca Henderson and Chu J. Hsiao and obstetrician Jody Steinauer followed "Kumar's (2013) call for scholarship that moves abortion work beyond a stigmatization framework, and Elisa Andaya and Joanna Mishtal's (2016) call for renewed anthropological attention to abortion in the United States in the face of new and vigorous anti-choice movements." These chapter authors also utilized the work of Joshua B. Barbour and John C. Lammers (2015) on the production of "deep professional identities," noting that "[p]rofessional identity is of vital importance in understanding how individuals enact and draw meaning from their work" and citing Jelena Zikic and Julia Richardson (2015) regarding that insight. Henderson, Hsiao, and Steinauer also noted that "professional identity is informed by diverse identifications and experiences, including those of race, ethnicity, gender, sexuality, and others." Citing the work of sociologist James R. Zetka (2011, 2020), these authors noted that for ob/gyns, "the growth of subspecialities, as well as new technologies such as laparoscopic surgical techniques, have caused a reexamination and redefinition of meaning and sense of professional self." Citing the work of Doyin Atewologun, Ruth Sealy, and Susan Vinnicombe (2016), Henderson, Hsiao, and Steinauer further acknowledged that identities are "intersectional." "Intersectionality" is a useful theoretical concept first developed by Black feminist author Kimberlé Crenshaw (1989, 1991):

who introduced the term to address the marginalization of Black women within not only antidiscrimination law but also in feminist and antiracist theory and politics . . . and to highlight the ways in which social movement organization and advocacy around violence against women elided the vulnerabilities of women of color, particularly those from immigrant and socially disadvantaged communities. (Carbado et al. 2013:1)

So important is this concept that Devon W. Carbado and colleagues (2013) created an entire special issue of the *Du Bois Review* around it. They noted that:

scholars and activists have broadened intersectionality to engage a range of issues, social identities, power dynamics, legal and political systems, and discursive structures in the United States and beyond. This engagement has facilitated intersectionality's movement within and across disciplines, pushing against and transcending boundaries, while building interdisciplinary bridges, and prompting a number of theoretical and normative debates. (Carbado et al. 2013:2)

In Chapter 3, series coeditor Ashish Premkumar used his "positionality" as both an MFM specialist and a medical anthropologist to provide, through vignettes, some understandings of what MFMs do that other ob/gyns don't, and of how they teach others. Ashish described his internalization of biomedicine's "hidden curriculum" as defined by anthropologists Lydia Dixon, Vania Smith-Oka, and Mounia El Kotni (2019:40) (see Series Overview, this volume), which, as Ashish noted, "often consists of non-evidence-based biomedical traditions." In his chapter, he considered "How my knowledge base as an MFM/anthropologist developed in tandem with engagement with biomedical and anthropological perspectives" and "How I embody this knowledge base within my surgical and procedural practices."

To ground his knowledge base within anthropology, Ashish drew on Donna Haraway's (1988) concept of "situated knowledges." Haraway defined this term as a means of understanding that all knowledge comes from positional perspectives, noting that an individual's positionality inherently determines what it is possible for that individual to know. Ashish saw this term as emphasizing "that knowledge itself, and the means of acquiring knowledge, are always partial, never universal. [Haraway] reached this conclusion by dissecting universal theories, historically proposed by Enlightenment thinkers who did not themselves acknowledge the racist, classist, and misogynistic roots from which their theories arose." Ashish situated his own knowledge within the "habitus" (Bourdieu 1977, 1997) of the biomedical space, which, as Ashish sees it, is "a cognitive space where group perceptions live, a space that they inhabit... The parameters of that space will be determined by the cultural capital of its inhabitants." Pierre Bourdieu (1986) argued that "cultural capital" involves familiarity with the dominant cultural codes in a society, yet social scientists have expanded that concept to define it "as an asset embodying cultural value" (Throsby 1999:3). Ashish noted that:

> Bourdieu (1997:141) further described the modalities of reproducing habitus, focusing on the effects of bodily practices: "We learn bodily. The social order inscribes itself in bodies through this permanent confrontation, which may be more or less dramatic but is always largely marked by affectivity [emotionality], and, more precisely, by affective transactions with the environment."

Ashish stated that "the crafting of an MFM configures a physician in a specific affective orientation with a pregnant person." He built on anthropologist Rachel Prentice's (2005, 2012) work on surgical training by focusing on how "affect" (feeling or emotion) is created during MFM procedures. He noted that "a hallmark of transitioning from an obstetrician/gynecologist to an MFM" involves "the ability to effectively produce and maintain an affective environment ... that emphasizes quietness, allowing simultaneously for the potential for calm to a patient, yet able to effectively allow for communication and coordination of multiple medical care teams—during difficult, and often traumatizing, situations."

Premkumar also noted that the orientation of the MFM involves creating the fetus as a "medical subject ... with a diagnosable pathology and need for medical intervention," even in utero. (Such an orientation could easily lead to the erasure of the pregnant person, yet Ashish does his best to ensure that it does not, as he describes in his vignettes.) During labor and birth, the obstetrician is responsible for the fetus only until the baby is born; after that, according to the segmentation of biomedical maternity care specialties, the pediatrician becomes responsible for the newborn's wellbeing. In contrast, the MFM is responsible for the wellbeing of the fetus with complications all the way through the perinatal process, while also being responsible for the wellbeing of the mother. To index this dual and full responsibility, Ashish noted that "the buck stops here" with the MFM. Deeply influenced by the work of world-famous medical anthropologist Paul Farmer (2010), Premkumar stated: "by focusing my scope of practice among highly marginalized populations who suffer from medical conditions that lead to higher risk of adverse pregnancy outcomes and early maternal mortality, I felt that my clinical work could help to improve the lives of vulnerable people." Ashish also took a "reproductive justice" (Ross and Solinger 2017) perspective in his praxes: "being able to counsel and provide options for contraception and abortion became my way of helping to enact reproductive justice." Ashish too referred to the concept of intersectionality: "By trying to treat each person who came to see me with dignity, kindness, and respect—regardless of intersectional forms of inequity—I sought to improve the highly disempowering experiences that mark most engagements with biomedical care."

Ashish brought up Robbie Davis-Floyd's definition of "holism" (see Series Overview, this volume) when he described a common problem that MFMs face:

> namely, the moments in which a care team must work on a pregnant woman to care for her fetus, not for her; this, at face value, contradicts the holistic ideological assumption that mother and baby are one, and that what is good for the mother is good for the baby (Davis-Floyd [1992] 2003, 2022). Yet, ontologically, this tenet of holism is not actually contradicted ... as [the pregnant person's] own best interests are served when her twin fetuses are rendered healthy, as our team attempted to do.

In Chapter 4, "Cold Steel and Sunshine: Ethnographic and Autoethnographic Perspectives on Two Obstetric Careers in the United States from across the Chasm," Kathleen Hanlon-Lundberg, also an MFM specialist/perinatologist, described the "chasm" she experienced as the gap between herself as an obstetrician and "the world of anthropology" she entered as she began to study medical anthropology—a field in which she found obstetricians critiqued and often vilified. But what she was reading and hearing about obstetricians from anthropological perspectives did not match her own perceptions of herself as an ob (obstetrician) nor of her ob colleagues. She stated:

> Largely maligned in reproductive anthropological literature as callous—if not brutal—self-serving effectors of the over-medicalization of childbirth, most obstetricians I know and have worked with are devoted to providing respectful, individualized care to their patients...
>
> Obstetricians are not a homogeneous group to be studied and "figured out." We have individual biologies and biographies, com-

plex motivations, a range of interpersonal skills and technical capabilities—or lack thereof . . . The responsibility of . . . obstetricians to promote good outcomes for mothers and babies cannot be overemphasized, but how that is accomplished is situated within the sociocultural conditions in which they learn, work, and live.

As we suggested in our Series Overview (this volume), may her words serve as an inspiration to social scientists who seek to malign obstetricians without studying their individualities and "complex motivations," as our chapter authors in Volumes II and III of this series (Davis-Floyd and Premkumar 2023a, 2023b) so carefully do. Kathleen described her training in ob/gyn "at a large, overcrowded, under-resourced public hospital that served a diverse population of low-income persons," likening this setting to those described by Khiara Bridges in *Reproducing Race* (2011), and to Erving Goffman's (1961) useful description of the "total institution," which, as Hanlon-Lundberg defined it, is "one that closes an individual off from other activities and situates daily routines and behaviors" within its walls.

In Chapter 5, obstetrician Jesanna Cooper described her "awakening" to humanistic practice, using no social science theories at all, but rather describing the traumas of her residency in terms of the Harry Potter books, which served her "as a solace during those four years." She said: "The Dementor's Kiss leaves its victims alive but soulless. I graduated residency a shell of my former self, as though kissed by a dementor. Intimidation, fatigue, and fear had extinguished my critical thinking abilities, joy, and love of service." Jesanna continued: "I exited training in June of 2007, a skilled medical professional with a cheerful bedside manner hiding innumerable terrors and anxieties. I practiced obstetrics and gynecology just as I was taught, driven by fear and seeking safety in conformity"—as indeed, many other obstetricians also, and understandably, do.

After describing the high price she paid for her "awakening," resultant practice changes, and efforts to change "the system," Jesanna concluded her chapter by asking "Why must we pay such a price for trying to humanize those systems?" The answers to that poignant question can be found in Robbie Davis-Floyd's (2023) chapter "Open and Closed Knowledge Systems, the 4 Stages of Cognition, and the Cultural Management of Birth" in Volume II of this series; a summary of that chapter is provided in the Series Overview at the beginning of this volume. To recap here in answer to Cooper's question, we note that the obstetric systems of hospitals around the United States are often Stage 1, silo-oriented, and fundamentalist systems designed to guard their epistemic boundaries and resist any substantive changes to their practices. Davis-Floyd (2023) argues that Stage 1 fundamentalist thinkers believe that "our way is the only right way," and often verge into the fanatical belief that "our way is so right that all who do not accept it should be either assimilated or eliminated." Said Ricardo (Ric) Jones, author of Chapter 7:

> my refusal to routinely perform "standard obstetric procedures" was part of this constructed image of a doctor who questioned the most basic foundations of the field of obstetrics, attacking the heart, the deeper structure, that sustains this medical specialty. In Robbie's terms, I was a Stage 4, humanistic obstetrician practicing within a Stage 1, silo-oriented, fundamentalist, and often fanatical obstetric system.... Thus, as I could not be assimilated, I was constantly a target for being eliminated.

Rosana Fontes agreed, saying in her chapter, "Like a Stage 1 . . . fundamentalist religious sect, technocratic obstetrics generates fear in its practitioners of searching for answers on their own. The punishment for those who follow another path is severe ostracism." And indeed, most of the Stage 4 humanistic chapter authors in this volume have been ostracized, shunned, and sometimes persecuted by their Stage 1 colleagues, as we further discuss below.

Ágnes (Agi) Geréb, coauthor of Chapter 8, is one of these; indeed, she is the author who experienced the greatest amount of persecution. She found Michel Foucault's analysis helpful in her comparison of "the prison-hospital nexus." She noted that her experiences in prison were "eerily familiar and stunningly reminiscent of the hospitals where I trained as a doctor and worked for nearly two decades":

> The rigidity of hierarchy separates the prisoners from the guards, although both are cut off from the outside world. This segregation reflects the insulation of staff from patients in hospitals. The power and information hierarchy are palpable, neatly separating the two classes. There is a clear pecking order within each of these institutions. ... The doctors' and prison guards' tight-knit communities are very much alike. Both prison guards and doctors cover for their colleagues, not only to maintain professional standards, but also for individual economic gain—similar to what Marsden Wagner (2008) describes as "tribal obstetrics." ...
>
> They oversee life and death; they can tell you what is wrong with you, treat you in whatever way they feel is appropriate, and tell you

when you can go home. All others—such as nurses, patients and their families in a medical facility, or prisoners and the visitors in a prison—lack this sanctified knowledge, elevated responsibility, and importance. I realized this in prison as I saw the guards acting as if they knew everything. No one could question what they did or how they did it. Prisoners must follow orders, just like patients.

Agi, who also employs Goffman's (1961) concept of the "total institution," found that her situation in prison felt "strangely and comfortingly familiar, yet totally alien." She had rejected this type of hierarchy and mode of communication after 17 years of practice at the Department of Obstetrics and Gynecology of the University of Szeged. Returning to Foucault, she noted that:

> Writing about France, Michel Foucault (1978) presented the emergence of the modern prison as a form of discipline enhanced by a new technological power that regulates the body and limits the questioning of power. He described this logic as applied to places such as schools, the military, and even hospitals, and my experiences in a Hungarian prison and in hospitals further highlight these parallels.

In this section describing the theoretical constructs and frameworks that our obstetrician authors found useful, and the lessons contained in them, we note that Rosana Fontes and Ricardo Jones of Brazil, Ágnes Geréb of Hungary, Evita Fernandez of India, and Marco Gianotti of the United States found series lead editor Robbie Davis-Floyd's delineations of "the technocratic, humanistic, and holistic paradigms of birth and health care" (described in the Series Overview, this volume) to be helpful both in making and in explaining the "paradigm shifts" they undertook from technocratic to humanistic—and often holistic—care. Rosana and Agi especially found useful Robbie's distinction between "superficial humanism"—which Agi called "painting the walls pink"—and the "deep humanism" that characterized both of their practices, along with many elements of the holistic model. Evita's midwifery trainees showed a distinct change in attitude "from a medicalized nursing mentality to the humanistic midwifery model of care." Ric Jones found Robbie's delineations of the three paradigms and her article on "Obstetric Training as a Rite of Passage" (Davis-Floyd 1987) useful for understanding that:

> The years of residency are the last part of a long transformative process . . . it is important that the obstetric resident who reaches the

end of his education reproduces, now as an obstetrician, the contents and . . . the values that guarantee meaning to and reinforce the social importance of the obstetric profession. These values, which are determined by technocratic ideology, stem from beliefs in the essential defectiveness of women, their inability to deal with their specific physiologic events—pregnancy, birth, breastfeeding—and the importance of biomedical professionals who will, above all, fix their defective body-machines.

Ric noted that Robbie's talk entitled "The Technocratic, Humanistic, and Holistic Paradigms of Birth" at the I International Congress on the Humanization of Childbirth in Brazil in 2000 "has shaped our discourse and our ways of thinking and practicing ever since." And he said that Robbie's book *Birth as an American Rite of Passage* (Davis-Floyd [1992] 2003) "had shown us precisely what was wrong with technocratic birth and *why* we needed to change"; that *From Doctor to Healer: The Transformative Journey* (Davis-Floyd and St. John 1998) had "showed us *how* we could change"; and that *Childbirth and Authoritative Knowledge* (Davis-Floyd and Sargent 1997) "gave us fresh perspectives on the fact that just because a given knowledge system is authoritative doesn't mean that it is correct." Ric also noted the resonance of Barbara Katz Rothman's (2021) naming of the "Biomedical Empire," which he often had to fight during his 34 years of home and hospital practice with his midwife and doula team, eventually losing that fight when his medical license was unfairly revoked by members of that "Empire."

Hakan Çoker, author of Chapter 10 on his teamwork model of "Birth with No Regret," used no social science concepts in his chapter, but rather found his grounding for the humanistic and holistic changes he and his team made in their practices in the pioneering works of Ferdinand Lamaze, Frédérick Leboyer, Grantly Dick-Read, and Michel Odent, and in Thomas Verny's *The Secret Life of the Unborn Child* (1982), along with many others, all of which he read voraciously in his desire to make his teamwork model as humanistic as it could possibly be, and to include the holistic concept of the baby as a conscious being both in utero and after birth. When he was attacked by other obs for his humanistic approach, he "read Grantly Dick-Read's *Birth without Fear* (1942) twice. I remember pages of him describing being attacked by his colleagues. I saw that nothing had changed since then."

Andrew Bisits, author of Chapter 11 on bringing vaginal breech births back in Australia, also used no social science concepts in his chapter, but rather biomedical ones. He referred to what a senior ob called "obstetric courage":

At first, I dismissed this as a slightly arrogant, "macho"-based quality. However, . . . I have come to think he meant that obstetricians need to develop a level of "steel" in order to deal with some of the difficult situations they are faced with. He further said that we need to rein in the level of "drama" that had increasingly become a feature of childbirth.

Bisits spoke of "problem-based learning," and of a module in a Clinical Epidemiology course called "Critical Reasoning": "The emphasis here was a thorough grounding in clinical epidemiology and the evolving area of evidence-based medicine, which included a rigorous approach to the critical appraisal of evidence." Bisits was strongly influenced by this emphasis on using evidence to guide clinical decisions, and by the publication of "the seminal textbook *Effective Care in Pregnancy and Childbirth* (Enkin, Kierse, and Chalmers 1989)":

This book became the foundation of evidence-based medicine, and eventually led to the current Cochrane Collaboration . . . [It] was a summary and synthesis of the most rigorous evidence in maternity care that could be used to justify clinical practice. This textbook was the first to use meta-analysis as a form of evidence synthesis, which until that time had mostly been a narrative and qualitative exercise.

In a commentary for a course project, Bisits discussed the role of "formal decision analysis" "as a way of helping women come to decisions about mode of birth when there is a breech baby at term." He extensively referenced a book by Harold C. Sox called *Medical Decision Making* (1988): "[t]he main thrust of this approach was to incorporate the patient's values and preferences in coming to a decision about any clinical care."

Bisits was delighted to discover a book by New Zealand midwife Maggie Banks, called *Breech Birth, Woman Wise* (1998):

Via emails, I discussed with her women adopting positions other than lithotomy for the births of breech babies. I commented to Maggie that obstetricians seemed to be psychologically locked into the lithotomy position . . . I therefore looked for the evidence behind other birthing positions at the critical time of pushing. If more gravity could be used, then upright positions could be more efficient ways to birth the breech baby—and hopefully to minimize hypoxia, which occurred more frequently in newborns after vaginal breech births.

Bisits additionally found helpful the work of Anne Frye: "In her textbook on holistic midwifery, Anne Frye (2005) provides a comprehensive description of normal and abnormal breech birth mechanics that is far superior to that in any obstetric textbook."

US ob Marco Gianotti, author of Chapter 12, grounded his ideology and practice "in both the technocratic and humanistic models, with the occasional incorporation of holistic modalities" such as aromatherapy. He noted that: "The practice of obstetrics presents a particular opportunity to incorporate doula support in hospitals, along with other humanistic modalities. My experience has shown that this can be done safely and with excellent clinical outcomes, even during a pandemic." Marco always encourages his patients "to come to our visits with a list of questions regarding the issues they want to address." He realized that "most biomedical physicians groan inside when a patient pulls out a paper with a list of questions or turns to the notes section of their smart phone," but he found that such lists "help to keep patients focused on their concerns, which keeps the conversation on topic without the patients having to ... remember their questions." He noted that "Many questions that revolve around more humanistic approaches, such as incorporating birth plans and doulas, can be more streamlined this way, and addressed in a manner that allows greater patient and provider satisfaction." Despite the humanistic elements that he has incorporated into his practice, which include encouraging his patients to labor and birth in upright positions, Marco revealed his still-technocratic orientation when he noted that he doesn't recommend trial of labor after cesarean and allows his laboring patients to drink broth and other clear liquids, but not to eat solid foods. He demonstrated that he is still in the process of transitioning to a more deeply humanistic model when he said:

> Although critiques of standard obstetric procedures such as those of series editor Robbie Davis-Floyd ... insist that laboring women should be allowed to eat actual foods if they wish, my hospital and I have not gone that far into "deeply humanistic" practice ... due to our perceptions of the danger of aspiration should the need for general anesthesia arise.

Yet Marco went on to note that:

> Despite our concerns, meta-analytic data would suggest that the risk for aspiration pneumonia isn't as high as we were taught ... more commentaries from maternal-fetal medicine specialists (MFMs) are suggesting that we should allow laboring women to eat as they

please ... Although this does remain a controversial topic, we continue to learn more with increasing data and research and to adjust accordingly.

And Marco reveals "deep humanism" when he describes that he and his staff chose to keep their practice open and continue to see patients in person during the COVID-19 pandemic when many other obstetric practices were shutting down, that he rejected telemedicine, and that he also continued to allow uninterrupted mother-baby contact when others were separating mothers and babies after birth.

Having presented the concepts and theoretical frameworks that our ob authors found useful, which include many important lessons to be learned, we now turn to summaries of these authors' motivations for becoming obstetricians, their experiences of obstetric training, their motivations for making a paradigm shift (if they did), the benefits they received as a result, and the heavy prices they often paid.

Motivations for Becoming Obstetricians

Not all of our chapter authors provided their motivations for becoming ob/gyns; we present the reports of those who did. For Scott Moses, who found, to his embarrassment, that he "really didn't like taking care of sick people":

> Obstetrics inspired me as the field that most dramatically fostered the care of patients on the upswing of life. As I forged my career path, perhaps I was trying to incorporate my experiences in seminary, where I witnessed clergy being granted the awesome task of stepping in during the most intense aspects of human experience. Likewise, I became energized by the privilege and opportunity of sharing in a patient's lifecycle events. The opportunity to attend the birth of a baby felt impossibly thrilling; that a patient would allow me to participate and a family would welcome me into the scene to me epitomized the privilege of care. These factors ultimately led me to only submit ob/gyn programs to the match for residency.

Ashish Premkumar:

> became drawn to obstetrics and gynecology, and particularly to MFM as a modality to combat everyday inequalities in the lives of the people I had come to see and know. In particular, by focusing

my scope of practice among highly marginalized populations who suffer from medical conditions that lead to higher risk of adverse pregnancy outcomes and early maternal mortality, I felt that my clinical work could help to improve the lives of vulnerable people.

Kathleen Hanlon-Lundberg "decided to specialize in obstetrics and gynecology as a balance of internal medicine and surgery, which would allow me continuity with my patients over their (my) lives." Her friend and colleague, whom she called "Emily," excelled at surgery, in part because of her long-held expertise in sewing—an expertise that she shared with Kathleen—but "did not want to enter general surgery." So, like Kathleen, she chose obstetrics and gynecology "as incorporating both internal medicine and surgery, and as perhaps being more accepting of female physicians." Jesanna Cooper "saw a career in obstetrics and gynecology (ob/gyn) as my passion and my destiny . . . I was convinced that, as an obstetrician/gynecologist, I would be given the opportunity to become a teacher and social advocate as well as a healer."

As a child, Rosana Fontes had "always regarded pregnancy as a magical and even supernatural event. When I was a kid, as the older cousin, I remember watching my aunts' tummies grow, and I stared at their puffy navels for long moments, wondering what was going on inside." After graduating from medical school, Rosana "decided on a residency in gynecology and obstetrics, motivated to discover what was going on inside those big tummies from my childhood."

Hakan Çoker at first thought that he chose obstetrics because it was a popular specialization in Turkey at the time, but later, after reading about transgenerational transmissions, "I now realize that I didn't really have a choice. My mother was a professional home and hospital midwife as was my aunt. Both of my grandmothers were village midwives." This realization that birth attendance was a family tradition made Hakan even more committed to his profession.

Obstetric Training as Experienced by Some of Our Chapter Authors

As with their motivations for becoming ob/gyns, some of our chapter authors did not speak about their training experiences, preferring to focus on other subjects. So here, again, we include only the ones who did. We begin with Jesanna Cooper, who reported her disillusionment with her training process, which she described above as experiencing the "Dementor's Kiss":

The personal statement that I wrote at age 24 illustrated the passion, idealism, and naïvete that many medical students possess when they begin their education. Medical training suppresses those qualities, replacing kindness with toughness, empathy with stamina, and intellectual curiosity with rigidity.... The cruelest moments were when we had poor outcomes. There was no "safe place" to "process," and they were not opportunities to learn and improve. Rather, we faced accusations and blame. I returned to the floor after a particularly bad shift and was told by the nurse that our patient from the previous night was in the ICU and that it was my fault. I had "killed her." I think back and remember that I was a trainee and that I had appropriately called my attending for help. Sometimes you do everything in your power and yet it ends badly. I wish someone had told me that. It would have helped to hear it.

As previously noted, Kathleen Hanlon-Lundberg "trained in obstetrics and gynecology at a large, overcrowded, under-resourced public hospital that served a diverse population of low-income persons" in what she called "battlefield-like conditions." During her residency, she "cared for persons seeking pregnancy and gynecologic care of all descriptions from around the world, whose commonality was poverty." Kathleen provided a raw, uncensored description of her residency experiences as she described that she and her fellow residents:

> cared for incarcerated women ... for wildly intoxicated laboring persons who clawed and screamed, birthing their growth-restricted babies through thick meconium ... I have delivered dead babies—tiny ones whose bodies have become rubbery yellow, bigger ones whose skin is slipping, recently demised fetuses who look like sleeping angels. I have delivered macerated bodies with disarticulated heads. I have seen a baby's scalp, stuck from shoulder dystocia, turn from pink to purple to blue as it died there on the mother's perineum, the obstetric team unable to either bring it forward or replace it into the uterus for cesarean delivery. I have seen women die of amniotic fluid embolism, infection, and trauma.

Kathleen's colleague Emily agreed, saying "Unexpected complications are what obstetricians have learned about, have witnessed in a myriad of unfortunate ways, have contended with through participation in many births, and have nightmares about." When social scientists critique obstetricians for their overly interventive practices, we must take such horrific experiences into account; given these, it is no wonder that obs so often focus on pathology and overly intervene "just in case."

Emily "trained in obstetrics and gynecology in a busy, well-respected community hospital program," in which "There was always a lot of surgery going on." Emily learned that "If a resident expressed interest, arrived earlier, and stayed later than the others, that individual saw, and was allowed to do, more." Emily described that "The high volume of routine and intensive cases in which residents on clinical rotations participate fosters expertise in caring for persons with a range of normal and pathological conditions and surgical challenges." Yet she also found that "continuity of care was often lacking . . . 'To be there twice for the same patient was very unusual.'"

Marco Gianotti completed his formal graduate training in obstetrics and gynecology in the summer of 1997:

> just before residency programs began to undergo a fundamental change from the very traditionalist biomedical training that had been the norm since the dawn of such training programs. Beginning in internship (now called first-year residency), unrestricted work hours and heavy caseloads were normative, and it was expected that residents would perform under these conditions. Training was very "patient-centered," consisting of heavy operative schedules in order to maximize learning during a relatively short training period; indeed, the amounts of on-call and work hours were taxing. Residents were just supposed to comply, no matter how exhausted they became.

Marco went on to note that:

> Since that time, training has shifted to a more "doctor-centered" model; there are now strict regulations and limitations on the number of calls a given resident is allowed to take and on the amount of time spent on direct patient care. Mandatory rest periods have been worked into residents' schedules to avoid the fatigue that often resulted in errors in judgment and, in turn, patient harm.

Yet Marco worries about the unintended consequences of this change, which, he believes, "may be fewer clinical situations and training opportunities experienced by each intern/resident, as the actual length of the training program has not changed in many years, and there is no possible way of including the same amount of training into a four-year program when restrictions on the amount of time spent training are in effect."

Marco continued by noting that "Subspecialty training has risen in an attempt to compensate for some of these shortfalls, adding an additional one to three years to training; however, many obstetric subspecialists (such as perinatologists) participate in more of a consultant role as opposed to delivering direct care the way generalists do."

Having presented the descriptions by some of our chapter authors of their experiences during and thoughts about obstetric training, we turn now to those who deliberately made a paradigm shift from technocratic to humanistic or holistic ideologies and practices, describing their motivations for making such a profound shift, the benefits they and their patients received, and the often extremely heavy prices they paid.

Motivations for Making a Paradigm Shift, Benefits Received, and Prices Paid

Motivations for Making a Paradigm Shift

Jesanna Cooper's motivation for making a paradigm shift came from her difficulties with breastfeeding her baby:

> The experience snapped me awake. Something was wrong. Why had my education left me with this huge knowledge deficit? If I was struggling with breastfeeding, then so were my patients. I didn't have the tools to help myself or the hundreds of women entrusting their care to me. If I didn't have the skills to medically support lactation, what other skills did I lack? I had failed to identify the power structures and biases shaping my education, training, and practice. I was lost. How could I find my way back?

Jesanna found her way back by remembering her girlhood zeal for activism; she said, "I had no business acting as a well-greased cog in the broken maternity care system of the United States. I needed to use my position as a platform for change. I would partner with midwives and doulas. I would create a culture and team characterized by understanding, compassion, and respect." And, over time, she did, despite the many challenges (described below) that she faced from her highly technocratic colleagues.

On making her paradigm shift, Rosana Fontes had these poignant words to say:

> When the obstetric humanistic paradigm ... found me, I had become disillusioned with the kind of obstetrics I practiced, seriously

planning to change careers... My exhaustion after long hours of attending births used to overwhelm both the patients and me. We both gave up. We had neither physical nor emotional support to endure this whole process, and we surrendered to cesarean surgery in the end. No one had taught me ... how to support women... In a country where cesarean births account for more than 56% of all deliveries, no one had explained to these women—nor to me—that it is natural to give birth. The interventions are numerous ... Every labor seemed to be a new battle to win. And victory hardly ever happened; my normal birth rate in private practice was 14% at most.

Ultimately, along with her dissatisfaction with her technocratic practice, Rosana's motivations for making a paradigm shift stemmed from two primary factors: (1) In 2013, she cared for a woman pregnant with twins who had joined the birth humanization movement in her region and had "a lot of contact with doulas." She came to Rosana because "she longed to have a VBAC (vaginal birth after cesarean), even with twins. She managed to give birth naturally and easily to her twin boys." From that time on, "women and doulas wanted me to be their ob, and we began a series of extraordinarily kind and trilateral growing relationships." (2) In 2014, Rosana attended a normal birth conference:

one of the few conferences here in Brazil at which an obstetrician can come into direct contact with evidence-based information about birth assistance and the people who are practicing it. This first conference changed my views of childbirth, women's power, corporate power, and the work of doulas and midwives. I intensely embraced this new universe I hadn't encountered in medical school, and it satisfied all my needs for the ability to make a professional change.

Ric Jones experienced "a thunderous epiphany" when he was called to attend the birth of a woman from the countryside who had walked into the hospital in labor and was squatting on the floor about to give birth when Ric entered the emergency room. Ignoring his exhortations to get up on the table, she gave birth "easily and naturally"—all Ric did was receive the baby and hand it off to a nurse. Later that day, reflecting on this birth, Ric realized that he had done nothing to help her and everything to try to stop her from giving birth as she wished—and there began his journey to his eventual home and hospital practice with a doula and midwife team.

For Agi Geréb of Hungary, who has attended more than 10,000 births during her careers as both an obstetrician and a midwife, her paradigm shift began during her 17 years of hospital practice, when she started to notice the lack of need for many of the routine interventions performed, and gradually stopped performing them, experiencing ostracism and negative sanctions as a result. She was also the first ob in Hungary to allow fathers into the labor and delivery rooms. Her paradigm shift was cemented after she resigned from her hospital practice yet found that many women still wanted her to attend their births, and since she no longer had hospital privileges, she had to attend these births in the women's homes. She said, "These early homebirth experiences in 1988 and 1989 formed the foundation of my practice" from then on, as did her attendance at multiple midwifery conferences, where she connected with other independent midwives who confirmed her beliefs about supporting and facilitating the flow of normal physiologic birth.

Hakan Çoker, author of Chapter 10, practiced technocratically for years until one day at a conference, he snuck into childbirth education workshop out of sheer curiosity, and, like Evita Fernandez (see below) was shocked to learn that his practices were not evidence-based. And there began his paradigm shift, which he continued by studying the "alternative childbirth" literature and attending workshops and midwifery conferences, eventually developing his "Birth with No Regret" model in Turkey, as he described in his chapter.

Evita Fernandez, who, like Hakan, started out practicing technocratically, described two "lightbulb moments" that motivated her to make a paradigm shift to humanistic practice: (1) In 2007, she invited Nutan Pandit, author of *Pregnancy: The Complete Childbirth Book* (2005) to teach a childbirth preparation course at Fernandez Hospital. Upon attending that course, "To my utter horror and dismay, I discovered that our practices in the labor and birthing rooms were out of sync with Nutans's teachings. I discovered that we were horribly interventional. We were not woman-centered." (2) Evita "began reading about maternal mortality and discovered that wherever midwifery care formed the backbone of maternity services, the ratios of maternal and infant mortality were low. Sweden, Denmark, the UK, and our neighbor, Sri Lanka, demonstrated this fact." Thence came her dream of introducing professional midwifery to India, starting with Fernandez Hospital in Hyderabad where she worked. Evita said:

> As obstetricians, a lot of what we were taught needed to be unlearned. We were trained to look at birth as a catastrophe waiting to happen.... Somewhere in our professional lives, we had forgotten

that a woman's body that holds and nurtures a baby could also birth that baby, if only we obstetricians would allow her to do so, if only we had the humility and conviction to step back and watch nature unfold itself in this sacred event. We had to unlearn and open our minds to re-learning the physiology of birth. We learned to look at birth in a whole new manner, taking a 180-degree turn in our approach.

Marco Gianotti did not make a paradigm shift per se, but he did come to incorporate many elements of humanism, and sometimes holism, in his otherwise technocratic practice. His motivations for doing so stemmed from being asked by his department Chair, during his third year of residency, to evaluate:

> many of the processes we were performing to determine if the cost was really justified and whether the procedures ... were likely to really change the care outcomes. For example, if a patient presents to labor and delivery and undergoes a precipitous delivery before an IV can be started, does she really need the IV at all? Why not give oxytocin intramuscularly—or not at all if she is doing well—immediately after she delivers? Do women with hypertensive disorders of pregnancy of varying degrees (which typically require delivery for resolution) really have to stay in a hospital bed until they deliver, regardless of gestational age? Could they not be in a home environment with outpatient monitoring or even home health visits?

For Marco,

> these simple questions, which were really on the cutting edge at that time, were the starting ideas in which technocratic and humanistic care would begin to blend in my practice into a more "hands-off" approach. At the time, this mode of thinking was received with mixed emotions by both residents and professors (attending physicians). After all, we were used to taking care of patients using more invasive approaches ... The idea of minimal intervention before and after delivery was a difficult one for most of us to incorporate into practice. Nonetheless, it was this novel approach that began to pave the way for the incorporation of more humanistic and holistic modalities in obstetric health care; we just didn't realize it at the time.

Starting in the 1970s, André Lalonde, author of Chapter 13, became a pioneer in paradigm-shifting in Canada. His motivations stemmed from the birth of his first child, during which he was allowed only very limited access to the labor room and was forbidden to touch his newborn because he was not "sterile":

> My wife was also separated from our son and we only saw him through the nursery window. No one talked to us about breastfeeding ... I also observed that the midwives (mostly from Europe) who acted as nurses in our labor ward had a great attitude and techniques to support laboring women ... Many nurses had similar great attitudes, yet were under the control of physicians and were rarely consulted on care changes.

Thus, when André became Chief of the Department of Obstetrics and Gynecology in a community hospital, he held a meeting at that hospital with doctors and nurses to ask "whether we could change current obstetric practice. I received positive support to look at how labor and delivery care was provided to women." Lalonde then created a committee of women whom he had cared for during labor and delivery "to advise me on changes that would make maternity services more women-friendly." Confronted with a flat refusal from pediatrics and pediatric nurses to his request to allow parents to visit their newborns in the nursery, he and 12 mothers stormed that nursery, and from then on, parental visits at will were allowed. Other humanistic changes ultimately achieved included allowing fathers/partners to be present; doing away with separate labor, delivery, and recovery rooms, and building rooms with flexible beds in which all women could labor, deliver, breastfeed, and recover in the same place; encouraging women to create birth plans that were then entered into their medical records and honored to the extent possible; allowing women to eat and drink during labor and to labor and deliver in positions of their choice; offering prenatal childbirth education classes; and attending VBACs and vaginal breech births. Lalonde was able to make these changes from a position of power, as he had become the President of the hospital board.

By the late 1980s, André was able "to propose and implement changes across Canada with the Society of Obstetricians and Gynecologists of Canada (SOGC)," because he "was recruited in 1990 to be the CEO of SOGC and accepted." From this new position of power: "I was then ideally placed to introduce many guidelines that would promote a more holistic approach to birthing ... that entailed many of the changes made in my community hospital." The national guidelines he introduced "included vaginal breech deliveries; VBACs; rural obstetrics; breastfeeding support; the promotion of single-room labor, birthing, and postpartum care; and risk management to reduce complications." Supporting the legalization and development of midwifery in Canada, he co-created programs to generate cooperation and collaboration among obstetricians, midwives, and nurses. A central goal of these ongoing programs "is to encourage the three professions to work as equals and to break down traditional silos and hierarchies."

Lalonde then commenced the international work that culminated in the development of *The International Childbirth Initiative* (ICI)*: 12 Steps to Safe and Respectful MotherBaby-Family Maternity Care* (which Hakan Çoker mentioned that he fully implements in his "Birth with No Regret" model). As Chair of the FIGO ICI committee, in his chapter André described the ICI and its ongoing implementations in birthing facilities large and small around the world, making clear his commitment to that Initiative and its transformative potential, and noting that a key feature of ICI implementation is the involvement of local advocates and groups. Lalonde went on to describe how to become an implementing hospital or practice, and listed the countries in which birthing facilities are implementing the ICI:

> To date (October 2022), the countries with facilities that have applied include Austria, Brazil, Canada, Chile, Colombia, Fiji, India, Indonesia, Kenya, Mongolia, Papua New Guinea, the Philippines, Rwanda, the Solomon Islands, Trinidad, Turkey, Uganda, and the United States. Countries that are initiating implementation (applications in progress) include Argentina, Australia, Burkina Faso, China, the Czech Republic, Germany, Honduras, Mexico, Nigeria, and Uruguay.

Robbie, who helped to wordsmith the ICI and sees it as the greatest hope for humanistic changes in maternity care practices worldwide, notes that research is urgently needed on the implementation processes, any barriers that arise, and on helping to find solutions to those barriers. If you are interested in conducting such research, please contact Robbie at davis-floyd@outlook.com.

The Positive Effects of These Paradigm Shifts: Working with Midwives

For all ob authors who made a paradigm shift, both their patients' satisfactions and their outcomes improved dramatically, as there was far less iatrogenic morbidity in the births they attended, and those who, like Kathleen Hanlon-Lundberg, Ricardo Jones, Evita Fernandez, Rosana Fontes, Hakan Çoker, André Lalonde, and Andrew Bisits worked collaboratively with midwives as colleagues found that the births attended by these midwives entailed even fewer interventions and thus fewer maternal and newborn morbidities. Andrew noted that "I learnt just as much from the midwifery staff as I did from the senior obstetricians, and I found this aspect of the learning very enjoyable. (It was also a very good ego-taming experience for me!)" When Andrew began to work more closely with midwives, he found that:

> In Newcastle, there was already a strong emphasis on midwifery, and the midwives were quite assertive. A number of midwives had established themselves as independent practitioners, which was quite revolutionary at the time ... These midwives taught me an enormous amount about childbirth. They helped me to understand the primary and pivotal role of midwifery in a woman's pregnancy, birth, and postnatal period.

Andrew learned from a midwife who was assisting the vaginal birth of a breech baby to be quiet at births and to simply sit and watch, and was greatly impressed by the minimal amount of hands-on interventions that this midwife performed to assist the breech baby's birth. Andrew also noted that this midwife had introduced a birthing stool into the labor and delivery rooms in their hospital:

> Since that time (1997), I have encouraged women to use the birth stool for vaginal breech births. The stool favors the efficient descent of the baby's body and encourages maximal expulsive effort from the woman. It has also resulted in a limited need for significant manipulations of the arms or the head. Since using this birth stool, I have not had to use forceps at all for the birth of the after-coming head.

In addition, Andrew noted that a senior midwife in the hospital where he worked had told him: "'Remember ... that what we do to these women during childbirth stays with them for the rest of their life.' These words of wisdom have stayed with me and have been a fundamental part of my approach to a woman who chooses to birth her breech baby vaginally."

Whereas Ric Jones based his practice on a teamwork model that included an obstetrician, a midwife, and a doula, Hakan Çoker's teamwork model of "Birth with No Regret" includes a midwife, a birth psychologist, and an obstetrician. The midwife also acts as a doula, providing continuous hands-on support for laboring women. The work of the birth psychologist is to monitor the energy in the room—what Ric (Jones

2009) has called the "psychosphere" of birth—and to provide emotional and psychological support to the birthing family and to the birth team. The success of this model was clearly demonstrated in the detailed statistics that Hakan provided in his chapter.

Kathleen Hanlon-Lundberg, who often worked with midwives, found that although some were "jaded," "difficult," and "callous," "most of the midwives strove to provide personalized, compassionate care to the single person under their watch at a time," leaving the rest of the births to the obstetric residents with their fear-based focus on pathology. Kathleen also noted that after completing her training, she worked at a large regional hospital "under a Chairman who was highly supportive of integrated, midwifery-based maternity and well-woman care. The midwifery staff embodied the best attributes of competent, compassionate healthcare professionals. Experiencing collaborative practice among midwives, family practitioners, and private and academic ob/gyns was the highlight of my career."

About working with midwives, Rosana Fontes of Brazil described:

> I remember when nurse-midwives were initially hired in my area... At that time, I was taking shifts in ... the only hospital in the area with a mission that encompassed humanistic values. In São Paulo, I had been used to working with nurse-midwives. Here, the obstetricians objected, saying that midwives would take their place and did not have the technical capacity to perform the same work. In fact, it was the opposite: there was so much work on the maternity ward that we obstetricians could not handle. After nurse-midwives did finally arrive, they took on a great deal of that work, and doctors remained resting in the break rooms while these midwives worked one-on-one with all laboring women. Midwives' inclusion in maternal and childcare was why, in our hospital, normal birth rates dramatically increased, and labor interventions decreased.

And Jesanna Cooper explained:

> I decided that my next step was to bring midwives to my practice and community. I was supporting women who wanted physiologic birth, and midwives are experts in physiologic birth ... As I write this in 2022, our hospital is the only one in Birmingham, [Alabama] with midwives on staff. We are in an underserved and socioeconomically depressed community, but boast the highest exclusive breastfeeding rates, lowest NTSV (nulliparous term singleton vertex—meaning a first-time mother with one baby in the head-down

position) cesarean birth rates, and highest VBAC (vaginal birth after cesarean) success rates in our state. In 2020, we were recognized by *Newsweek* as one of the nation's best maternity programs based on JCAHO (Joint Commission on Accreditation of Healthcare Organizations) quality outcome scores. My practice has added more midwives, which enabled us to implement group prenatal care, which decreases preterm and early term birth rates.

Jesanna went on to state that the doula community in her area noticed their humanistic policies and practices and "began to encourage clients to deliver at our hospital." Her commitment to breastfeeding support had led her to question all "routine" labor interventions that might affect lactation success. She now asked "Why?" rather than "Where are we on the curve?" before starting IV fluids or Pitocin, and rarely artificially broke membranes. She no longer treated "active management of labor" as the gold standard:

> My newly adopted, critical approach to obstetric protocols was embraced by women seeking a physiologic birth. I began to see birth in ways that I never had before. I began to see myself and my role in a birthing person's room differently. During labor, I became an ancillary player only. However, my medical degree meant that I must play more than a supporting role when it came to advocating for the space and support for these normal, physiologic births.

Yet despite such benefits—which were what kept them going—as previously noted, several of our chapter authors found that there were also high prices to pay for having made their paradigm shifts.

Challenges Faced and Prices Paid: The High Costs to Obstetricians of Humanistic Practice

For Jesanna, Rosana, Ric, Agi, and Hakan, these very steep costs included ostracism, verbal attacks, and sometimes bullying and outright persecution by their technocratic ob colleagues, and often also by the hospitals in which they worked and by the obstetric establishments in their respective regions—all part of the "Biomedical Empire" (Rothman 2021). For example, some years after his development of the model of "Birth with No Regret," Hakan Çoker was attacked by other obstetricians:

> for teaching doula classes to non-healthcare professionals; for blaming other obstetricians for not treating women humanistically; for

making birth into a business and making too much money from it ... I was the "charlatan." I was stealing couples' money through "useless" childbirth education. I was teaching unacceptable human rights in childbirth ... I had no right to teach childbirth education classes because I had no university degree. I had no right to train doulas; they were useless and dangerous.

Hakan responded to these attacks not by blaming those who blamed him, but by seeing each attack:

> as an opportunity to write about evidence-based birth, women's preferences, informed consent, humanistic and respectful birthing environments, delayed cord clamping, the safety of non-interventionist, Mother-Friendly approaches, and MotherBaby-Friendly Cesareans. The more I wrote respectfully in responding to their concerns, the more obstetricians started being interested not only in what I wrote but also in how I wrote. Later many came to our courses secretly, saying that they had been affected by my respectful answers, even though I was still being viciously attacked by other obs.

Most sadly, Hakan was also attacked by midwives who saw the doulas he was training as "threats to their profession." He stated, "Because I train doulas, about half of the midwives in Turkey do not like me and often attack me."

As Jesanna Cooper began to work with midwives, she:

> underestimated the knee-jerk resistance of the biomedical establishment when it comes to change. I thought that presenting safety data on midwifery outcomes while demonstrating an increase in patient volumes related to our policy changes would convince the hospital administration and the medical executive committee [to hire midwives]. I was wrong. I was called out for "insubordination" and had my medical license threatened. It took three years of advocating, politicking, and coalition-building to credential our hospital's first midwife.

Asking, "What drives obstetricians to live like this and practice the way we do?" Jesanna responded:

> obstetricians are strong and want birth environments that allow us to be brave. We want birth settings that allow self-control and respect, both for our patients and for ourselves. But, like our patients,

we are limited by maternity care systems that impede our ability to realize our potential. Obstetricians work in a professional setting of fear. We fear being "wrong." We fear lawsuits. We fear professional ostracism. We fear bullying. We fear disappointing our patients. We fear disappointing ourselves. We fear the consequences of not meeting standards set by courts, hospital governance bodies, and insurance companies. We fear not being able to support our families financially and emotionally. Alongside our patients, obstetricians suffer from flawed and dehumanizing biomedical training and maternity care systems.

In Jesanna's distressing yet honest words, we see how obstetricians are constrained by these fears, and, like so many obs, we perceive the difficulties of making positive, humanistic changes within those "flawed and dehumanizing" maternity care systems. Given these systemic flaws, we find it rather amazing that obstetricians like Jesanna have nevertheless managed to create humanistic changes, which is easier to do in private practice and much harder to do when working hospital shifts. In contrast, André Lalonde experienced battles in making his changes, but no outright persecution, because, as previously noted, he worked from positions of leadership and power.

The challenges faced by Ric Jones and Agi Geréb were overwhelming persecutions, which ultimately resulted in Ric's losing his license to practice as an ob due to a neonatal death that was not his fault, but was used by the obstetric establishment—the "Biomedical Empire"—to finally force him out of practice after 34 years of home and hospital birth attendance with outstanding outcomes, including a cesarean birth (CB) rate of 16.5% in a city with a CB rate of 75%. And Agi's persecutions resulted in a 77-day imprisonment, three years of home confinement, and a ten-year prohibition on practicing (she was 67 at the time). These are the two most extreme examples of the results of obstetric persecutions among our ob chapter authors.

The costs of such paradigm shifts unfortunately often also included stress, exhaustion, and burnout, as these humanistic obs were frequently sought out by pregnant people who wanted "natural" births; thus, since they were usually the only—or one of a few—obs willing to provide that kind of woman-centered care, they often had to be on-call 24/7. Rosana Fontes said, with emphasis, "I learned that what is humanizing for laboring women is not always humanizing for their obstetricians; it's not a two-way street—as Jesanna Cooper explains in more detail in the preceding chapter." Jesanna, whose entirely humanistic practice with midwives "fills me with pride and gives me the sense of professional accomplishment and fulfillment that had been lacking in my career for so many years" said "I wish it were enough." But it wasn't enough; Jesanna explained that:

> Helping others achieve empowering and beautiful birth experiences is all-consuming, but it does not lead to a fulfilling life... I am tired. Over the past eight years, I have tried, unsuccessfully, to add ob/gyn partners to share in the call load. Hospitals generally aid practices financially in these efforts, but mine wouldn't. Even if they had been willing, how does one find an ob/gyn willing to work more hours for less money practicing in a way that they had not trained for? The obstetrics and family practice physicians at my hospital refuse to share call or to back up my midwife partners—though they enjoy advertising our hospital's strong outcomes, which are due to the midwifery model of care. The compromises that I have made with nursing and hospital administration to credential midwives to practice in this hospital have led to taxing in-person call requirements that do not make business sense for our practice and contribute to my mental and physical exhaustion. My hospital requires my presence in-house most of the times the midwives are working. The personal toll is significant. I have missed innumerable family events, children's school productions, and athletic games. I can't commit to attending family members' weddings. I work when sick with the flu because I have no coverage. I haven't been to the dentist or gotten a mammogram in years. I struggle with depression. I am overweight, have chronic back pain, and never exercise. I continue working under these conditions because my residency trained me to do so. I'm an obstetrician. I can work impossible hours without collapsing, so I do. I realize that I am functional, but not ok. I am cracking.

Kathleen Hanlon-Lundberg and Rosana Fontes were "cracking" too, so they both left obstetrics for a time, returning only once they were fully rested, and then only practicing minimally compared to the over-full practices they had left behind in favor of more balanced lives in which they could spend more time with their families. (Upon reading Jesanna's chapter, Rosana emailed us to say "I wonder when Jesanna will reach that place, as I have." And she did; she sold her clinic in 2021, and is now retired.) Ric Jones did enjoy a balanced life, as he and his midwife and doula team only took on a few births per month, most of which were home births; thus, unless these births clustered (meaning occurring back-to-back), they rarely experienced overstress and burnout. And so it is with Hakan Çoker, whose "Birth with No Regrets" team attends only three to five births per month, and who receives full support from his team and from the satisfied couples who leave their births with no regrets, as did Ricardo Jones and his midwife and doula team before he was forced to stop practicing.

The challenges that Evita Fernandez and her colleagues faced in introducing professional midwives and the midwifery model of care to the Fernandez Hospital in Hyderabad, and later to the whole country, did not result in ostracism or persecution, as Evita, like André Lalonde, was working from a position of power—in Evita's case, as Head of the Fernandez Hospital, which her parents had founded. Her challenges did include "facing the fears and prejudices" of her obstetric colleagues," and "combating the age-old tradition of doctors attending every birth," for which Evita and her like-minded colleagues had to "crack" the "solid patriarchal environment . . . as the midwifery trainees empowered with evidence-based practices began to question old beliefs," and to teach obs and midwives to work together as colleagues "with mutual respect and trust."

We hope that it is with "mutual respect and trust" among our readers and ourselves that we conclude this volume, which, again, is part of a three-volume series on *The Anthropology of Obstetrics and Obstetricians: The Practice, Maintenance, and Reproduction of a Biomedical Profession*. This present book is Volume I of that series. Volume II is titled *Cognition, Risk, and Responsibility in Obstetrics: Anthropological Analyses and Critiques of Obstetricians' Practices* (Davis-Floyd and Premkumar 2023a). Volume III is called *Obstetric Violence and Systemic Disparities: Can Obstetrics Be Humanized and Decolonized?* (Davis-Floyd and Premkumar 2023b). We hope that our readers will now turn to Volumes II and III!

Robbie Davis-Floyd Adjunct Professor, Dept. of Anthropology, Rice University, Houston, Fellow of the Society for Applied Anthropology, and Senior Advisor to the Council on Anthropology and Reproduction is a cultural/medical/reproductive anthropologist interested in transformational models of maternity care, an international speaker, and author, coauthor, or lead editor of multiple articles, encyclopedia entries, book chapters, and books, the latest of which is the solo-edited *Birthing Techno-Sapiens: Human-Technology Co-Evolution and the Future of Reproduction* (2021). She also serves on the Board of the International MotherBaby Childbirth Initiative, in which capacity she helped to create the *International Childbirth Initiative* described above. Email: davis-floyd@outlook.com.

Ashish Premkumar is an Assistant Professor of Obstetrics and Gynecology at the Pritzker School of Medicine at The University of Chicago and a doctoral candidate in the Department of Anthropology at The Graduate School at Northwestern University. He is a practicing maternal-fetal medicine subspecialist. His research focus is on the intersections of the social sciences and obstetric practices, particularly surrounding the issues of risk, stigma, and quality of health care during the perinatal opioid use disorder epidemic of the 21st century. E-mail: premkumara@bsd.uchicago.edu.

References

Andaya E, Mishtal J. 2016. "The Erosion of Rights to Abortion Care in the United States: A Call for a Renewed Anthropological Engagement with the Politics of Abortion." *Medical Anthropology Quarterly* 31(1): 40–59.

Atewologun D, Sealy R, Vinnicombe S. 2016. "Revealing Intersectional Dynamics in Organizations: Introducing 'Intersectional Identity Work.'" *Gender, Work & Organization* 23(3): 223–247.

Banks M. 1998. *Breech Birth, Woman Wise*. Hamilton NZ: Birthspirit Books.

Barbour JB, Lammers JC. 2015. "Measuring Professional Identity: A Review of the Literature and a Multilevel Confirmatory Factor Analysis of Professional Identity Constructs." *Journal of Professions and Organization* 2(1): 38–60.

Bourdieu P. 1977. *Outline of a Theory of Practice* (R. Nice, Trans.) Cambridge: Cambridge University Press.

———. 1986. "Forms of Capital." *Handbook of Theory and Research for the Sociology of Education*, ed. Richardson JG, 241–258. New York: Greenwood.

———. 1997. *Pascalian Meditations*. Stanford, CA: Stanford University Press.

Bridges K. 2011. *Reproducing Race: An Ethnography of Pregnancy as a Site of Racialization*. Berkeley: University of California Press.

Carbado DW, Crenshaw KW, Mays VM, Tomlinson B. 2013. "Intersectionality: Mapping the Movements of a Theory." *Du Bois Review* 10(2): 303–312.

Crenshaw K. 1989. "Demarginalizing the Intersection of Race and Sex: A Black Feminist Critique of Antidiscrimination Doctrine." *University of Chicago Legal Forum* 1989: 139–168.

———. 1991. "Mapping the Margins: Intersectionality, Identity, and Violence against Women of Color." *Stanford Law Review* 43(6): 1241–1300.

Davis-Floyd R. 1987. "Obstetric Training as a Rite of Passage." *Medical Anthropology Quarterly* 1(3): 288–318.

———. (1992) 2003. *Birth as an American Rite of Passage*, 2nd edn. Berkeley: University of California Press.

———. 2022. *Birth as an American Rite of Passage*, 3rd edn. Abingdon, Oxon: Routledge.

———. 2023. "Open and Closed Knowledge Systems, the 4 Stages of Cognition, and the Cultural Management of Birth." In *Cognition, Risk, and Responsibility in*

Obstetrics: Anthropological Analyses and Critiques of Obstetricians' Practices, ed. Davis-Floyd R, Premkumar A, Chapter 1. New York: Berghahn Books.

Davis-Floyd R, Premkumar A, eds. 2023a. *Cognition, Risk, and Responsibility in Obstetrics: Anthropological Analyses and Critiques of Obstetricians' Practices*. New York: Berghahn Books.

———. 2023b. *Obstetric Violence and Systemic Disparities: Can Obstetrics Be Humanized and Decolonized?* New York: Berghahn Books.

Davis-Floyd R, Sargent C, eds. 1997. *Childbirth and Authoritative Knowledge: Cross-Cultural Perspectives*. Berkeley: University of California Press.

Davis-Floyd R, St. John G. 1998. *From Doctor to Healer: The Transformative Journey*. New Brunswick NJ: Rutgers University Press.

Dick-Read G. 1942. *Childbirth without Fear: The Principles and Practice of Natural Childbirth*. London: Heinemann Medical Books.

Dixon LZ, Smith-Oka V, El Kotni M. 2019. "Teaching about Childbirth in Mexico: Working across Birth Models." In *Birth in Eight Cultures*, ed. Davis-Floyd R, Cheyney M, 17–48. Long Grove IL: Waveland Press.

Enkin M, Kierse MJC, Chalmers I. 1989. *Effective Care in Pregnancy and Childbirth*. Oxford: Oxford University Press.

Farmer PE. 2010. *Partner to the Poor: A Paul Farmer Reader*, ed. Sussey H. Berkeley: University of California Press.

Foucault M. 1978. *Discipline and Punish: The Birth of the Prison*. New York: Pantheon Books.

Frye A. 2005. *Holistic Midwifery: A Comprehensive Textbook for Midwives in Homebirth Practice. Volume 2, Care During Labor and Birth*. Portland OR: Labrys Press.

Goffman E. 1961. *Asylums: Essays on the Condition of the Social Situation of Mental Patients and Other Inmates*. Garden City NY: Anchor Books.

Haraway D. 1998. "Situated Knowledges: The Science Question in Feminism and the Privilege of Partial Perspective." *Feminist Studies* 14(3): 575–599.

Heschel AJ. 1945. "Prayer." *Review of Religion* 9(2): 153–168.

Hunter KM. 1991. *Doctor's Stories: The Narrative Structure of Medical Knowledge*. Princeton NJ: Princeton University Press.

Jones R. 2009. "Teamwork: An Obstetrician, a Midwife, and a Doula in Brazil." In *Birth Models that Work*, ed. Davis-Floyd R, Barclay L, Daviss BA, Tritten J, 271–304. Berkeley CA: University of California Press.

Kumar A. 2013. "Everything Is Not Abortion Stigma." *Women's Health Issues* 23(6): e329–331.

Parker W. 2017. *Life's Work: A Moral Argument for Choice*. New York: Atria Books.

Prentice R. 2005. "The Anatomy of a Surgical Simulation: The Mutual Articulation of Bodies in and through the Machine." *Social Studies of Science* 35(6): 837–866.

———. 2012. *Bodies in Formation: An Ethnography of Anatomy and Surgery Education*. Durham, NC: Duke University Press.

Ross LJ, Solinger R. 2017. *Reproductive Justice: An Introduction*. Berkeley: University of California Press.

Rothman BK. 2021. *The Biomedical Empire: Lessons Learned from the COVID-19 Pandemic*. Stanford CA: Stanford University Press.

Shah M. 2020. *You're the Only One I've Told: The Stories behind Abortion*. Chicago IL: Chicago Review Press.

Sox HC. 1988. *Medical Decision Making*. Stoneham MA: Butterworth Publishers.
Throsby D. 1999. "Cultural Capital." *Journal of Cultural Economics* 23: 3–12.
Turner V. 1969. *The Ritual Process*. New York: Penguin Books.
Van Gennep A. 1960. *The Rites of Passage*. Chicago IL: University of Chicago Press.
Wagner M. 2008. *Born in the USA: How a Broken Maternity System Must be Fixed to Put Women and Children First*. New York: Penguin.
Zetka JR. 2011. "Establishing Specialty Jurisdictions in Medicine: The Case of American Obstetrics and Gynaecology." *Sociology of Health & Illness* 33(6): 837–852.
———. 2020. "Innovation, Professional Identity, and Generational Divides in Medicine: The Case of Gynecologic Laparoscopy in the USA." *Social Science & Medicine* 266: 113350.
Zikic J, Richardson J. 2015. "What Happens When You Can't Be Who You Are: Professional Identity at the Institutional Periphery." *Human Relations* 69(1): 139–168.

Index

abortion, 2, 10, 14, 26, 262, 267
  abortion-only providers, 38
  and professional identity. See under professional identity
  anti-abortion, 23, 37, 40
  as "dirty work," 32
  "conversion" to performing, 19, 263
  criminalization of, 35
  emotions while performing, 15–18, 24
  ethics (morality) of. See under ethics
  feelings of loss, 16–17, 21–23
  feminism and, 35, 39, 42, 48
  in Israel, 25
  in the USA, 25
  late term, 22
  methods, 30n13
  mifepristone used in, 30n12
  prenatal screening and, 85–86
  Roe v Wade, 2, 27, 32, 35, 37–38, 50–51, 51n1
  stigmatization of providing, 33, 39–40, 45
  unsafe, 37
Active Birth (Balaskas), 194, 196, 207
Adorno, Theodor, 113
AIDS (HIV), 55
ambulance services for newborns, 168n2
American Medical Association (AMA), 40, 49
anthropology, xii, 12, 17, 88–91, 139, 159, 263, 265, 267
  activism in, 88
  American Anthropological Association, 88

Anthropology of Obstetrics and Obstetricians: The Practice, Maintenance, and Reproduction of a Biomedical Profession, 290
  attitude toward obstetricians, 3–4, 88
  autoethnography, 55, 73
  biomedicine and, 89–90, 267
  ethnocentrism, xx–xxi
  history of, xii–xiv
  medical, xv, 1, 54, 72, 88, 265, 267
  of birth and of midwifery, xiii, 72, 130
  of obstetrics and obstetricians, xii, xxix, 3, 32, 55, 111, 130, 267
  sources for, xiii–xiv
  of reproduction, xiii, 72
Aquinas, Thomas, 17, 26
Arendt, Hannah, 113
Arslan, Laurence Issele, 196
Association for Prenatal and Perinatal Psychology and Health (APPPAH), 208n2
Australia, 210
  "Becoming a Breech Expert" (BABE), 221
  Health Insurance Holdings (HIH), collapse of, 217
  midwives in, 215
  Newcastle Medical School, 213, 220
  influenced by McMaster University (Canada), 214
  vaginal breech birth in, 214–215
autopsy, 75–76

Baby-Friendly Hospital Initiative (BFHI), xxiv

Balaskas, Janet, 196
Banks, Maggie, 215, 272
Barnes, William, 36
Baswal, Dinesh, 184
Beckingham, Andy, 174
Benincasa, Miria, 107
Between the Ears: Birth Stories (Jones), 130
biomedicine, 33–34, 123, 229
  conservative forces in, 139
  defined, 33
  ethnography and, xv, 32, 89–90
  "hidden curriculum" of, 55
  obstetrics as a branch of, xiii
  technocratic, 228
birth
  "alternative birth practice," 159
  amniotic fluid embolism during, 79, 131–132, 141n2, 276
  and poverty, 79–80, 276
  "as a catastrophe waiting to happen," 178, 280
  as disease, 102, 110
  as "rite of passage" (Davis-Floyd), 112
  attending a, 13
  being quiet at, 216, 266, 284
  "birth plan," 181, 233–239, 248–250, 273, 282
    and hospitals, 236
    defined, 234–235
    obs reactions to a, 235–236
  birthing room. *See under* hospital
  breech (including vaginal breech delivery, VBD), 7, 77, 181, 183, 210, 247–248, 284
    and cesarean procedure, 215
    Breech without Borders website, 221
    electronic heart monitoring during, 213
    forceps used during, 212
    global percentage having, 210
    International Term Breech Trial. See International Term Breech Trial
    international study of, 217–218
    Lovset's maneuver, 212–213
    new studies of VBB, 220
    optimizing safety in, 218–219, 222–223
    positions during, 215
    practices involving breech births, 210–213, 221
    PREMODA study of VBB, 218–219
    preterm babies and, 224n1
    Vaginal Breech Initiative, 220
  complications and procedures. *See under* medical procedures used during birth
  cross-cultural differences on, xiii, xvi, xxii, xxv, xxx, 1, 26–27, 94, 112
  cultural models of, 5, 73, 89–91, 140
  father/partner's presence during, xxiv, 129, 149, 159, 166, 200, 206, 246, 280, 282
  global childbirth scene (summary), xxi–xxvii
  high thrombocyte count in mother, 156
  home, xv, xxv, xxviii, xxx, 6, 100, 109, 134–139, 146–166, 168n1, 176, 250, 280, 289
    Dutch system, 135
    Hungarian system, 145
    outcomes for, 136
    requiring hospitalization, 156
    "the soul of home birth," 145
  humanization of, 103–111, 125–129, 131–135
  humanization movement, 6, 103, 117–118, 279
  Network for the Humanization of Birth. *See under* Brazil
  hypoxia, 105, 156, 215, 272
  labor, xvii, xxii, 5, 8, 82, 97, 102–111, 126, 131, 134, 136–137, 148, 156, 171, 174, 186, 192–193, 197–200, 203, 218, 222, 233–242, 245–251, 266, 273, 279, 281
    "active management of labor," 98

contractions, 58, 84, 131, 148, 197
eating and drinking during, xvii
induction or augmentation of, xxvii, 206, 259n1
intervention in, xvi, xxii, 98, 102–107, 110, 205, 212, 285–286
latent, xxiv
pain of, xxiv, 110, 194
preterm, 58
"standard procedures" applied to, xxvii
treating people undergoing, xv, 196, 282
miscarriage, 16, 22–23, 26, 118, 231, 241
"MotherBaby-Family" triad, 254
moxibustion and, 194
normal viewed as "vaginal birth + epidural," 128
pool, 162
positions during, xvii–xviii, xxii, 136, 181, 185–186, 215, 237, 247, 249, 279
lithotomy position, 129, 186, 205, 212
postpartum period, xvii, 80, 97, 107, 147, 172, 193, 199, 242
baby-friendly, xxiv
care during the, 61, 97, 162, 246, 282–283
depression. See under women
issues within the, xxii, 66, 247–251
premature rupture of membranes (PROM), 95
prenatal exercise, 194
procedures. See medical procedures used
psychologist, role of the, 198–201
"psychosphere" of (Jones), xvii, 133, 285
"soft factors" in, 134
"risks" of, 28, 46, 107, 211–212, 215, 219, 221
shoulder dystocia, 79, 82, 145–149, 156, 216, 276
"skin-to-skin." See under newborn(s)

"smoothing birth" (Jones), 135
stool, 215–216, 223, 284
tachypnea after, 137
twin delivery, 15, 55–66, 68n8, 69n15, 73, 77, 108, 130, 145, 149, 156, 197, 267, 279
twin-to-twin transfusion syndrome. See twin-to-twin transfusion syndrome
unpredictability of, 132, 239
vaginal birth after cesarean (VBAC), 82, 98, 103, 162, 181, 234, 248–249, 279, 286
in France, 249
"trial of labor after a cesarean" (TOLAC), 234
inducing with prostaglandins, 248, 259n1
vaginal or abdominal delivery, 21, 84, 110
water birth, 76, 129, 181, 194–197
Birth as an American Rite of Passage (Davis-Floyd), 130, 271
Birth Models That Work (Davis-Floyd et al.), 130
Birth without Fear (Dick-Read), 203, 271
Birthing Models on the Human Rights Frontier: Speaking Truth to Power (Daviss and Davis-Floyd), 195
Black Lives Matter movement, 50
Bonaro, Debra Pascali, 251
Bourdieu, Pierre, 55, 266
Brazil, 4, 5, 101, 123
Acaiá team, 109, 116
arrest of Lula da Silva
birth rates in, 102–103
Brazilian Ministry of Health, 108
Bolsonaro, Jair, 139
cesarean rates in Brazil, 125
"Floydettes," 130
Health Psychology Graduate Program, São Paulo Methodist University, 107
high cesarean birth rate, 110
home birth rate, 109

International Conference for the Humanization of Childbirth I, 129
Mátria Clinic, 106–109, 117
  birth outcomes at, 109
  new legion of professional midwives in, 140
  nurse-midwives in, 102
  ob/gyns in, 101
  Orelhas de Vidro (Ricardo Jones' blog in Portuguese), 140, 141n3
  Regional Council of Medicine, São Paulo, 109
  ReHuNa (Network for the Humanization of Birth), 112, 129, 140
  São Francisco de Assis Hospital, Jacareí, Brazil, 102
  SIAPARTO (São Paulo, Brazil), 103
  study of outcomes, 108
  training of ob/gyns in, 141n1
  transdisciplinary birth care team, 128
  University of São Paulo Midwifery School (Brazil), 106
  vestibular (university entrance exam), 123
  "witch hunt" against humanistic ob/gyns in, 139
breastfeeding (lactation), xxiv, 4, 95–99, 107, 119, 124, 141, 156, 181, 193, 197, 200, 206, 242, 246–249, 278, 282, 284, 286
  and newborn care courses, 197
  consultant, 106, 242
Breastfeeding: Scientific Bases (de Carvalho), 130
Breech Birth, Woman Wise (Banks), 215, 272
Bridges, Khiara, 268

Canada, 245
  all-birthing room maternity ward, 249
  Family Centered Maternity and Newborn Care (Canadian government guidelines), 250, 253
  Hôpital Général La Salle (Montreal), 245
  midwifery in, 250–252
  legalization of non-nurse midwifery, 250
  offering VBACs in, 248–249
  Royal Victoria Hospital (McGill University), 245
  Society of Obstetricians and Gynecologists of Canada (SOGC), 249, 250, 282
Carbado, Devon W., 264
"Carry It On" (Joan Baez), 154
Childbirth and Authoritative Knowledge (Davis-Floyd and Sargent), 130, 271
Coalition for Improving Maternity Services (CIMS), 130
Cochrane Collaboration, 214, 272
Coelho, Paulo, 175
contraception, xxx, 28, 29n1, 56, 57, 251
  intrauterine devices (IUDs), 118
COVID-19 pandemic, 50, 101, 107, 116, 187, 228–231, 240–243, 273
  telemedicine during, 243
Czene, Ágnes, 146

Davis, Elizabeth, 194
Davis-Floyd, Robbie E., xv, xxxii, 8, 55, 57, 100n1, 111–112, 115, 124, 129, 133, 165, 195, 196, 228, 233–234, 237, 252, 267, 270–272, 283
Daviss, Betty-Anne, 195, 219, 220
death (fetus, baby, mother), xxii, 13, 22–23, 64, 72, 79, 84, 132–133, 136, 138, 146, 156, 171–172, 219, 276
  sudden infant death syndrome (SIDS), 146
  preventable, 171
DeLaurentis, Kelly, 43
"Dementor's kiss" (from Harry Potter novels), 95, 268, 276

298 ♦ Index

Dick-Read, Grantly, 135, 194, 203, 204, 207, 272
Domján, Kati, 160
doulas. *See* midwives and doulas
drugs, 126
   birth without, 180
   epidural, 63, 78, 84, 95, 128, 180, 206, 211, 246
   mifepristone. *See under* abortion
   opioid use disorder during pregnancy, 68n6
   oxytocin, 119, 141, 149, 233, 287
      Pitocin (synthetic oxytocin), xxii, 98, 104, 147–148, 235
   pain management, 83, 105
   prostaglandins, 248
   respiratory effects of cocaine use on newborns, 80
Duarte, Ana Cristina, 103
Du Bois Review, The, 264–265

Effective Care in Pregnancy and Childbirth (Enkin, Kierse, and Chalmers), 211, 214, 272
embodiment, the importance of, 66–67, 72
"Embrace" [Phase-Change Material (PCM)], 181
Encyclopedia Britannica, 229
Enning, Cornelia, 104
Ernst, Kitty, 160
ethics, 1–2, 12, 33–34, 44, 49, 68n1, 68n9, 154, 262
   clinical, 17
   cognitive dissonance and, 263
   compassion, 94
   "imperative of conscience" (Jones), 140
   lawsuits, xxiv, 4, 212
   master's degree in medical, 29n2
   medical, 12, 18, 29n2, 263
   "narrative ethics" (Hunter), 11, 263
   "obstetric violence," 129
   of abortion, 10, 14–15, 17–19, 21–25
   "patient autonomy," 22
   patient's struggle with, 18–19

persecution of humanistic ob/gyns. *See under* politics and power
practice without judgment, 20
prayer, 264
reproductive rights and justice, xvii, 2, 21–23, 27–28, 32, 55, 205, 253–254, 267
   "Texas Heartbeat Act," 28
social injustice, 94, 96, 145, 203
training, 11, 17, 263
violence against women. *See under* politics and power
unfair legal prejudice, 155
European Court of Human Rights, 152, 165
European Union's Petitions Committee (Brussels), 150
Evans, Jane, 220
"evidence-based" medicine practices, 55, 68n4

family planning, xxxiii, 14, 16, 18, 28, 55–57, 68n2, 118, 291
   contraception. *See* contraception
Farmer, Paul, 266–267
fathers in delivery room. *See under* hospitals
fear, 4, 32, 95, 99–104, 165, 210–211, 215, 263
   "adrenaline cycle" (Dick-Read), 135
   and birth, xviii, 115, 156, 198, 204
   and critical thinking, 268
   and Stage 1, 165
   doctors instilling, 155
   of being wrong, 4, 100
   of home birth, xxx, 136
   of imprisonment, 166
   of lawsuit, xxiv, 28, 100
   of losing self, 118–119
   of pandemic, 240
   of reprisals and repercussions, 4, 28, 100, 109, 156, 178, 288
   overcoming, 18, 290
   technocratic obstetrics and, 104, 269, 285
fetus, 55, 60, 68n1, 68n8, 103, 237
   as patient, 54, 61, 68n1, 266

cross-cultural perspective on, 26–27
electronic fetal monitoring (EFM).
  See under medical procedures
fetoscopy. See under medical
  procedures
hypoxia, 105
loss of, 14–16, 22, 23
personhood of, 10
problems defining, 26–27, 69n11
Floyd, Peyton Elizabeth, 129
Fondello, Milena, 106
forceps. See under medical procedures
"formal decision analysis" (Bisits),
  214–215
Foucault, Michel, 64, 155, 269
*From Doctor to Healer: The
  Transformative Journey*
  (Davis-Floyd and St. John),
  130, 271
Frye, Anne, 220, 272
Fuchtner, Carlos, 252

Ganguly, Kadambini, 172
Gaskin, Ina May, xviii, 129, 172
gender, 35–36, 80, 81, 85–86, 94, 211, 264
  doctor vs. nurse, 73
George Washington University, 220
Ginsburg, Faye, xii
Glezerman, Marek, 219
Goffman, Erving, 268, 270
Gramsci, Antonio, 110
Grihyasutra (Paraskara), 27, 30n15
Guidelines on Midwifery Services (India), 6
Gunn, David, 40
gynecology, gynecologists (gyn). See
  ob/gyn

Haber, Bea, 158
"habitus" (Bourdieu), 55, 65, 266
  defined, 65
Hannah, Mary, 216
Haraway, Donna, 55, 60–61, 265
Harper, Barbara, 196
Harris, Lisa, 22, 29n6
Hart, Gail, 194

healthcare industry, 81, 97–100,
  135–136, 152
Healthy Beginnings (Lalonde et al.), 249
Held, Rabbi Shai, 23
Hellen Diller Medical Center
  (University of California San
  Francisco), 220–221
HELLP syndrome, 108
Henderson, Rebecca, 35
Herschderfer, Kathy, 252
Heschel, Abraham Joshua, 24, 264
Hodnett, Ellen, 207
holistic paradigm. see under
  technocratic, humanistic, and
  holistic paradigms
home birth. See under birth
hospitals, xxvi–xxvii, 73, 75, 77, 79,
  236–237, 289
  academic, 84–86
  anesthetists, 248
  birthing room, 246
    conversion from delivery room,
    248
  Catholic, run by nuns, 251
  Chair of the Ob-Gyn Department,
    154
  delivery room, 79
  different levels of care in, 68n7
  husbands (fathers, partners) in
    delivery room, 158, 240,
    245–246
  insistence upon use of nursery, 246
  labor and delivery unit, 84
  like prisons, 154
  midwives on staff of, 98–99
  prenatal classes at, 247
humanistic (bio-psycho-social)
  paradigm. See under
  technocratic, humanistic, and
  holistic paradigms
Hungary, 5, 144
  Alternatal Alapítvány a Háborítatlan
    Születésért, Szülésért
    (Alternatal Foundation for
    Undisturbed Birth), 147, 160
  anyasági támogatás (maternity
    benefit), 148

as a "grey society," 160
authoritarianism. *See under* politics and power
Budapest municipal prison, 144
Egészségügyi Tudományos Tanács (Healthcare Scientific Council), 145
En God Start i Livet (A Good Start to Life), 150
Faculty of Health Sciences, Semmelweis University, 146
Fővárosi Ítélőtábla (Court of Appeals), 145
Fővárosi Fellebbviteli Főügyészség (Prosecutor's Office), 145
háborítatlan (undisturbed) birth, 152
home birth movement in, 155–161
hospitals, 150
Kúria (Supreme Court), 145
legalizing home birth in, 162
Mérce Egyesület (a NGO), 161
Napvilág (Birth House), 147, 156, 160
Nemzetközi konferencia a születésro (International Conference on Childbirth), 160
nurse-practitioners in, 158
obstetric midwife in, 160
Pediatric Clinic of Semmelweis University (Budapest), 148
President János Áder of, 145
Prime Minister Viktor Orbán of, 150
struggle for independent midwifery in, 149
Szabadon szülni, szabadnak születni (2012 film by Frigyes Fogel), 168n3
Szent István Hospital, 147
Társaság a Szabadságjogokért (Hungarian Civil Liberties Union), 152
University of Debrecen, 146
University of Szeged Hospital, 146, 158
"witch hunt" against humanistic ob/gyns in, 165
women's protests and marches for change, 152, 164

HypnoBirthing (the Mongan method), 195, 207

India, 6, 171
Accredited Social Health Activist (ASHA), 184
Auxiliary Nurse Midwife (ANM) in, 173
Calcutta Medical College, 172
District Hospital defined, 183
Federation of Obstetric and Gynecological Societies of India (FOGSI), 182
Fernandez Foundation, 182, 187–188, 189n3
Fernandez Hospital (Hyderabad), 173, 280
antenatal childbirth preparation course in, 174
birth suites at, 181
Professional Midwifery Education and Training (PMET) Program at, 176
General Nursing and Midwifery (GNM), 173
Guidelines on Midwifery Services in India (Ministry of Health and Family Welfare), 186, 189n4
Indian Nursing Council (INC), 174, 182, 187–188
Institute of Public Health (IPH), 184
"Janani Suraksha Yojana," the, 189n1
launch of midwifery in Telangana State, 182–186
maternal mortality ratio (MMR), 171
midwife defined, 189n2
midwife-led care unit (MLCU), 188
Ministry of Health and Family Welfare, 182, 184, 187–188
National Midwifery Task Force (NMTF), 182
National Nursing and Midwifery Commission, 189n5
Nurse Practitioner in Midwifery in, 174–175

PROMISE campaign, 176
Scope of Practice for Midwifery Educator and Nurse Practitioner Midwife, 188
training in, 174–175
"trouser-and-shirt" ladies, 184
UNICEF All-India Conclave, 182
"informed relativism" (Davis-Floyd), 112
insurance industry and protocols, 82, 87, 100, 110, 117, 162, 210–211, 217
International Childbirth Initiative (ICI), xxiv, 8, 208n3, 251–255, 283
12 steps of, 255
countries and facilities associated with, 257–258
how to join, 255
implementation of, 254–256
International Childbirth Initiative (ICI): 12 Steps to Safe and Respectful Mother Baby-Family Maternity Care, xxiv, 199, 202, 251
official languages of, 256
principles of, 253–255
International Term Breech Trial (Hannah et al.), 216–218
critiques of, 219

Jackson, Louellen, xvii
Joffe, Carole, 35
Johnson, Ken, 224n5
Joint Commission on Accreditation of Healthcare Organizations (JCAHO), 98
Jones, Ricardo, 112
Jordan, Brigitte, 89
Journal of Obstetrics and Gynecology of Canada, 249

Karabekir, Neşe, 195, 197
Kaur, Inderjeet, 182
Kelly, Sally, 194
Király, Ági, 145
Kitzinger, Sheila, 128, 160
Königsmarkova, Ivana, 165

labor. *See under* birth
lactation. *See* breastfeeding
Lamaze, Ferdinand, 272
Lamaze method (training), 130, 194–195, 252
six Lamaze practices, 208n1
Lancet, The, 216, 217
Leboyer, Frédérick, 194, 272
laborists ("deck docs"), 83–84
Learn to Give Birth Like the Indians (Paciornik), 140
LGBTQQA1+ movement, 50
Life's Work: A Moral Argument for Choice (Parker), 19
"liminality" (Turner), 12, 263

Maimonides, 12
Malawi, 49
maternal-fetal medicine (MFM), 54, 237, 265–266, 267
affective environment, 65, 266
high risk patients, 55, 56–57, 267
Society for Maternal-Fetal Medicine, 54
training of MFM specialists, 54–57, 68n2, 265
Medicaid, 238
Medical Decision Making (Sox), 215
medical ethics. *See under* ethics
"medical gaze" (Foucault), 65
medical procedures used, 3, 108, 276
aromatherapy, 237
Bluetooth technology, 237
cesarean, xiv, xxiii, 6, 62–64, 85, 98, 102, 107–108, 110, 125, 129, 131, 136, 172, 181, 192, 202, 206, 212–213, 215, 218
"once a cesarean, always a cesarean," 248
vaginal birth after cesarean (VBAC). *See under* birth
continuous IV, 235–236
saline lock, 236
cutting the umbilical cord, 163, 195, 203, 206
dietary protocols, 237, 248, 273
drugs. *See* drugs

302 ◆ Index

epidural. *See* drugs
episiotomy, xxii, 103, 114, 126, 129, 154, 195, 203
  perineal lacerations, 114
evaluating the efficacy of, 233, 281–282
fetal heartrate monitoring [electronic fetal monitoring (EFM)], xxvii, 105, 108, 233, 235
fetoscopy, 58
forceps, use of, 79, 103, 126, 212
induction (artificial) of, xxvii, 199, 206
intrauterine pressure catheters, 233
Kristeller maneuver (pressure on mother's abdomen), 104, 126, 129, 148
practices involving breech births. *See under* birth
science-based (evidence-based) practices of, 107, 111, 135, 214–215
spotlights, use of, 203
stirrups, use of, 176
surgery, 3, 12–13, 16, 24, 30n13, 58, 63–64, 66, 68n2, 77, 80, 81, 86, 107, 119, 275, 277
tubal ligations, 249
ultrasound, xiii, 58, 221
unnecessary, 104, 125, 127, 129, 133, 158, 172, 205
uterine cavity revision, 147
vacuum suction (extractor), 103, 148, 197, 206
medical school, 76, 123
  academic medicine, 84–86
  MD-PhD programs, 88
Memoirs of the Man Made of Glass: Reminiscences of a Humanistic Obstetrician (Jones), 130
Midwifery Today, 130
  conferences, 194
midwives and doulas, xv, xxi, xxv, 5–6, 80, 85, 98–99, 103–108, 117, 126, 147, 171–173, 192–194, 211–215, 234, 238, 250–252, 273, 278, 283–289
  as "agents of change," 183
  as competing with doctors, 154, 204
  as "natural birthers," 203
  as "quackery" (in Hungary), 146
  "Birth with No Regret" (Çoker), 7, 195, 198, 280, 284
    principals of, 199–200
  caseload, 168n1
  in Uganda, Guatemala, Haiti, Papua New Guinea, 250
  International Confederation of Midwives (ICM), 175, 187
  International Day of the Midwife, 186
  listening to, 96, 106, 176, 194–195, 211–215, 284
  maternal morbidity low with, 174
  midwives vs. doulas, 204, 287
  mistakes by, 117
  model of childbirth, 126
  nurse-midwifery programs, 160, 173, 183, 245, 285
  ob/gyn training as, 146, 158
  outcomes, 178–185, 283–284
  Professional Midwifery Education and Training (PMET), 6
  subordination to ob/gyns, 162, 203–204
  training 175–178, 182–186
  traditional midwives/traditional birth attendants (TBAs), 6
Miller, Suellen, 111

National Abortion Federation (NAF), 40
National Health Service (NHS) in UK, 176, 182
newborn(s), neonatal, 177, 181
  as conscious beings, 205
  "golden hour" after childbirth, 242
  separation from mother, xvi, xxiv, xxvi, 197
  "skin-to-skin," 96–98, 181, 195, 199, 203
  streptococcal infection in, 148
"not so much to sea, not so much to earth" (Portuguese proverb), 117

Index ♦ 303

nulliparous term singleton vertex (NTSV), 98
nurses, nursing, xiii, xv, 6, 237–238
  nurse-midwifery. See under midwives
  "nurses' aide," 74–75
  "nursing home," 74–75

ob/gyns (obstetricians, gynecologists), xiv, 32, 72
  Accreditation Council for Graduate Medical Education, 232
  adapting to technocratic practice, 96, 113, 157, 229–230
  American College of Obstetricians and Gynecologists (ACOG), 218, 230
  and family practitioners, 82
  and nurses/midwives, 96, 102, 125, 245, 248, 283–286
  as neonatologist, 83, 138
  as advocates and activists, 38, 39, 45, 49, 50, 99, 114, 182, 200–204, 287
  American College of Obstetricians and Gynecologists (ACOG), 40, 49, 68n3, 203–204, 234
  Association of Professors of Obstetrics and Gynecology, 50
  Family Planning Fellowship, 10, 13, 29n1, 41, 50
  attending home births, 134–135
  burn-out, 289
  care that is "too little, too late" (TLTL), 82
  challenges to providing good care, 87, 128, 178, 202–203
  changing practice style, 96, 99–100, 106, 114–118, 128, 157, 178, 229–231, 239, 246, 252–254, 273, 283–286
  childhood experiences of, 93, 123
  clinical epidemiology and, 214
  compared with prison guards, 155
  during COVID pandemic. See COVID-19
  dedication of, 90
  divorce rate for, 86
  drugs used by. See drugs
  ethics. See ethics
  fear of change and authority. See fear
  history of changes in care, 35, 37, 50, 79, 176, 210–211
  humanistic ob/gyns banned from hospitals, 109
  "I am a God syndrome," 84, 198
  imprisonment of. See under politics and power
  International Federation of Gynecology and Obstetrics (FIGO), 203–204, 251
    International Safe Motherhood Committee, 251
    Mother-Baby Friendly Birthing Facilities guidelines, 251
    Safe Motherhood Newborn Health (SMNH) committee, 251
  LGBTQ care, 42, 46–47
  lifestyle of (private life of), 86, 93, 99, 114–115, 123
  motivations for becoming an (summarized), 274–275
  motivations for making a paradigm shift (summarized), 278–283
  naïveté of young, 96, 119
  narratives by, 11–32, 36, 39, 44, 54, 73, 93, 152–155, 192, 210, 232–234, 245
  oaths taken by, 30n8, 44
  obstetric disrespect, violence, and abuse (DVA), xxviii–xxix, 104
  ostracized by fellow, 125–128, 132–133, 138, 203, 269, 280
  summarized, 286–290
  "pay attention to details," 77
  perinatology, xiii, xiv, 2, 84–85, 87–88
    maternal-fetal medicine. See maternal-fetal medicine
  persecution of humanistic ob/gyns. See under politics and power
  poor outcomes, 95, 212, 276
  practices around breech births. See under birth

pressure to conform, 103–105, 202, 218, 233, 286–290
private practice, 81, 118, 234
procedures used by. *See under* medical procedures used
professional identity. *See* professional identity
racial disparities in practice, xxviii, 46–47
"right amount at the right time in the right way" (RARTRW), 111, 119
sued for negative outcomes, 205–206
  steps to avoid being, 205–206
"shared decision making," 20
scorn for "Indigenous" childbirths, 125
"speak for themselves," 1
technological innovations and, 229–232
  internet, 229–232
  See also social media
"The buck stops here" (President Truman), 67
training, xv, 12–15, 37, 41, 66, 72–73, 95–98, 104, 124, 192–194, 245–246, 268
  as a midwife, 146, 173, 211–215, 221, 232–234
  "doctor-centered," 232, 277
  summarized, 275–278
"tribal obstetrics" (Wagner), 154, 269
unnecessary procedures by. *See under* medical procedures
what we have learned from, 262
who provide abortion, 32, 36
"obstetric courage," 271
"obstetric paradox," xxvi
obstetrics, obstetricians (obs). *See* ob/gyn
Odent, Michel, 129, 160, 194, 207, 272
O Renascimento do Parto (*Birth Reborn*), 131
Orgasmic Birth (documentary), 131

Paciornik, Moysés, 140
Page, Lesley, 129

Pandit, Nutan, 173, 280
Parker, Willie, 19–20, 263
Parks, Rosa, 172
patients. *See under* women
perinatology (maternal-fetal medicine). *See under* ob/gyn
pharmaceutical industry, 73, 82, 87, 105
pharmaceuticals. *See* drugs
Planned Parenthood, 94
politics and power, xxix, 211
  biopolitics, xiv, 35
  capitalism and patriarchy, 135
  "discipline and punish" (Foucault), 133
  gender, 211
  "hegemony," xxvi, 110, 119, 165
  ideologies and, 110, 115
  Hungarian authoritarianism, 150
  "nature of power and evil" (Arendt), 113
  persecution of humanized ob/gyns, 132–133, 138–141, 144–150
    Ágnes Geréb's imprisonment, 144–155
  summary of, 286–290
polarization, 116
power, 103, 279
  empowerment of women, 97, 249
  medicine's control over women's bodies, 111–113, 165
  "Mothers' Revolution," 152
  women retrieving their, 119, 156–157
"social totality" (Adorno), 113
"The freedom of a country can be measured by the freedom of birth" (Geréb), 165
"total institution" (Goffman), 155, 268, 270
violent control of human birth and women's bodies, xxvii, xxix, 113, 204, 264
postpartum depression. *See under* women
postpartum period. *See under* birth
pregnancy. *See under* women

Pregnancy: The Complete Childbirth Book (Pandit), 173, 280
Premkumar, Ashish, xxxiii, 9
Prentice, Rachel, 65, 266
Preston, Charles, 30n15
professional identity, 32–35, 38–39, 46–48, 77, 264
　abortion and, 33–34, 50
　cultural change in, 33–34, 48
　"deep" (Barbour and Lammers), 264
　ideals, values, beliefs, norms, attitudes, morals and, 33, 44
　"intersectionality" (Crenshaw), 264
　"Professional Identity Formation" (PIF), 33
　race, ethnicity, gender, sexuality and, 35, 47
Promoting Normal Birth (Donna), 130
psychodramatic roleplay, 197

race, racial, xxviii, 35, 42, 67, 78, 96, 264
"radical amazement," 2
Rapp, Rayna, xii
rebozo (shawl), 194
Reed, Becky, 176
religion, 10, 17, 19, 26
　Buddhist, 27
　Catholic, 17, 26, 251
　Hindu, 26–27
　Jewish, 11–12, 24, 26, 29n4
Reproducing Race (Bridges), 78, 268
Re-Thinking the Physiology of Vaginal Breech Birth (Daviss), 224n3
Reynolds, Peter, xxvii
Rites of Passage, The (van Gennep), 12, 263
rituals, xx, xxvii, 23–26, 30n10, 30n14, 30n15, 111–112, 140
　baptism, 23, 26, 77
　in utero, 26
　Baruch Dayan HaEmet (Jewish blessing), 25, 30n11
　circumcision, 26
　defined, xxvii
　enact a culture's core values, xvi, xxvii, 2, 112

obstetric procedures as, xxvii, 12
"marking the event," 24
meditation, 27
Mikvah (Jewish), 23
Mizuko Kuyo (Japanese), 27
"rite of passage." *See under* birth
Ronque, Natalia, 115
Rothman, Barbara Katz, 110, 139, 271
Rousseff, Dilma, 139
Royal College of Obstetricians and Gynecologists (RCOG) guidelines, 221

Salomão, Dayane, 106
"see one, do one, teach one," 60, 69n12
Shah, Meera, 20, 263–264
Sherry, Gilbert, 195
Simon Williamson Clinic (Birmingham), 97
"situated knowledges" (Haraway), 55, 60, 65, 265
social media, 202, 229–231, 235
　Google, 229–230
Society of Obstetricians and Gynecologists of Canada (SOGC) guidelines, 221
Soros Foundation, 161
Sox, Harold, 215
Spinning Babies (Tully's method, classes), 103, 181, 194
stages of cognition (Davis-Floyd), xx–xxi, 1, 104–105, 109, 113
　reflective thinking, 114
　Stage 1 (concrete thought), xx, 113, 165, 268–269
　Stage 2 (ethnocentrism), xx–xxi
　Stage 3 (cultural relativism), xx–xxi
　Stage 4 (global humanism), xx, 115, 133
　"substage," xx–xxi, 1, 115, 119
Steinauer, Jody, 36, 39
　Medical Students for Choice, 41
Stringer, Kate, 183
Stromerova, Zuzana, 165
Summa Theologica (Aquinas), 17
surgery. *See under* medical procedures
Swedas, Jurgita, 165

technocratic, humanistic, and holistic
paradigms (Davis-Floyd), xvi–
xix, Table 0.1, 111, 228, 270
balancing/blending the three
paradigms, 228, 233, 237–239,
247–248, 273
challenges of changing the status quo,
xxvii, 157
fear of paradigm change. *See* fear
holistic paradigm, xvi, 1, 157, 267
principles of connection and
integration, xvii
humanistic (bio-psycho-social)
paradigm, xvi, 1, 102, 119,
238, 253, 268, 282
imprisonment for practicing in
Hungary, 6, 144
meeting patient for first time, 231
principle of connection, xvii
superficial and deep humanism,
xvii, 160–161, 270
"painting the walls pink"
(Geréb), 162, 270
three principles of, 108
indigenous model of childbirth,
125–127
"list of six principles" of (Jones),
126
"paradigm shift," xvi, xxviii, 4–5, 101,
104, 112, 119, 129, 274, 278
costs to ob/gyns for (summarized),
286–290
motives for making (summarized),
278–283
positive effects of (summarized),
283–286
redefined as "technocratic-
superficially humanistic-
deeply humanistic-holistic,"
xvii
technocratic paradigm, xvi, xxvii, 1,
104, 107, 124, 134–135
"Biomedical Empire" (Rothman),
139, 271, 286
birth services in, 198
"body as a machine," xvi–xviii,
xxvii, 111, 124

first-time pregnancy considered
"high risk," 148
"1-2 Punch" (Reynolds), xxvii, 111
principle of separation, xvi
repercussions of home birth on,
135–136
summary of, xvi–xxix
"The Emperor is naked!" (Jones),
140
"there are no births without risk,"
109
Ternovszky, Anna, 152, 165
The Secret Life of the Unborn Child
(Verny), 195, 271
Thorpe, Nick (BBC), 160
"threshold" (Weir), 61
Tritten, Jan, 194
Tully, Gail, 181, 194
Turkey, 7, 192
10 Steps for the Mother-Friendly
Hospitals of Turkey, 202
birth psychology in, 201
"Birth with No Regret" team in,
197–198, 286
Hand to Hand for Birth Association,
207
humanistic birth in, 201–202
*International MotherBaby Childbirth
Initiative (IMBCI): 10 Steps
to Optimal MotherBaby
Maternity Services*, 202, 251
International MotherBaby Childbirth
Organization (IMBCO), 202
Istanbul Birth Academy, 197
Ministry of Health Mother-Friendly
Hospital Committee, 202
technocratic birth services in, 198
Turner, Victor, 12, 253
twin-to-twin transfusion syndrome
(TTTS), 55, 57–64
amnioreduction, 58–60
fetoscopic laser obliteration, 58
hydrops fetalis, 62, 69n14
polyhydramnios, 68n8

ultrasound. *See under* medical
procedures

United Nation's Convention on the Elimination of All Forms of Discrimination against Women (CEDAW), 150
University of Central Lancashire, 187
University of São Paulo School of Medicine, 101
unnecessary procedures. *See under* medical procedures

Vakati, Karuna, 182
van Gennep, Arnold, 12, 263
Varlık, Serpil, 195
"view from somewhere," 55, 60
Vilar, Jose, 129

Wagner, Marsden, 129, 154, 269
Walker, Shawn, 181
Wax, J. R., 135
Weir, Lorna, 61
Wendland, Claire, 49
WhatsApp, 116
women (pregnant, "patients," mothers), 106
 Adriana's childbirth, 133–134
 centered, 21, 171, 175, 181
  "woman-centered" care, 253
  "recipient-centered" care, 253
 Centering Pregnancy, 107, 112
 choice, 83, 215, 248
 economically vulnerable, 118
 emotional support team for, 109, 203–206
 empowerment of. *See under* politics and power
 gratefulness of, 242
 inflated expectations of, 89
 leading role in childbirth experience, 128
 marginalized, 55, 118
 Melanie's case, 57–64
  death of Caleb, 64
 Miriam's case, 55
 patient-centered mode, 81
 patient-doctor relationship, 231, 238
 patient's lists, 231, 273
 patients' narratives, 11, 18–19
 postpartum depression, 156, 206
 pregnancy, pregnant people, xii, xv–xvii
  antenatal care, 183
  childbirth education classes, 7, 183, 194–198, 200–201
  empowerment of xxviii
  hypertensive disorders of, xxviii
 prepare patients for birth and motherhood, 97
 pressure on care-givers, 87, 116, 128, 235–238
 respect by caregivers for, 126–127, 253–254
 satisfaction surveys, 81, 83, 177
 seen as persons, 81, 215, 246
 sources of information, 230
 sterilization, 249
 Vania's death, 132–133, 136
 Zita's death, 146
World Health Organization (WHO), 108, 129
 "WHO Recommendations: Intrapartum Care for a Positive Childbirth Experience," 199, 204

You're the Only One I've Told (Shah), 20, 263

Zetka, James R., 50, 264

www.ingramcontent.com/pod-product-compliance
Lightning Source LLC
Chambersburg PA
CBHW070906030426
42336CB00014BA/2314